Methods in Molecular Biology

Series Editor
John M. Walker
School of Life and Medical Sciences
University of Hertfordshire
Hatfield, Hertfordshire, AL10 9AB, UK

For further volumes:
http://www.springer.com/series/7651

Methionine Dependence of Cancer and Aging

Methods and Protocols

Edited by

Robert M. Hoffman

AntiCancer, Inc., San Diego, CA, USA; Department of Surgery, University of California, San Diego, CA, USA

Humana Press

Editor
Robert M. Hoffman
AntiCancer, Inc.
San Diego, CA, USA

Department of Surgery
University of California
San Diego, CA, USA

ISSN 1064-3745 ISSN 1940-6029 (electronic)
Methods in Molecular Biology
ISBN 978-1-4939-8795-5 ISBN 978-1-4939-8796-2 (eBook)
https://doi.org/10.1007/978-1-4939-8796-2

Library of Congress Control Number: 2018960767

This Humana Press imprint is published by the registered company Springer Science+Business Media, LLC part of Springer Nature.
The registered company address is: 233 Spring Street, New York, NY 10013, U.S.A.

Dedication

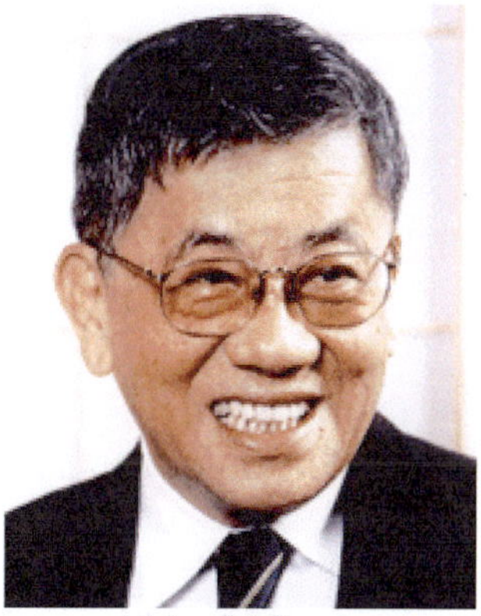

Takashi Sugimura

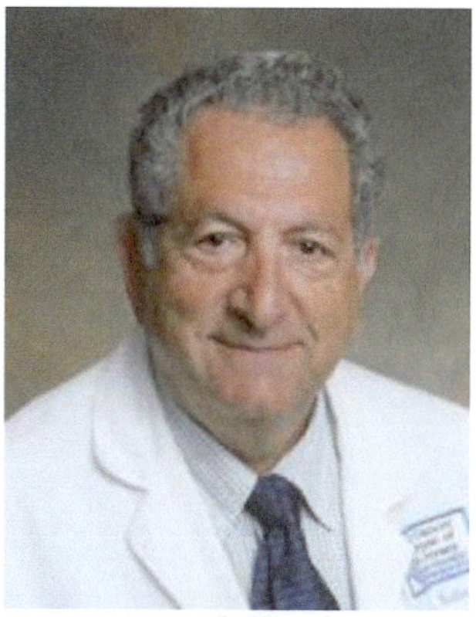

Joseph Bertino

Fathers of the field of methionine dependence of cancer

"We were interested in learning if L5179Υ cells, a mouse lymphoblastic leukemia cell line, required methionine for growth and if methionine depravation inhibited the effect of methotrexate. The basis for the study came from studies by others that showed that two cell lines, L1210 and Walker 256, required methionine for growth, while Hela and HEp2-cells were able to grow if supplied with homocysteine and vitamin B_{12}, required for the synthesis of methionine. Our studies showed that L5178Υ cells were very sensitive to methionine deprivation and log phase cells began dying as early as 6 h. and 90% were dead by 24 h. L5178Υ cells were also sensitive to methotrexate, but pretreatment with a methionine-free medium partially rescued these cells from methotrexate cell kill. Given the fact that this work was published in 1975, and that there is a methionine-degrading enzyme now available, clinical studies in tumors that show methionine auxotrophy are warranted."

Joseph R. Bertino, M.D.
American Cancer Society Professor
Rutgers Cancer Institute of New Jersey
University Professor of Medicine and Pharmacology
Rutgers Robert Wood Johnson Medical School

Preface

During the writing and editing of the present *Methionine Dependence of Cancer and Aging: Methods and Protocols* volume, I asked the 91-year-old eminent professor and oncologist, Eugene P. Frenkel, to write a chapter. He thought about it a while and said "Robert, you have missed the train, methioninase should have gone to the clinic 15 years ago."

However, as this present exciting volume shows, there are many more trains coming and that targeting methionine with methioninase can not only greatly improve cancer therapy, it may also slow aging.

The present volume tells many stories from the past to the future of targeting methionine for cancer and aging. We will learn how Sugimura [1] almost 60 years ago observed that rat tumors slowed when methionine was restricted in their diet, the first hint that methionine is a target in cancer. We will learn that the elevated requirement of cancer cells for methionine in order to proliferate is not due to the inability of cancer cells to synthesize methionine [2] but is due to the cancer cells excess use of methionine, possibly for aberrant transmethylation reactions [3, 4] which could be the basis of malignancy itself.

We will learn how methioninases were developed over the past 45 years [5–10] to target cancer. Intriguing chapters describe the selective cell-cycle arrest of cancer cells in the late S/G_2 phase by methionine restriction [11–15] and how this has been exploited for the development of methionine-restriction-based chemotherapy, enabling selective elimination of cancer cells in the presence of normal cells in vitro and in vivo.

We will learn about the latest in the molecular biology of changes in the cancer cell when methionine is restricted.

We will also read about the major role methionine restriction is playing in extending lifespan of many species of animals and the potential to do so in humans [16–19], possibly with a drinkable methioninase!

Science often proceeds with "starts and stops." Sometimes there are discoveries made "ahead of their time" before they can be widely understood or applied. It took 40 years before the "scientific community" realized that Mendel discovered genetics [20]. Another example is bacterial-based therapy of cancer, discovered 100 years too early [21]. But now is the time to exploit methionine restriction for cancer and aging! Please see for yourself in reading the present volume which I hope will be enjoyable and rewarding.

San Diego, CA, USA — ***Robert M. Hoffman***

References

1. Sugimura T, Birnbaum SM, Winitz M, Greenstein JP (1959) Quantitative nutritional studies with water-soluble, chemically defined diets. VIII. The forced feeding of diets each lacking in one essential amino acid. Arch Biochem Biophys 81:448–455
2. Hoffman RM, Erbe RW (1976) High *in vivo* rates of methionine biosynthesis in transformed human and malignant rat cells auxotrophic for methionine. Proc Natl Acad Sci USA 73:1523–1527
3. Stern PH, Hoffman RM (1984) Elevated overall rates of transmethylation in cell lines from diverse human tumors. In Vitro 20:663–670

4. Judde JG, Ellis M, Frost P (1989) Biochemical analysis of the role of transmethylation in the methionine dependence of tumor cells. Cancer Res 49:4859–4865
5. Kreis W, Hession C (1973) Biological effects of enzymatic deprivation of L-methionine in cell culture and an experimental tumor. Cancer Res 33:1866–1869
6. Tan Y, Xu M, Tan X-Z, Tan X-Y, Wang X, Saikawa Y, Nagahama T, Sun X, Lenz M, Hoffman RM (1997) Overexpression and large-scale production of recombinant L-methionine-α-deamino-γ-mercaptomethane-lyase for novel anticancer therapy. Prot Exp Purification 9:233–245
7. Takakura T, Mitsushima K, Yagi S, Inagaki K, Tanaka H, Esaki N, Soda K, Takimoto A (2004) Assay method for antitumor L-methionine γ-lyase: comprehensive kinetic analysis of the complex reaction with L-methionine. Anal Biochem 327:233–240
8. Takakura T, Ito T, Yagi S, Notsu Y, Itakura T, Nakamura T, Inagaki K, Esaki N, Hoffman RM, Takimoto A (2006) High-level expression and bulk crystallization of recombinant L-methionine γ-lyase, an anticancer agent. Appl Microbiol Biotechnol 70:183–192. doi: 10.1007/s00253-005-0038-2
9. Takakura T, Takimoto A, Notsu Y, Yoshida H, Ito T, Nagatome H, Ohno M, Kobayashi Y, Yoshioka T, Inagaki K, Yagi S, Hoffman RM, Esaki N (2006) Physicochemical and pharmacokinetic characterization of highly potent recombinant L-methionine γ-lyase conjugated with polyethylene glycol as an antitumor agent. Cancer Res 66:2807–2814
10. Kudou D, Misaki S, Yamashita M, Tamura T, Takakura T, Yoshioka T, Yagi S, Hoffman RM, Takimoto A, Esaki N, Inagaki K (2007) Structure of the antitumour enzyme L-methionine γ-lyase from *Pseudomonas putida* at 1.8Å resolution. J Biochem 141:535–544
11. Hoffman RM, Jacobsen SJ (1980) Reversible growth arrest in simian virus 40-transformed human fibroblasts. Proc Natl Acad Sci USA 77:7306–7310
12. Guo HY, Herrera H, Hoffman RM (1993) Unchecked DNA synthesis and blocked cell division induced by methionine deprivation in a human prostate cancer cell line. In Vitro Cell Dev Biol 29A:359–361
13. Yano S, Takehara K, Zhao M, Tan Y, Han Q, Li S, Bouvet M, Fujiwara T, Hoffman RM (2016) Tumor-specific cell-cycle decoy by *Salmonella typhimurium* A1-R combined with tumor-selective cell-cycle trap by methioninase overcome tumor intrinsic chemoresistance as visualized by FUCCI imaging. Cell Cycle 15:1715–1723
14. Yano S, Li S, Han Q, Tan Y, Bouvet M, Fujiwara T, Hoffman RM (2014) Selective methioninase-induced trap of cancer cells in S/G_2 phase visualized by FUCCI imaging confers chemosensitivity. Oncotarget 5:8729–8736
15. Orentreich N, Matias JR, DeFelice A, Zimmerman JA (1993) Low methionine ingestion by rats extends life span. J Nutr 123:269–274
16. Ables GP, Hens JR, Nichenametla SN (2016) Methionine restriction beyond life-span extension. Ann N Y Acad Sci 1363:68–79
17. Lee BC, Kaya A, Gladyshev VN (2016) Methionine restriction and life-span control. Ann N Y Acad Sci 1363:116–124
18. Grant L, Lees EK, Forney LA, Mody N, Gettys T, Brown PA, Wilson HM, Delibegovic M (2016) Methionine restriction improves renal insulin signalling in aged kidneys. Mech Ageing Dev 157:35–43
19. https://www.nobelprize.org/nobel_prizes/medicine/laureates/1946/muller-lecture.html
20. Hoffman RM (ed) (2016) Bacterial therapy of cancer: methods and protocols. Methods in Molecular Biology 1409. Walker, John M., series ed. Humana Press (Springer Science+Business Media New York)
21. Coley WB (1891) Contribution to the knowledge of sarcoma. Ann Surg 14:199–220

Contents

Contributors

WADDAH AL-REFAIE • *AntiCancer, Inc., San Diego, CA, USA; Department of Surgery, University of California, San Diego, CA, USA*

N. YU. ANISIMOVA • *Laboratory of Combined Treatment, N.N. Blokhin Cancer Research Center, Moscow, Russia*

S. V. BAZHENOV • *State Research Institute of Genetics and Selection of Industrial Microorganisms, Moscow, Russia; Laboratory of Molecular Genetics, Moscow Institute of Physics and Technology, Dolgoprudny, Moscow Region, Russia*

JOSEPH R. BERTINO • *Rutgers Cancer Institute of New Jersey, New Brunswick, NJ, USA*

STACEY L. BORREGO • *Department of Biological Chemistry, University of California, Irvine, Irvine, CA, USA*

N. V. BULUSHOVA • *State Research Institute of Genetics and Selection of Industrial Microorganisms, Moscow, Russia*

SHUSHMA CHATURVEDI • *Rutgers Cancer Institute of New Jersey, New Brunswick, NJ, USA*

DENNIS W. COALSON • *Anesthesia and Critical Care, University of Chicago Medicine, Chicago, IL, USA*

VINCENT L. CRYNS • *Department of Medicine, University of Wisconsin Carbone Cancer Center, University of Wisconsin School of Medicine and Public Health, Madison, WI, USA*

D. ZH. DAVYDOV • *Laboratory of Combined Treatment, N.N. Blokhin Cancer Research Center, Moscow, Russia*

C. DOUGLAS WALLACE • *Rady Children's Hospital, San Diego, CA, USA*

RICHARD W. ERBE • *Pediatrics and Medicine, University at Buffalo, Buffalo, NY, USA; Division of Genetics, The Women and Children's Hospital of Buffalo, Buffalo, NY, USA*

EUGENE P. FRENKEL • *Department of Internal Medicine, Division of Hematology/Oncology, University of Texas at Dallas, Southwestern Medical School, Dallas, TX, USA*

WEIYAN GUO • *AntiCancer, Inc., San Diego, CA, USA*

QINGHONG HAN • *AntiCancer, Inc., San Diego, CA, USA*

ROBERT M. HOFFMAN • *AntiCancer, Inc., San Diego, CA, USA; Department of Surgery, University of California, San Diego, CA, USA*

YASUNORI HOSHIYA • *Department of Surgery, Keio University, Tokyo, Japan*

KENTARO IGARASHI • *AntiCancer, Inc., San Diego, CA, USA; Department of Surgery, University of California, San Diego, CA, USA*

KENJI INAGAKI • *Department of Biofunctional Chemistry, Graduate School of Natural Science and Technology, Okayama University, Okayama, Japan*

PETER KAISER • *Department of Biological Chemistry, University of California, Irvine, Irvine, CA, USA*

KEI KAWAGUCHI • *AntiCancer, Inc., San Diego, CA, USA; Department of Surgery, University of California, San Diego, CA, USA*

DEMETRIUS M. KOKKINAKIS • *Department of Pathology and the Cancer Institute, University of Pittsburgh, Pittsburgh, PA, USA*

V. Y. KOTOVA • *State Research Institute of Genetics and Selection of Industrial Microorganisms, Moscow, Russia*

DAIZOU KUDOU • *Department of Biofunctional Chemistry, Graduate School of Natural Science and Technology, Okayama University, Okayama, Japan*

SHUKUAN LI • *AntiCancer, Inc., San Diego, CA, USA*
DA-WEI LIN • *Department of Biological Chemistry, University of California, Irvine, Irvine, CA, USA*
DAVID MACHOVER • *Hopital Paul Brousse, Villejuif Cedex, France*
DMITRY MALIN • *Department of Medicine, University of Wisconsin Carbone Cancer Center, University of Wisconsin School of Medicine and Public Health, Madison, WI, USA*
I. V. MANUKHOV • *State Research Institute of Genetics and Selection of Industrial Microorganisms, Moscow, Russia; Laboratory of Molecular Genetics, Moscow Institute of Physics and Technology, Dolgoprudny, Moscow Region, Russia*
KILMER S. MCCULLY • *Department of Pathology, Harvard Medical School, Boston, MA, USA; Pathology and Laboratory Medicine Service, VA Boston Healthcare System, Boston, MA, USA*
KENJI MIKI • *AntiCancer, Inc., San Diego, CA, USA; Department of Surgery, University of California, San Diego, CA, USA*
TAKASHI MURAKAMI • *AntiCancer, Inc., San Diego, CA, USA; Department of Surgery, University of California, San Diego, CA, USA*
V. S. POKROVSKY • *Laboratory of Combined Treatment, N.N. Blokhin Cancer Research Center, Moscow, Russia; Department of Biochemistry, People's Friendship University (RUDN University), Moscow, Russia*
HARISHA RAJANALA • *Department of Medicine, University of Wisconsin Carbone Cancer Center, University of Wisconsin School of Medicine and Public Health, Madison, WI, USA*
JULIAN E. SPALLHOLZ • *Departments of Nutritional Sciences, Texas Tech University, Lubbock, TX, USA*
PETER H. STERN • *AntiCancer, Inc., San Diego, CA, USA*
ELENA STREKALOVA • *Department of Medicine, University of Wisconsin Carbone Cancer Center, University of Wisconsin School of Medicine and Public Health, Madison, WI, USA*
TOMOAKI TAKAKURA • *Discovery Research Laboratories, Shionogi & Co., Ltd., Hyogo, Japan*
AKIO TAKIMOTO • *Discovery Research Laboratories, Shionogi & Co., Ltd., Hyogo, Japan*
YUYING TAN • *AntiCancer, Inc., San Diego, CA, USA*
MINGXU XU • *AntiCancer, Inc., San Diego, CA, USA*
SHIGEO YAGI • *AntiCancer, Inc., San Diego, CA, USA*
ZHIJIAN YANG • *AntiCancer, Inc., San Diego, CA, USA*
SHUYA YANO • *AntiCancer, Inc., San Diego, CA, USA; Department of Surgery, University of California, San Diego, CA, USA*
JORGE ZAVALA SR • *Comprehensive Cancer Center of Northwest Mexico, Tijuana, Mexico*
JORGE ZAVALA JR • *Comprehensive Cancer Center of Northwest Mexico, Tijuana, Mexico*
G. B. ZAVILGELSKY • *State Research Institute of Genetics and Selection of Industrial Microorganisms, Moscow, Russia*

Chapter 1

Methods to Study the Role of Methionine-Restricted Diet and Methioninase in Cancer Growth Control

Shushma Chaturvedi and Joseph R. Bertino

Abstract

Cancer cells require exogenous methionine for survival and therefore methionine restriction is a promising avenue for treatment. The basis for methionine dependence in cancer cells is still not entirely clear. While the lack of the methionine salvage enzyme methylthioadenosine phosphorylase (MTAP) is associated with methionine auxotrophy in cancer cells, there are other causes for tumors to require exogenous methionine. Restricting methionine by diet or by enzyme depletion, alone or in combination with certain chemotherapeutics, is a promising antitumor strategy.

Key words Methionine, Methioninase, Homocysteine, Suspension cultures, Adherent cells

1 Introduction

Methionine dependency of tumor cells is a promising avenue for treatment of cancers. Methionine-dependence phenotype (MDP) refers to the reduced ability of cells to proliferate when methionine is restricted and/or replaced by its immediate precursor homocysteine. MDP is a characteristic of some human tumor cell lines, human tumors in vivo, and normal somatic tissue in some individuals. However, given the variety of possible approaches and their complex and sometimes unpredictable effect on the host, it is important to identify an ideal anticancer diet that targets most deregulated metabolic pathways of cancer cells, without significantly affecting healthy tissues. Methioninase, a methionine scavenger enzyme, degrades methionine, and inhibits growth of a variety of cancer cells in culture as well as solid tumors and leukemia in animals [1]. As an alternative to dietary depletion of methionine, the potential use of methioninase has been studied by several investigators. In laboratory animals with Lewis lung carcinoma, synergistic antitumor activity was demonstrated between methioninase and the chemotherapy drug 5-fluorouracil [2]. Similar

Robert M. Hoffman (ed.), *Methionine Dependence of Cancer and Aging: Methods and Protocols*, Methods in Molecular Biology, vol. 1866, https://doi.org/10.1007/978-1-4939-8796-2_1,

results were found with colon cancer [3] and brain cancer models [4]. Dietary methionine restriction and methioninase, alone or in combination with certain chemotherapeutics, present a promising antitumor strategy to inhibit cancer growth in methionine-dependent tumors. Recombinant methioninase, a homotetrameric pyridoxal 5′-phosphate enzyme (MW172 kilodaltons), is generated recombinantly in *E. coli*. In an orthotopic lung cancer model, recombinant methioninase plus methioninase gene therapy was effective in suppressing cancer [5]. This chapter highlights methods that are commonly used to test in vitro and in vivo methionine deficiency in the treatment of cancer (*see* **Notes 1–4**).

2 Materials and Instrumentation

2.1 Cell Lines and Growth Conditions

Cancer cell lines from ATCC are grown in the media recommended by ATCC.

2.2 Materials

- Culture vessels containing suspension/adherent cells.
- Tissue culture flasks, plates, or dishes.
- Disposable, sterile 15 mL tubes.
- 30 K Amicon filter (Lexington, MA, USA).
- Balanced salt solution such as Dulbecco's phosphate-buffered saline (DPBS), containing no calcium, magnesium, or phenol red.
- Dissociation reagent such as trypsin or TrypLE™ Express, without phenol red.
- Complete growth medium, pre-warmed to 37 °C.
- RPMI 1640 (GIBCO Thermo Fisher Scientific) with glutamine and vitamin B_{12}.
- RPMI-1640 Medium without methionine (MET) A1451701 (Fisher Scientific)—The corresponding type of MET-free media supplemented with 0.005 mg/L vitamin B_{12}.
- L-Homocysteine (HCY) (Sigma Chemical Co., St. Louis, MO).
- 50 mL 10% dialyzed fetal bovine serum (FBS).
- Bovine serum albumin (MW 66,000) (Sigma, Louis, MO, USA).
- Sweet potato β-amylase (MW 200,000) (Sigma, Louis, MO, USA).
- Kaleidoscope Prestained Protein Standards (Bio-Rad, Hercules, CA, USA).
- 5 mL 10,000 U/mL penicillin/10,000 μg/mL streptomycin.
- L-Methionine.

- Dithiothreitol.
- Polyoxyethylene.
- Sorbitan monooleate (Tween 80).
- Isopropyl-β-D-thiogalactopyranoside (IPTG).
- 3-Methyl-2-benzothiazolinone hydrazone hydrochloride monohydrate (MBTH).
- L-Ethionine.
- L-Homoserine.
- Polypropylene glycol No. 2000.
- PLP (Sigma Aldrich).
- Lowry Protein Reagent kit (Sigma).
- All other chemicals from Sigma Chemical Co. (St. Louis, MO).
- Trypan blue.
- *P. putida* ATTCC 8209 (American Type Culture Collection, Rockville, MD).
- PT7Blue T-vector (Novagen, Madison, WI).
- Limulus amebocyte lysate (LAL).

2.3 Instrumentation

- 37 °C Incubator with humidified atmosphere of 5% CO_2.
- Cavitator-type homogenizer (Microfluidics Corp., Newton, MA, USA; model HC 8000).
- HPLC-L-6200A Intelligent pump (Hitachi, Ltd., Tokyo, Japan) with a Supelco Progel-TSK column (G3000 SWXL, 30 cm × 7.8 mm).
- Spectrophotometer (Hitachi U2000).
- DEAE Sepharose FF (Pharmacia, Uppsala, Sweden).
- ActiClean Etox column, 25 × 60 (Sterogene, CA).
- Countess® II FL Automated Cell Counter, trypan blue, and/or Coulter Counter® (Beckman Coulter).
- BioRad Bench Microplate reader.

2.4 Media

- Complete RPMI 1640 medium (Thermo Fisher Scientific)—To make 500 mL, mix 50 mL dialyzed FBS and1% penicillin (5000 IU/mL)/streptomycin (5 mg/mL) to 445 mL of RPMI medium. Store at 4 °C.
- RPMI 1640 special medium without methionine (Thermo Fisher Scientific)—For MET deprivation, formulate the medium by supplementing RPMI-1640 special medium with additional nutrients to closely match the original medium for each cell line, without addition of 15 mg/MET. Store at 4 °C.

- MTS(3-(4,5-dimethylthiazol-2-yl)-5-(3-carboxymethoxyphenyl)-2-(4-sulfophenyl)-2H-tetrazolium) stock solution, 5 mg/mL in PBS.

3 Steps

3.1 Dietary Methionine Restriction Therapy for Cancer Growth Control In Vitro

3.1.1 Suspension Cells (e.g., CCRF–CEM, Leukemia T Cells)

- Grow suspension cells in a 75 cm^2 bottle to late log phase (80% confluence) in complete RPMI medium. Routinely passage cells weekly and maintain in 5% CO_2 at 37 °C.
- Transfer the cells to a 15 mL centrifuge tube and centrifuge at 1200 × *g* for 5 min at room temperature.
- Aspirate the medium and wash cells twice with 2 mL PBS pre-warmed to 37 °C.
- Resuspend cells in RPMI medium with dialyzed FBS.
- Incubate cells for 24 h at 37 °C.
- Plate (1–5 × 10^5/mL) cells, depending on the type of cell line and the size of the cells for 24 h.
- After 24-h incubation, divide groups in the following manner: One control group for each tumor-cell type is maintained in complete medium. Another group is placed in MET-depleted homocysteine (HCY) containing (MET^-HCY^+) medium to study the effects of HCY substitution for MET. Seed cells into 3 mL MET^+HCY^- or MET^-HCY^+ medium plus dialyzed FBS in 6-well plates or in 10 mL of medium in T25 flasks.
- Incubate cells at 37°in 5% CO_2 atmosphere.
- All experiments are carried out in triplicate, and the rate of growth is assessed at 0 and 24 h, 2, 4, and 6 days, by cell counting.

3.1.2 In Vitro Proliferation Assay for Adherent Cells (e.g., 3T3, Fibroblast Cells)

- Detach the cells with trypsin-EDTA solution and determine the cell number and cell viability using a Vi-CELL XR Cell Counter.
- Plate (10^5) cells/mL per well in triplet in 200 μL dialyzed RPMI media in a 96-well tissue culture plate.
- Incubate overnight at 37 °C in a humidified atmosphere under 5% CO_2.
- The next day, wash the cells with PBS, and then treat the control group with complete RPMI medium and the test group with MET^- RPMI-1640 medium.
- Incubate cells at 37 °C in a 5% CO_2 atmosphere.
- After 24 h remove culture media from the cells and replace with 180 μL fresh media.
- Add 20 μL MTS solution containing phenazine methosulfate (PMS) to each well and incubate for 1–4 h at 37 °C.

- Measure the absorbance at 490 nm using a microtiter plate reader at 0, 24 h, 2, 4, and 6 days.
- Express cell viability as the percentage of viable cells compared with control cells in complete medium.

3.2 Dietary Methionine Restriction Therapy for Cancer Growth Control In Vivo

3.2.1 Animals

Maintain 5-week-old male or female NOD-SCID gamma (NSG) mice in quarantine for 1 week prior to the initiation of the experimental protocol. Throughout the quarantine period, house all animals in a conventional animal facility in groups of three in solid-bottomed cages lined with wood chips, with free access to food (standard laboratory rodent chow) and acidified water, and maintain on a 12-h light/dark cycle, 50% humidity, and 21 °C temperature. Record body weights weekly.

3.2.2 Diets

Use a diet lacking MET with other amino acids, minerals, vitamins, carbohydrates, and lipids. The control diet is similar but with MET added. One week after the acclimation period on a normal diet, at 6–7 weeks of age, inject cancer cells intraperitoneally (i.p.) and when tumor is palpable randomize mice into two groups, the MET-deficient diet in one group and the MET-replete diet in the second group. Use a minimal of eight animals per group to achieve statistical significance ($p < 0.05$).

Monitor the body weight, tumor size, and food consumption twice weekly. Alternatively use a luciferase or fluorescent-protein-transfected tumor, and measure tumor growth after luciferin administration and bioluminescence imaging or fluorescence imaging, respectively. Five weeks after the final treatment, sacrifice mice from both the control and methionine-restricted (MR) groups, and remove and photograph the tumor for analysis of cell proliferation.

3.3 Dietary MR Therapy for Cancer Growth Control Using Methioninase (METase)

METase from *Pseudomonas putida*, which degrades extracellular MET to α-ketobutyrate, ammonia, and methanethiol, has been demonstrated to have antitumor efficacy in vitro and in vivo [6].

3.3.1 Bacteria and Gene Vectors

- *P. putida* ATTCC 8209, American Type Culture Collection (Rockville, MD).
- PT7Blue T-vector, Novagen (Madison, WI).

3.3.2 Preparation of Recombinant Methioninase (rMETase) from Pseudomonas putida

This procedure is according to Muharram [7].

Cloning of the L-methioninase gene from *Pseudomonas putida* using *Escherichia coli* JM109 using the PT7Blue T-vector:

- Amplify the MET gene cloned from *P. putida* with PCR using the pAC-1 rMETase plasmid as a template and two primers

5'GCCGGTCTGTGGAATAAGCT3′ and 5'CCAGGGTCGA CTCCAGCGCC3'.

- The steps in the PCR reaction are as follows:
- Denature at 95 °C for 10 min, then 5 cycles of denaturation at 94 °C for 30 s, annealing at 60 °C for 30 s, and extension at 72 °C for 2 min.
- 25 cycles of denaturation at 94 °C for 30 s and 60 °C for 30 s, then extension at 72 °C for 1.5 min, and then a final extension at 72 °C for 10 min.
- Purify the PCR-amplified product 1365 bp band and sequence.
- Amplify the METase gene.
- Ligate the amplified METase gene to the PT7Blue T-vector at the EcoRV T-cloning site.
- Introduce the plasmid PT7-METase to *E. coli* DH5-α using standard transformation procedures.
- Use *E. coli* JM109 cells as host strain for expression of recombinant METase.
- For an overexpression vector, use the PT7-METase as a template DNA with the primers 5'GGAATTCCATATGCACGGC TCCAACAAGC-3′ and 5'AGTCATGGATCCTCAGGCACTC GCCTTGAGTGC-3' for the PCR reaction. Collect and purify the PCR-amplified product (1220 bp), which contains the METase gene with sites modified for the NdeI and BamH I restriction enzymes.
- Digest the DNA sequence with the NdeI and BamH I enzymes and ligate into the pT7-7 vector at the NdeI- and BamH I-cloning sites using standard protocols.
- Transform the resulting plasmid into *E. coli* BL21 (DE3) competent cells.
- Select positive clones from ampicillin-containing plates.
- After storage at 4 °C for 24 h, monitor for high levels of rMETase with a distinct yellow-orange color due to high enrichment of the pyridoxal phosphate-containing rMETase.
- Select the clones by their color and then by activity assay. Classify all yellow-orange colonies as positive for METase and noncolored clones as METase negative.

Fermentation

- Place 10 μL isopropyl-β-D-thiogalactopyranoside (IPTG)-induced *E. coli* cells, harboring the vector, PT7Blue T-vector, into 5 mL LB medium with 100 μg/mL ampicillin in a flask and grow at 37 °C at 400 rpm overnight.

- Transfer this culture to 800 mL terrific broth (TB) in 6 L flasks and grow overnight at 37 °C at 400 rpm (OD_{600} should be approximately 10).
- Transfer 800 mL cultures into 10,800 mL TB medium cultures in 6 L flasks and grow at 37 °C at 400 rpm for 16 h (OD_{600} should be approximately 10).
- Change the medium with fresh TB and incubate for another 6 h.
- When the OD_{600} reaches 20, harvest the bacterial cells by centrifugation at 4000 × *g* at 4 °C for 10 min.

Enzyme Purification

- Suspend the pellet in extraction solution containing 20 mM potassium phosphate, pH 9.0, 10 mM pyridoxal phosphate, and 0.01% β-mercaptoethanol.
- Lyse the culture with a cavitator-type homogenizer.
- Carry out heat treatment of the homogenate at 50 °C for 1 min.
- Centrifuge the suspension at 8000 × *g* and 4 °C for 30 min.
- Collect the supernatant and purify rMETase by ultrafiltration using a Millipore with buffer (10 mM potassium phosphate, pH 8.3).
- Adjust the pH to 7.2 by ultrafiltration.

Chromatographic Conditions

This procedure is according to Tan et al. [8]. Purify rMETase by three different steps using DEAE Sepharose FF and ActiClean Etox columns, the latter is designed for eliminating endotoxin.

- First column: DEAE Sepharose FF (pH 7.2). The first column is 100 mm in diameter and 30 cm in height, with a volume of 2400 mL of DEAE Sepharose FF. The elution flow rate is 15–50 mL/min.
- Apply 40–80 g of total protein (10–20 mg/mL) on the column.
- After loading, prewash the column with 40 mM potassium chloride in PPM buffer (10 mM potassium phosphate, pH 7.2, containing 10 mM PLP and 0.01% β-mercaptoethanol) for approximately 10 vol, until the OD_{280} drops below 0.1. Elute the protein with a linear gradient of 40–300 mM potassium chloride in PPM buffer.
- Collect elution fractions and identify the fractions containing rMETase by yellow color and activity assay.
- Second column: DEAE Sepharose FF (pH 8.3). The height of the second column (XK 50/30) is 25 cm, with a volume of 500 mL. The elution flow rate is 6–8 mL/min.
- After 24-h dialysis in 80 mM potassium chloride and 10 mM potassium phosphate (pH 8.3), apply 5–10 g of total protein (2–5 mg/mL) on the second column.

- After loading, prewash the column with 80 mM potassium chloride and 10 mM potassium phosphate (pH 8.3) for approximately 4 vol, until the OD_{280} drops below 0.1.
- Elute rMETase with a linear gradient of 80–300 mM potassium chloride in 10 mM potassium phosphate buffer (pH 8.3).
- Collect elution fractions containing rMETase and identify by yellow color and activity assay.
- Third column: ActiClean Etox. To eliminate endotoxin, purify rMETase (10–20 mg protein/mL), in a volume of 200–300 mL and apply on an 800 mL ActiClean Etox column (25 × 60) with a bed height of 40 cm.
- Elute the protein with elution buffer (0.12 M sodium chloride in 10 mM sodium phosphate, pH 7.2), at a flow rate of 1 mL/min.
- Collect the enzyme fractions and identify by yellow color and activity assay.
- Concentrate the final eluant with 30 K Amicon Centriprep concentrators by centrifugation at 4000 × *g* for 30 min at 4 °C.
- Perform sterilization with 0.2 μm nylon filter (Nalgene).

Formulation of rMETase

- rMETase in solution consists of 0.12 M sodium chloride and 10 mM sodium phosphate buffer (pH 7.2), at a concentration of 10–20 mg/mL.

rMETase Lyophilization

- Freeze rMETase in solution on dry ice and acetone and then lyophilize at −80 °C, under a vacuum of 100 millibar for 72 h.

Analysis of rMETase

- Load a sample of 20 μL (0.1–0.5 mg/mL) and elute with elution solution (0.12 M sodium chloride in 10 mM sodium phosphate buffer, pH 7.2) at a flow rate of 1.0 mL/min.
- Identify the protein-containing fractions with a spectrophotometer at a wavelength of 280 nm.
- Use bovine serum albumin (MW 66,000) and sweet potato β-amylase (MW 200,000) as MW standards.

Electrophoresis

- Carry out the electrophoresis in 7.5% polyacrylamide-precast plates in 0.2 M Tris–glycine buffer, pH 8.3, both with and without 0.1% SDS.
- Use Kaleidoscope Prestained Protein Standards as molecular weight standards.

Activity Assay

- Carry out the assay in a 1 mL vol of 50 mM phosphate buffer, pH 8.0, containing 10 μM PLP and 10 mM MET for 10 min at 37 °C, with different amounts of enzyme.
- Stop the reaction by adding 0.5 mL 4.5% TCA.

- Centrifuge the suspension in an Eppendorf centrifuge at 13 k rpm for 2 min.
- Add 0.5 mL supernatant to 0.5 mL 0.05% 3-methyl-2-benzothiazolinone hydrazone in 1 mL 1 M sodium acetate, pH 5.2, and incubate at 50 °C for 30 min.
- Determine the amount of reaction product by spectrophotometry at OD_{335}.
- Determine the amount of protein with the Lowry Reagent kit (Sigma) with bovine serum albumin as a standard.
- Calculate the specific activity as units/mg protein, with one unit of enzyme defined as the amount that catalyzes the formation of 1 μmol of α-ketobutyrate.

Endotoxin Assay

- The endotoxin level is measured by the limulus amebocyte lysate (LAL) test.
- Mix the sample with the LAL and incubate at 37 °C for 10 min. Mix the sample with the substrate solution supplied with the kit and incubate at 37 °C for additional 6 min.
- Stop the reaction with stop reagent supplied with the kit.
- Determine the absorbance of the sample with a spectrophotometer at 410 nm.
- Plot the standard curve from the endotoxin supplied in the kit at concentrations from 0.1 EU/mL to 1 EU/mL.
- Calculate the concentration of endotoxin from the standard curve.

3.3.3 In Vitro Growth Inhibition Effect of rMETase on Human Cancer Cell Lines

- Plate (2000 cells/well) cells in 100 μL culture medium containing 10% dialyzed bovine serum in a 96-well culture plate.
- Twenty-four hours later, treat the cells with a purified serial twofold dilution of rMETase (100 μL) to each well.
- Incubate for 3 days in a CO_2 incubator.
- After 3 days incubation with rMETase, determine cytotoxicity and the IC_{50} value with the MTT assay (0.2 μg/μL). Incubate for 2 h.
- Measure the absorbance at 540 nm in a BioRad Bench Microplate reader using 1 cm path-length plastic spectrophotometer cells.
- Express the growth inhibition as the percentage of absorbance of treated cells with respect to untreated cells.

3.3.4 Antitumor Efficacy of rMETase on Patient-Derived Orthotopic Xenografts (PDOX) in Nude Mice

This procedure is according to Murakami et al. [9].

- Randomly divide the PDOX model mice ($n = 8$) into an rMETase treatment group ($n = 4$) and an untreated control group ($n = 4$).
- When tumor volume reaches 60 mm^3, administer rMETase (100 units) by intraperitoneal injection, every 24 h for 14 consecutive days.
- Measure the tumor length, width, and mouse body weight twice a week.
- Collect blood samples at 24 h after the last rMETase administration for L-MET determination and sacrifice all the mice on day 15.
- Calculate tumor volume with the formula: Tumor volume (mm^3) = length (mm) × width (mm) × width (mm) × 1/2. Tumor volume ratio is defined as the ratio of volume on each measurement day relative to day 0.

Plasma L-MET Levels

- Treat a mouse without tumor with 100 units rMETase by i.p. administration.
- Collect 50 μL blood from the retro-orbital plexus in heparinated capillary tubes before treatment and 3, 6, 12, and 24 h after treatment.
- Centrifuge the blood at 4000 rpm for 5 min to obtain plasma.
- Measure the plasma L-MET levels with an HPLC after derivatization of serum amino acids with the fluoraldehyde reagent *o*-phthaldialdehyde (OPA).
- Measure tumor protein levels to standardize tumor L-MET measurements. Express L-MET levels as the percentage of the initial plasma L-MET level.

Tumor Protein-Level Measurement

- Place each PDOX tumor briefly in1 mL phosphate-buffered saline (PBS).
- Sonicate tumors on ice for 30 s and subsequently centrifuge at 12,000 rpm for 10 min.
- Collect the supernatants and dilute to concentrations ranging from 200 to 1500 μL/mL.
- Prepare fourfold dilution of protein assay reagent and add sonicated tumor supernatants to each tube.
- Measure the absorbance of 595 nm with a U-2000 spectrophotometer.
- Calculate protein levels from a standard curve obtained with bovine serum albumin (BSA) used as a protein standard.

- Calculate the standardized MET levels using the following formula: standardized L-methionine level (nmol/mg protein) = L-methionine level (nmol/mL)/protein level (mg protein/mL).

4 Notes

1. MET metabolism.

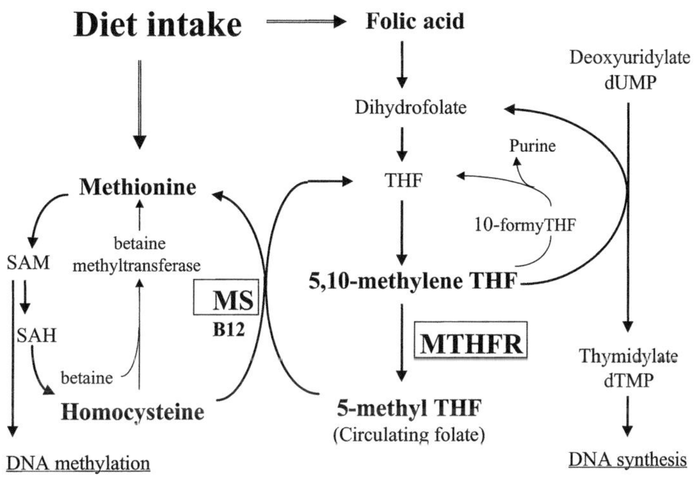

2. MET auxotrophy (dependence) of tumors may be detected clinically by a high signal using [^{11}C] methionine PET imaging.
3. The antitumor effects of MET deficiency may be augmented with cell-cycle-specific chemotherapy.
4. As dietary restriction is usually not well accepted by patients, enzymatic MET restriction using methioninase may be more effective and better tolerated than dietary restriction and should be explored further in clinical trials, alone or in combination with other therapies.

References

1. Hoffman RM (2015) Development of recombinant methioninase to target the general cancer-specific metabolic defect of methionine dependence: a 40-year odyssey. Expert Opin Biol Ther 15:21–31
2. Yoshioka T, Wada T, Uchida N, Maki H, Yoshida H, Ide N, Kasai H, Hojo K, Shono K, Maekawa R, Yagi S, Hoffman RM, Sugita K (1998) Anticancer efficacy in vivo and in vitro, synergy with 5-fluorouracil, and safety of recombinant methioninase. Cancer Res 58 (12):2583–2587
3. Tan Y, Sun X, Xu M, Tan X-Z, Sasson A, Rashidi B, Han Q, Tan X-Y, Wang X, An Z, Sun F-X, Hoffman RM (1999) Efficacy of recombinant methioninase in combination with cisplatin on human colon tumors in nude mice. Clin Cancer Res 5:2157–2163

4. Kokkinakis DM, Hoffman RM, Frenkel EP, Wick JB, Han Q, Xu M, Tan Y, Schold SC (2001) Synergy between methionine stress and chemotherapy in the treatment of brain tumor xenografts in athymic mice. Cancer Res 61:4017–4023
5. Miki K, Xu M, An Z, Wang X, Yang M, Al-Refaie W, Sun X, Baranov E, Tan Y, Chishima T, Shimada H, Moossa AR, Hoffman RM (2000) Survival efficacy of the combination of the methioninase gene and methioninase in a lung cancer orthotopic model. Cancer Gene Ther 7:332–338
6. Tan Y, Xu M, Guo H, Sun X, Kubota T, Hoffman RM (1996) Anticancer efficacy of methioninase in vivo. Anticancer Res 16 (6C):3931–3936
7. Muharram MM (2016) Recombinant engineering of L-methioninase using two different promoter and expression systems and in vitro analysis of its anticancer efficacy on different human cancer cell lines. Pak J Biol Sci 19 (3):106–114. https://doi.org/10.3923/pjbs.2016.106.114
8. Tan Y, Xu M, Hoffman RM (2010) Broad selective efficacy of recombinant methioninase and polyethylene glycol-modified recombinant methioninase on cancer cells in vitro. Anticancer Res 30(4):1041–1046
9. Murakami T, Li S, Han Q, Tan Y, Kiyuna T, Igarashi K, Kawaguchi K, Hwang HK, Miyaki K, Singh AS, Nelson SD, Dry SM, Li Y, Hiroshima Y, Lwin TM, DeLong JC, Chishima T, Tanaka K, Bouvet M, Endo I, Eilber FC, Hoffman RM (2017) Recombinant methioninase effectively targets a Ewing's sarcoma in a patient-derived orthotopic xenograft (PDOX) nude-mouse model. Oncotarget 8 (22):35630–35638. https://doi.org/10.18632/oncotarget.15823

Chapter 2

Altered Methionine Metabolism in Cancer Cells

Robert M. Hoffman, Peter H. Stern, Dennis W. Coalson, C. Douglas Wallace, and Richard W. Erbe

Abstract

Many different types of cancer cells have been shown to be methionine (MET) dependent. Cancer cells, unlike normal cells, grow poorly or not at all when MET is restricted. Cancer cells have an elevated requirement for exogenous MET for growth, despite high levels of endogenous synthesis. This requirement reflects increased utilization of MET by cancer cells, analogous to increased utilization glucose by cancer cells (Warburg effect). To answer the critical question of whether MET-dependent cancer cells synthesize normal amounts of MET, we determined the levels of MET, S-adenosylmethionine (AdoMET), and S-adenosylhomocysteine (AdoHCY) that were synthesized by MET-dependent cancer cells under conditions of MET restriction. We demonstrated that MET-dependent cells synthesize a normal amount of endogenously synthesized MET but are still deficient in AdoMET. In contrast, exogenously supplied MET results in normal AdoMET levels. The ratio of AdoMET to AdoHCY is low in MET-dependent cells growing in MET-restricted medium but is normal when MET is supplied. Under conditions of MET restriction, the low AdoMET/AdoHCY ratio probably limits proliferation of MET-dependent cancer cells. The amount of free MET is also low in MET-dependent cancer cells under MET restriction. The elevated MET requirement for cancer cells may be due to enhanced overall rates of transmethylation compared to normal human cells. Thus, MET-dependent cancer cells have low levels of free MET, low levels of AdoMET, and elevated levels of AdoHCY under conditions of MET restriction probably due to overuse of MET for transmethylation reactions ("Hoffman effect"), thereby blocking cellular proliferation.

Key words Cancer, Methionine dependence, Methionine restriction, Methionine synthase, Free methionine, Homocysteine, S-adenosylmethionine, S-adenosylhomocysteine, Transmethylation, 3-Deazaadenosine

1 Introduction

Sugimura et al. made the initial observation that cancer cells require excess methionine (MET) when tumors in rats slowed their growth on MET-restricted diets [1]. L5178Y mouse leukemia cells neither grew nor survived in folate- and vitamin-B_{12}-supplemented medium in which MET was replaced by its precursor DL-homocysteine (HCY) [2]. Walker-256 rat breast carcinoma (W-256) and L1210 murine lymphocytic leukemia [3] showed a

Robert M. Hoffman (ed.), *Methionine Dependence of Cancer and Aging: Methods and Protocols*, Methods in Molecular Biology, vol. 1866, https://doi.org/10.1007/978-1-4939-8796-2_2,

similar MET requirement. Normal cells proliferated well under these conditions [3–6].

It has been shown by us and others [2–10] that a large number of cancer cells grown in culture are MET dependent. That is, these cells, unlike normal cells, do not grow or grow poorly in MET-restricted medium. Cancer cell lines in culture that demonstrate the MET-dependent phenotype include rat mammary tumors [2, 8], mouse leukemic cells [7], human leukemic cells [9], human adenocarcinoma of the breast [11], human neuroblastoma [11], and simian virus 40 (SV40)-transformed human cells [2] and numerous other cancer cell types [12–16]. Cells taken directly from rat sarcomas and murine leukemias have shown MET dependence when put in primary culture [17].

The generality of MET dependence suggests that it is a basis of oncogenic transformation itself [18].

Thus, the cancer cells are MET "auxotrophs," which have nutritional requirements not observed in the genetically related normal cells. It was originally suggested that the MET auxotrophy of the malignant cells resulted from diminished in vivo activity of 5-methyltetrahydropteroyl-L-glutamate:L-homocysteine *S*-methyltransferase (EC 2.1.1.13) (MET synthase), the enzyme which catalyzes the terminal reaction in MET biosynthesis [19].

This chapter demonstrates that cancer cells synthesize as much as or greater amounts of MET than normal cells, and have normal levels of MET synthase, despite their large requirement for exogenous MET. The biochemical basis of MET dependence has remained controversial. We review in this chapter that cancer cells overuse MET, possibly for aberrant transmethylation reactions, and therefore arrest growth under conditions of MET restriction.

2 Materials

1. Normal human skin fibroblast strains, such as MGF316 and MGF323 [8].
2. SV80 [9] and W18VA2 [10] human cell lines transformed by simian virus 40 (SV-40), kindly provided by Drs. D. M. Livingston and P. H. Black, or other cancer-cell types.
3. The Walker-256 (W-256) rat breast carcinoma line [3], obtained from the American Type Culture Collection, Rockville, MD.
4. Eagle's minimal essential medium (MEM, GIBCO, Grand Island, NY).
5. Dialyzed fetal calf serum.

6. Fetal calf serum (Microbiological Assoc., Farmington Hills, MI).
7. Hydroxocobalamin (OH-Cbl) (Schwarz/Mann).
8. Minimal essential medium (MEM) lacking MET but containing 1.5 μM OH-Cbl and 0.1 mM folic acid (Sigma), and supplemented with 10% dialyzed fetal calf serum.
9. MEM with MET and 15% fetal calf serum.
10. DL-homocysteinethiolactone-HCl (Sigma, St. Louis, MO).
11. 100 mm Petri dishes.
12. Coulter counter.
13. [5-^{14}C]Me-H_4-PteGlu (57.7 Ci/mol, Amersham, Piscataway, NJ).
14. Phosphate-buffered saline (PBS).
15. Hanks' balanced salt solution (GIBCO).
16. Aquasol (New England Nuclear), containing 5% acetic acid, 8% water, and 0.2 mL 1 M KH_2PO_4.
17. Gel filtration column.
18. Beckman amino acid analyzer.
19. Sulfosalicylic acid.
20. Eppendorf tubes.
21. Beckman microfuge.
22. Dithiothreitol.
23. *N*-ethylmaleimide.
24. HCl.
25. 3-Deazaadenosine (Sigma).
26. Ninhydrin-cadmium acetate.
27. Scintillation vials.
28. 3 mL absolute methanol.
29. Beckman LS-100 scintillation counter.
30. [^{35}S]MET (Amersham) at a specific activity of 1420 Ci/mmol (1 Ci = 3.7×10^{10} becquerels).
31. [^{35}S]HCY thiolactone synthesized by a modification of the procedure of Baernstein [20].
32. Altex programmable chromatograph for HPLC with a VYDAC strong-cation-exchange column (Separations Group, Hesperia, CA) or other HPLC apparatus.
33. Camag or other high-voltage electrophoresis apparatus.

3 Methods

3.1 Determination of Cancer Cell Proliferation Under MET Restriction

1. Grow cells in Eagle's MEM supplemented with 1.5 MM hydroxocobalamin (OH-Cbl) and 15% fetal calf serum.
2. For growth experiments, use MEM lacking MET but containing 1.5 μM OH-Cbl and 0.1 mM folic acid, and supplemented with 10% dialyzed fetal calf serum.
3. Add various amounts of homocysteine (L-HCY) in the form of DL-HCY lactone-HCl.
4. Grow cells in duplicate 100 mm petri dishes containing 10 mL medium. Refeed on day 5 and every 2 days thereafter or daily where indicated.
5. Enumerate cells in a Coulter counter.

3.2 Determination of MET Synthesis

1. For radioactivity uptake experiments, inoculate 5–8 $\times$ 10^5 cells into 60 mm petri dishes with 5 mL of MEM containing 1.5 M OH-Cbl and supplement with 15% fetal calf serum.
2. Two days later, wash the dishes three times with 2 mL warm medium consisting of MEM but lacking serum, folic acid, HCY, and MET.
3. Replace the final wash media with 2 mL solution consisting of 1.6 mL MEM containing 1.5 μM OH-Cbl and 0.90 μCi [5-^{14}C] methyl-H_4-folic acid (57.7 Ci/mol, Amersham) but lacking MET and unlabeled folic acid; 0.2 mL of dialyzed fetal calf serum; and 0.2 mL of Dulbecco's phosphate-buffered saline (PBS) containing HCY.
4. Incubate the cells at 37 °C for 26 h after which the dishes are washed quickly four times with 2 mL aliquots of ice-cold Hanks' balanced salt solution (GIBCO).
5. Dissolve the cells in 1.0 mL 0.1 M NaOH in 2% Na_2CO_3, and add a 0.5 mL portion to 10 mL of Aquasol containing 5% acetic acid, 8% water, and 0.2 mL of 1 M KH_2PO_4.
6. Measure radioactivity in a Beckman liquid scintillation spectrometer or equivalent.
7. Dissolve an additional aliquot of cells for protein determination [21].

3.3 Incubation and Preparation of Cells for Amino Acid Analysis

1. Incubate normal diploid cells at subconfluent levels, and incubate the SV40-transformed cells or other cancer cells at subconfluent or confluent amounts.
2. Incubate cells with 100 μM [^{35}S]MET in MET-containing medium (30 μCi/mL for 17 h at 37 °C in 95% air/5% CO_2) or with 100 μM [^{35}S]HCY lactone in MET restricted (MR) medium (25 μCi/mL for 24 h at 37 °C under similar conditions) [18].

3. After incubation, wash the cells three times with cold phosphate-buffered saline and add 5% sulfosalicylic acid.
4. Scrape the cells off the dish, incubate on ice for 15 min, and then centrifuge in a Beckman Microfuge or equivalent for 5 min.
5. Use the supernatant for high-pressure liquid chromatography (HPLC) and amino acid analysis.
6. Dissolve the pellet in 300 μL 0.1 M NaOH and analyze for protein content by the method of Lowry et al. [21].

3.4 Measurement of Free Cellular MET and HCY

1. Add 50 μL supernatant extracted from the cells to an Eppendorf tube containing 10 mg disodium phosphate.
2. Agitate the mixture to dissolve the phosphate.
3. Add MET and HCY standards at a concentration of 3 mg/mL each as well as 0.1 M dithiothreitol in a 5 μL solution to the 50 μL cell extract.
4. Keep the solution at room temperature for 15 min with occasional agitation.
5. Allow the mixture to react for 15 min with saturating amounts of *N*-ethylmaleimide before acidification with 1 N HCl [22].
6. To separate the derivatized sulfur amino acids, perform high-voltage electrophoresis using a 6% formic acid buffer or equivalent [22].
7. Place 10 μL of each sample on buffer-wetted paper that can accommodate up to six samples on a single sheet.
8. Effect the separation for 30 min at 3500 V and 110 mA.
9. Dry the paper for 15 min in an oven, spray with ninhydrin-cadmium acetate, and heat for an additional 5 min.
10. Cut the spots identified by the standards as containing derivatized HCY and MET into small strips, place in scintillation vials, and extract for 30 min with 3 mL absolute methanol.
11. Determine the amount of radioactivity in the vials on a Beckman LS-100 scintillation counter or equivalent using a toluene-based scintillation fluid.
12. This method has been demonstrated to separate MET and HCY from each other and the rest of the cellular sulfur-containing amino acids and peptides [23].

3.5 HPLC Analysis of AdoMET and AdoHCY

1. Use an Altex programmable chromatograph for HPLC with a VYDAC strong-cation-exchange column (Separations Group, Hesperia, CA) or equivalent. Use the method modified by Chiang and co-workers [24–27].

2. Inject an aliquot (100 μL) of the above supernatant into the HPLC, which is set at a flow rate of 2.5 mL/min.
3. For the first 10 min, elute the material with a linear gradient of 0–15% 0.8 M ammonium formate/100–85% 0.01 M ammonium formate, pH 4.
4. From minutes 10–30, increase the 0.8 M buffer by a gradient from 15 to 25%, and from minutes 30–40, by a gradient to 100%, and maintain to minute 55.
5. Collect fractions at 30-s intervals in an LKB fraction collector between minutes 12 and 25 and at 1-min intervals or equivalent between minutes 40 and 55.
6. Calibrate the machine with authentic AdoHCY, which is eluted between minutes 15 and 20, and with authentic AdoMET, which is eluted between minutes 45 and 50 [18].

3.6 Amino Acid Analysis of Cellular Proteins

1. Hydrolyze the pelleted sulfosalicylic acid pellet in 6 M HCl at 110 °C for 24 h.
2. Analyze this hydrolysate for MET with a high-voltage electrophoresis apparatus [22].

3.7 Scintillation Counting

1. Use a toluene-based scintillation fluid for all HPLC fractions and amino acid analysis, and assay radioactivity on a Beckman LS-100 counter or equivalent [18].

3.8 Measurements of Transmethylation Rates

1. Measure the transmethylation rate in MET-containing medium.
2. Plate cells at a density of 10^6 cells/35 mm plate in MET-containing medium and 24 h later add 100 μM [^{35}S] MET (25 μCi/mL).
3. Replace the same concentration of unlabeled MET.
4. After 24 h of labeling, add freshly prepared periodate-oxidized 3-deazaadenosine to give a final concentration of 10 μM, an amount which we have demonstrated to block the hydrolysis of AdoHcy.
5. Prepare oxidized 3-deazaadenosine as follows: 10 μL of a 0.1 M solution of sodium periodate in water is added to 90 μL of an 11 mM solution of 3-deazaadenosine in 0.11 M acetate buffer, pH 4.
6. Allow the mixture to stand protected from light for 1 h at room temperature and then add to 9.9 mL ice-cold cell culture medium.
7. In the presence of the inhibitor, measure the time-dependent accumulation of AdoHcy as the indicator of the rate of AdoMET-dependent transmethylation.
8. Measure a point each half hour for a period of 2½ h [28].

9. Measure the transmethylation rate in MR medium.
10. Follow similar procedures except replace the [^{35}S]MET medium with 1 mL MR medium containing 25 μCi 100 μM [^{35}S]HCY 1 h prior to addition of 3-deazaadenosine.

4 Results

4.1 High MET Synthase Activity in MET-Dependent Cancer Cells

Methionine transmethylation metabolism is outlined in Fig. 1. When HCY replaced MET in folate- and hydroxocobalamin (OHCbl)-supplemented media, the normal human fibroblasts MGF323 and MGF316 grew throughout the 2–3-week test period, while W-256 cancer cells and the two SV-40-transformed human cancer cell lines ceased growth after the initial 0.2–1.5 divisions (Fig. 2) [7, 8].

However, MET synthase was similar in the malignant and SV-40-transformed cells and the normal cell lines [2]. When incubated in OH-Cbl-supplemented media lacking both MET and folic acid, all cell types took up radioactive label added to the medium as [5-^{14}C]Me-H_4-PteGlu, the methyl donor in the MET synthase reaction. Uptake of [5-^{14}C]Me-H_4-PteGlu was highly stimulated by HCY, the methyl group acceptor in MET biosynthesis (Fig. 3).

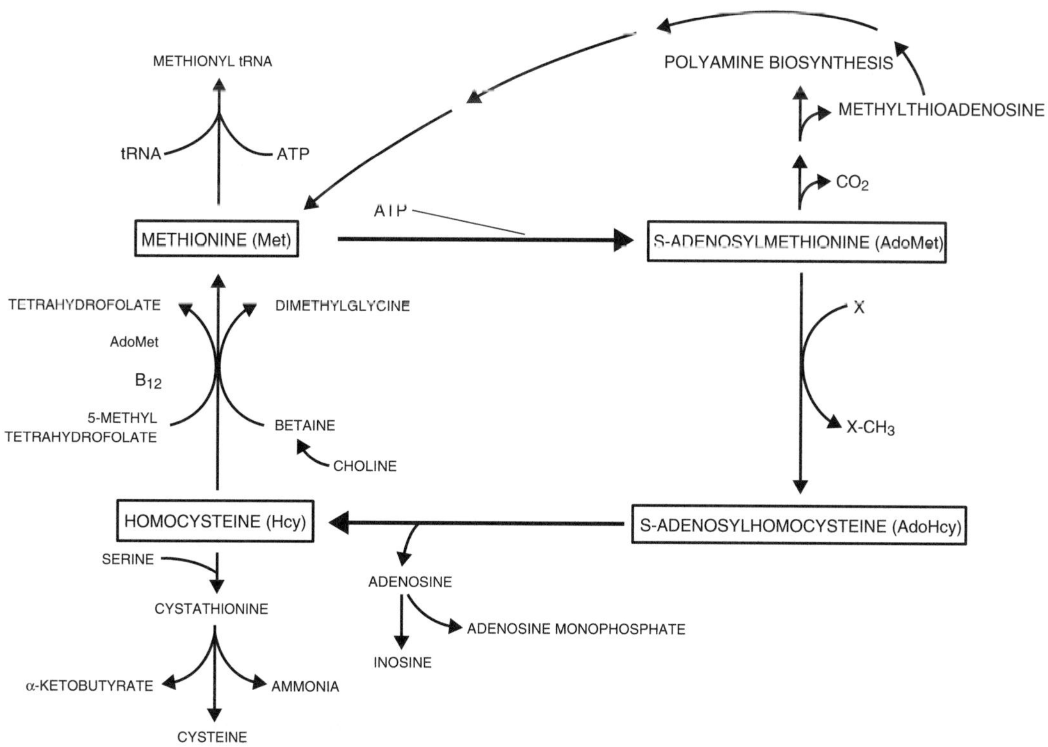

Fig. 1 Pathway of methionine/transmethylation metabolism [28]

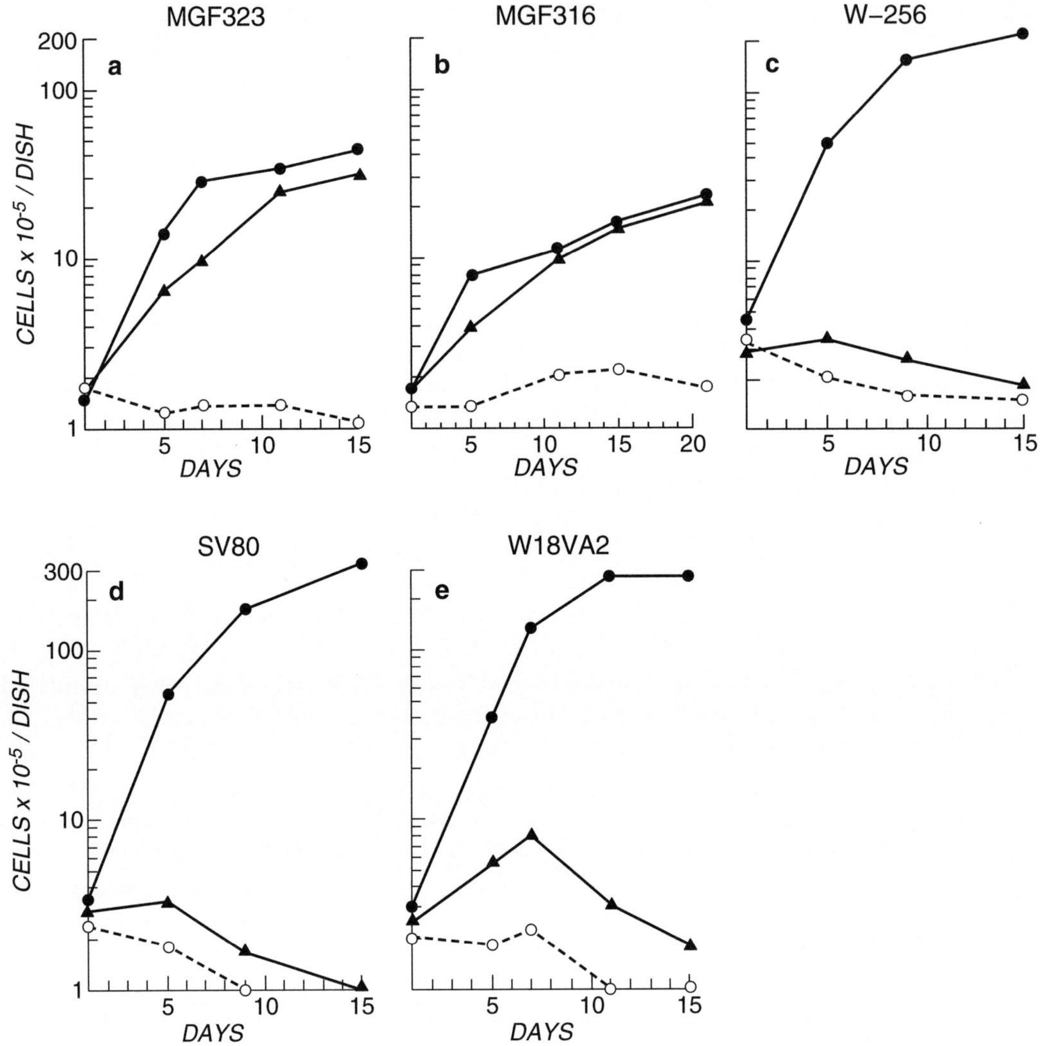

Fig. 2 Growth of normal, malignant, and transformed cells in OH-Cbl-supplemented media with or without methionine. Cells were inoculated and grown in 100 mm petri dishes containing 10 mL MEM lacking methionine and supplemented with 10% dialyzed fetal calf serum and either 0.1 mM L-methionine plus 7.5 MM OH-Cbl (filled circle) or 0.1 mM homocysteine plus 7.5 AM OH-Cbl (filled triangle) or 7.5 MM OH-Cbl alone (open circle). Cells in duplicate dishes were counted on the days indicated in the graphs [2]

The rate of uptake by the malignant and the two transformed lines was high and in the case of transformed SV80 cells was substantially higher than in either normal cell line. When the growth medium contained 0.1 mM HCY, the uptake of label from [5-^{14}C] Me-H_4-PteGlu increased to between 4.2- and 10.6 (SV-80 cells)-fold [2].

Amino acid analysis demonstrated that the majority of the radioactive label from [5-^{14}C]Me-H_4-PteGlu taken up by both normal and malignant cells was incorporated into MET. The cancer

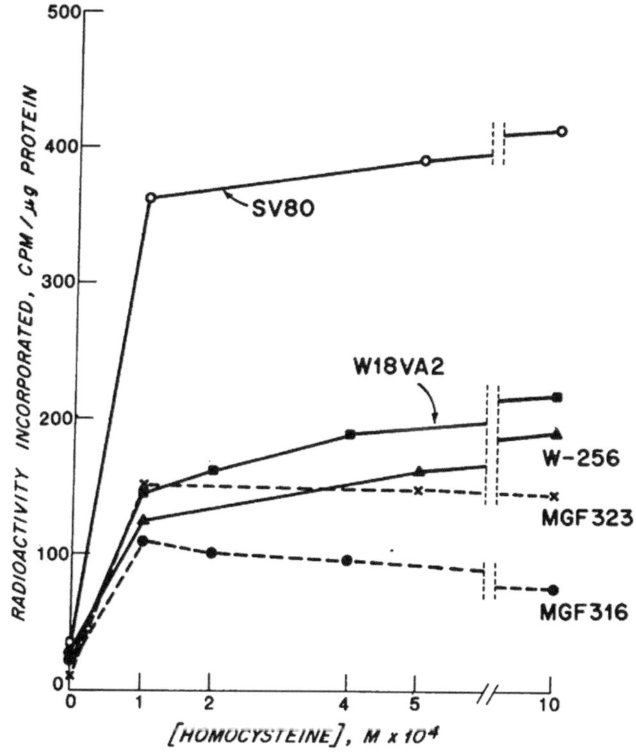

Fig. 3 Effect of homocysteine on the cellular uptake of radioactive label from [5-^{14}C]Me-H_4PteGlu. The medium in which the cells were incubated contained homocysteine at the concentration indicated on the abscissa but lacked methionine. After 26 h, intracellular radioactivity was measured as described in Methods. Each point is the average of two determinations. Dashed lines, normal fibroblast strains. Solid lines, malignant and transformed cell lines. (Open circle) SV80; (filled square) W18VA2; (filled triangle) W-256; (×) MGF323; (filled circle) MFG316 [2]

cells synthesized at least as much MET as normal cells which grew well under conditions of MET restriction [2].

The malignant cells were unable to grow on HCY alone, but grew rapidly on HCY when otherwise limiting amounts of MET were added. In normal cells, HCY and small amounts of MET had an additive effect. The presence of a small amount of MET resulted in disproportionately greater growth of the malignant cells compared to normal cells. At MET concentrations ranging from 1 μM, which was distinctly limiting, to 100 μM HCY exerted a growth-stimulating effect on the cancer cells (*see* **Note 1**) [2].

Folate repletion studies yielded further evidence of high in vivo MET synthase activity. Cells were depleted of folates by growth in folate-deficient medium containing 0.1 mM MET until division ceased. 5-Me-H_4-PteGlu (1–100 μM) restored normal growth rates in normal fibroblasts and cancer cells (*see* **Note 1**) [2].

The maximal growth rates did not distinguish the normal cells from cancer cells in MET-containing medium. These results suggest the inability of transformed and malignant cells to grow in MR medium is due neither to a more rapid growth rate nor reduced MET synthase (*see* **Note 3**) [2].

4.2 AdoMET Levels in MET-Dependent Cancer Cells in MR Medium

Normal human fibroblasts BA and AF2 had large amounts of AdoMET compared with adenosylhomocysteine (AdoHCY) in MR medium. MET-dependent SV40-transformed human cell lines P5 and P1 had very low AdoMET compared to AdoHCY in MR medium (*see* **Note 4**). However, MET-independent revertants R5 and RI isolated from P5 and P1, respectively, showed normal AdoMET/AdoHCY ratios (*see* **Notes 2** and **4**) [18].

The calculated AdoMET/AdoHCY ratios were much lower in the very MET-dependent cancer cell lines compared to those that could grow when MET was replaced by HCY averaging 0.842 and 8.1, respectively [29].

Since the pool of free MET is the precursor of AdoMET and the pool of free HCY is an important precursor of AdoHCY, these pool sizes were measured to determine the relationship between these four metabolites and their relationship to MET dependence. There was a significant reduction in the MET pool size of MET-dependent SV0-transformed fibroblasts relative to MET-independent diploid fibroblasts in MR medium. There was no significant difference between the HCY pool sizes for either group [23].

Thus, MET-dependent cells did not seem deficient in MET biosynthesis as mentioned above, but rather they are deficient in the steady-state concentration of free MET [23].

There was an over tenfold reduction in the amount of AdoMET with a concomitant reduction in the AdoMET/AdoHCY ratio in MET-dependent compared to MET-independent cells as mentioned above. Thus, in MR medium, the MET-dependent cells are specifically deficient in free MET and in AdoMET [23].

In MET-containing medium, the AdoMET and AdoHCY levels are similar in MET-dependent and MET-independent cells. This is in contrast to the highly reduced AdoMET levels and AdoMET/AdoHCY ratios in MET-dependent cells in MR medium [23].

5 Elevated Transmethylation in Cancer Cells

To measure the overall rates of cellular transmethylation, the following strategy was followed: (1) AdoHCY hydrolysis was blocked by periodate-oxidized 3-deazaadenosine, as mentioned above

5.1 Rates of Transmethylation in Cancer and Normal Cells

(2). With AdoHCY hydrolysis blocked, the time-dependent accumulation of AdoHCY should reflect the rate of transfer of methyl groups from AdoMET and thereby its conversion to AdoHCY (3). Since transmethylation rates are dependent on the amounts of AdoMET and inversely proportional to the amount of AdoHCY accumulated, rates were normalized by multiplying the amount of cellular AdoHCY present by the AdoHCY/AdoMET ratio present at each time point measured. Therefore, transmethylation rates could be directly compared in the various cell types normalized at each time point for their AdoMET and AdoHCY amounts [28].

Figure 4 demonstrates the transmethylation rates in 18 human tumor cell lines and 4 normal human fibroblast cell strains in $HCY^{-}MET^{+}$. All of the cancer cell lines tested have rates of transmethylation that are greater than those of normal fibroblasts [28].

It has been demonstrated that a number of human and animal tumors have elevated levels of tRNA methyltransferase [24], an excess and unbalanced tRNA methylation, and elevated levels of methylated bases excreted [25] (*see* **Note 3**). It would seem that enhanced transmethylation rates in the cancer cells we have

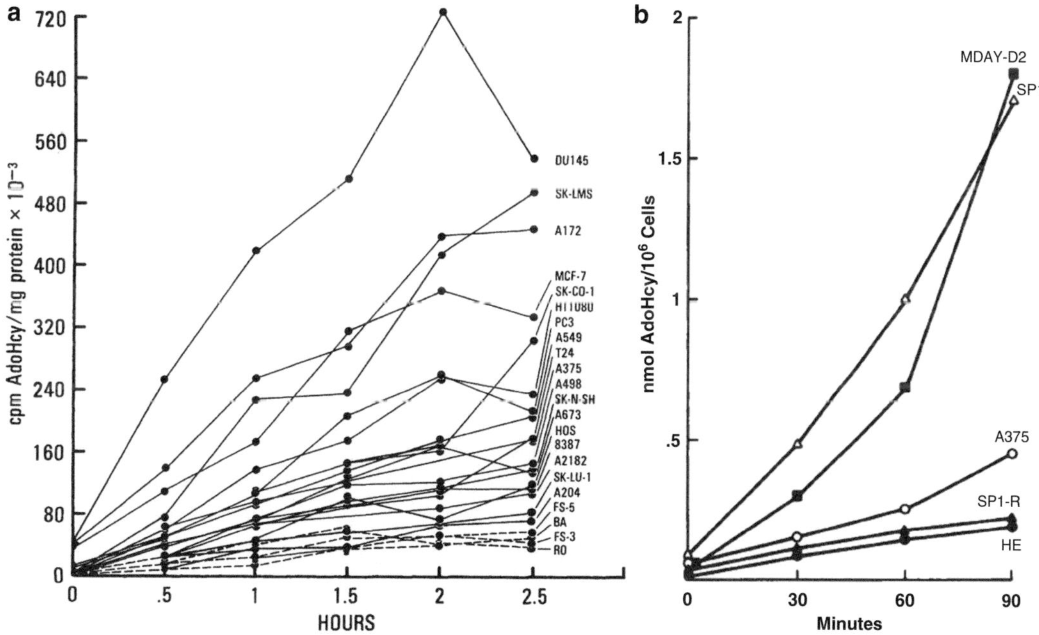

Fig. 4 Rates of transmethylation of human tumor cell lines and normal human fibroblast cell strains. All cells, with the exception of malignant melanoma A375 and rhabdomyosarcoma A204, were plated for 24 h at a density of 10^6 cells/35 mm petri dish. A375 and A204 were plated at a density of 2.5×10^5 cells/60 mm petri dish. All cells were labeled with 100 μM [^{35}S]-methionine (25 μCi/mL) for 24 h. Periodate-oxidized 3-deazaadenosine was added to a concentration of 10 μM and the accumulation of [^{35}S]AdoHCY was measured at half-hour intervals for 21/2 h as described in Methods. Values are counts/min (cpm) ^{35}S/mg cellular protein. Solid lines are human cancer cell lines. Dashed lines are human normal cell strains [28] (**a**); or nmol AdoHcy/10^6 cells [30] (for identifying of cells please *see* Fig. 5) (**b**)

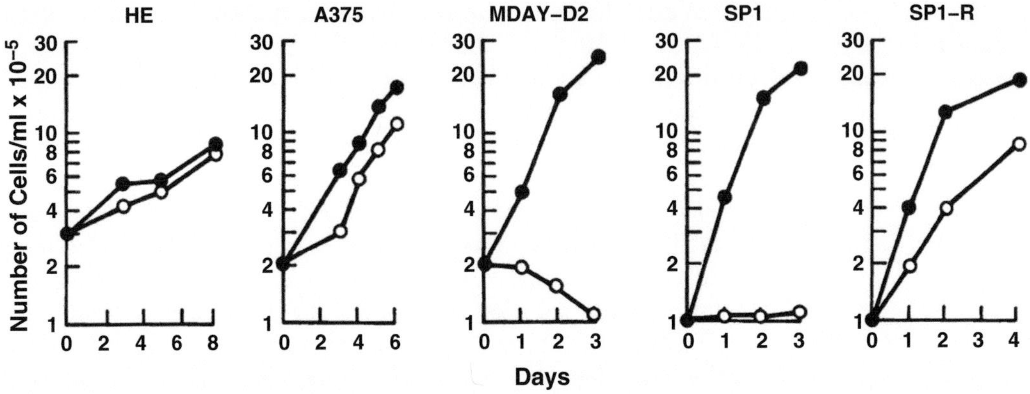

Fig. 5 Growth of the cell lines in $MET^{+}HCY^{-}$ (filled circle) and MET^{-} HCY^{+} (open circle) media. HE human lung embryo fibroblasts (filled circle), A375 human melanoma (open circle), SP-1 mouse mammary carcinoma (open triangle), and MDAY-D2 lymphoma (filled square) cells were placed in MET^{+} HCY^{-} medium and SP1-R which reverted to MET independence from SP1 revertant cells (filled triangle) in $MET^{-}HCY^{+}$ medium [30]

observed are responsible at least in part for MET dependence of cancer cells. In support of this hypothesis, Judde et al. [30] found that MET-independent revertants (SP1-R) (Fig. 5) reduced their rate of transmethylation compared to their MET-dependent parental cancer cells (SP1) (Fig. 4b).

Possibly certain transmethylations are enhanced at the expense of others. For example, we have found that many of the same cancer cell lines characterized in this chapter have deficient DNA methylation [31]. It is noteworthy that immortalized lymphoblasts which may be considered partially oncogenically transformed have higher rates of transmethylation than stimulated or quiescent lymphoblasts [28].

6 Conclusion

It should be emphasized, that all the human cancer cell lines tested demonstrate a defect in methionine metabolism, in that all have a very low free-MET pool compared to normal cells in MR medium. The MET-dependent cancer cells are additionally defective in their AdoMET/AdoHCY ratio. The low free MET in cancer cells despite high levels of MET synthase are likely due to enhanced aberrant transmethylation in the cancer cells [29] (*see* **Note 6**).

7 Notes

1. Three lines of evidence indicated high in vivo activity of MET synthase in malignant cells. First, the levels of MET synthase activity did not distinguish the normal from the malignant or transformed cells. Second, the uptake of radioactive label from

[5-^{14}C]Me-H_4PteGlu, the methyl donor in MET biosynthesis, was greatly stimulated in both normal and malignant or SV40-transformed cells by HCY (Fig. 1), the methyl group acceptor in MET biosynthesis. A majority of the radioactive label taken up from [5-^{14}C]Me-H_4PteGlu was recovered as MET as measured by amino acid analysis of hydrolyzates of normal and malignant cells. Third, in the presence of otherwise limiting amounts of exogenous MET, HCY stimulated growth of the malignant and transformed cells [2].

2. Tisdale [32, 33] also has reported a reduction of AdoMET levels in MET-dependent Walker-256 rat breast cancer cells.
3. Growth in MR medium is directly correlated with the AdoMET/AdoHCY ratio, implying that this ratio, which determines the ability of cells to methylate [34, 35], is critical for cell growth and that its reduction is symptomatic of MET dependence [18].
4. A general metabolic defect in human cancer cells affecting the MET pathway is suggested, since all of the diverse human cancer cell lines tested are altered in at least one aspect of MET metabolism [29].

References

1. Sugimura T, Birnbaum SM, Winitz M, Greenstein JP (1959) Quantitative nutritional studies with water-soluble, chemically defined diets. VIII. The forced feeding of diets each lacking in one essential amino acid. Arch Biochem Biophys 81:448–455
2. Hoffman RM, Erbe RW (1976) High *in vivo* rates of methionine biosynthesis in transformed human and malignant rat cells auxotrophic for methionine. Proc Natl Acad Sci U S A 73:1523–1527
3. Hoffman RM, Jacobsen SJ, Erbe RW (1978) Reversion to methionine independence by malignant rat and SV40-transformed human fibroblasts. Biochem Biophys Res Commun 82:228–234
4. Hoffman RM, Jacobsen SJ, Erbe RW (1979) Reversion to methionine independence in simian virus 40-transformed human and malignant rat fibroblasts is associated with altered ploidy and altered properties of transformation. Proc Natl Acad Sci U S A 76:1313–1317
5. Jacobsen SJ, Hoffman RM, Erbe RW (1980) Regulation of methionine adenosyltransferase in normal diploid and SV40-transformed human fibroblasts. J Natl Cancer Inst 65:1237–1244
6. Hoffman RM, Jacobsen SJ (1980) Reversible growth arrest in simian virus 40-transformed human fibroblasts. Proc Natl Acad Sci U S A 77:7306–7310
7. Chello PL, Bertino JR (1973) Dependence of 5-methyltetrahydrofolate utilization by L5178Y murine leukemia cells in vitro on the presence of hydroxycobalamin and transcobalamin II. Cancer Res 33:1898–1904
8. Halpern BC, Clark BR, Hardy DN, Halpern RM, Smith RA (1974) The effect of replacement of methionine by homocystine on survival of malignant and normal adult mammalian cells in culture. Proc Natl Acad Sci U S A 71:1133–1136
9. Kreis W, Goodenow M (1978) Methionine requirement and replacement by homocysteine in tissue cultures of selected rodent and human malignant and normal cells. Cancer Res 38:2259–2262
10. Kreis W, Baker A, Ryan V, Bertasso A (1980) Effect of nutritional and enzymatic methionine deprivation upon human normal and malignant cells in tissue culture. Cancer Res 40:634–641
11. Kreis W (1979) Tumor therapy by deprivation of L-methionine: rationale and results. Cancer Treat Rep 63:1069–1072
12. Hoffman RM (2015) Development of recombinant methioninase to target the general cancer-specific metabolic defect of methionine dependence: a 40-year odyssey. Expert Opin Biol Ther 15:21–31

13. Tan Y, Sun X, Xu M, Tan X-Z, Sasson A, Rashidi B, Han Q, Tan X-Y, Wang X, An Z, Sun F-X, Hoffman RM (1999) Efficacy of recombinant methioninase in combination with cisplatin on human colon tumors in nude mice. Clin Cancer Res 5:2157–2163
14. Kokkinakis DM, Hoffman RM, Frenkel EP, Wick JB, Han Q, Xu M, Tan Y, Schold SC (2001) Synergy between methionine stress and chemotherapy in the treatment of brain tumor xenografts in athymic mice. Cancer Res 61:4017–4023
15. Mecham JO, Rowitch D, Wallace CD, Stern PH, Hoffman RM (1983) The metabolic defect of methionine dependence occurs frequently in human tumor cell lines. Biochem Biophys Res Commun 117:429–434
16. Yoshioka T, Wada T, Uchida N, Maki H, Yoshida H, Ide N, Kasai H, Hojo K, Shono K, Maekawa R, Yagi S, Hoffman RM, Sugita K (1998) Anticancer efficacy *in vivo* and *in vitro*, synergy with 5-fluorouracil, and safety of recombinant methioninase. Cancer Res 58:2583–2587
17. Koziorowska J, Pieńkowska K, Tautt J (1980) Dependence on exogenous methionine of rat sarcoma and murine leukemia cells in culture. Arch Immunol Ther Exp (Warsz) 28:709–416
18. Coalson DW, Mecham JO, Stern PH, Hoffman RM (1982) Reduced availability of endogenously synthesized methionine for S-adenosylmethionine formation in methionine dependent cancer cells. Proc Natl Acad Sci U S A 79:4248–4251
19. Ashe H, Clark BR, Chu F, Hardy DN, Halpern BC, Halpern RM, Smith RA (1974) N5-methyltetrahydrofolate: homocysteine methyltransferase activity in extracts from normal, malignant and embryonic tissue culture cells. Biochem Biophys Res Commun 57:417–425
20. Baernstein HD (1945) The determination of catechol, phenol, and hydroquinone in urine. J Biol Chem 161:685–692
21. Lowry OH, Rosebrough NJ, Farr AL, Randall RJ (1951) Protein measurement with the Folin phenol reagent. J Biol Chem 193:265–275
22. Jonas AJ, Schneider JA (1981) A simple, rapid assay for cysteamine and other thiols. Anal Biochem 114:429–432
23. Stern PH, Mecham JO, Wallace CD, Hoffman RM (1983) Reduced free-methionine in methionine-dependent SV40-transformed human fibroblasts synthesizing apparently normal amounts of methionine. J Cell Physiol 117:9–14
24. Chiang PK, Cantoni GL (1979) Perturbation of biochemical transmethylations by 3-deazaadenosine in vivo. Biochem Pharmacol 28:1897–1902
25. Guranowski A, Montgomery JA, Cantoni GL, Chiang PK (1981) Adenosine analogues as substrates and inhibitors of S-adenosylhomocysteine hydrolase. Biochemistry 20:110–115
26. Johnson GS, Chiang PK (1981) 1-methylnicotinamide and NAD metabolism in normal and transformed normal rat kidney cells. Arch Biochem Biophys 210:263–269
27. Bader JP, Brown NR, Chiang PK, Cantoni GL (1978) 3-Deazaadenosine, an inhibitor of adenosylhomocysteine hydrolase, inhibits reproduction of Rous sarcoma virus and transformation of chick embryo cells. Virology 89:494–505
28. Stern PH, Hoffman RM (1984) Elevated overall rates of transmethylation in cell lines from diverse human tumors. In Vitro 20:663–670
29. Stern PH, Wallace CD, Hoffman RM (1984) Altered methionine metabolism occurs in all members of a set of diverse human tumor cell lines. J Cell Physiol 119:29–34
30. Judde JG, Ellis M, Frost P (1989) Biochemical analysis of the role of transmethylation in the methionine dependence of tumor cells. Cancer Res 49:4859–4865
31. Leodolter A, Alonso S, González B, Ebert MP, Vieth M, Röcken C, Wex T, Peitz U, Malfertheiner P, Perucho M (2015) Somatic DNA hypomethylation in H. pylori-associated high-risk gastritis and gastric cancer: enhanced somatic hypomethylation associates with advanced stage cancer. Clin Transl Gastroenterol 6:e85
32. Tisdale MJ (1980) Changes in tHNA methyltransferase activity and cellular S-adenosylmethionine content following methionine deprivation. Biochim Biophys Acta 609:296–305
33. Tisdale MJ (1980) Effect of methionine deprivation on methylation and synthesis of macromolecules. Br J Cancer 42:121–128
34. Johnston JM, Kredich NM (1979) Inhibition of methylation by adenosine in adenosine deaminase-inhibited, phytohemagglutinin-stimulated human lymphocytes. J Immunol 123:97–103
35. Hoffman DR, Marion DW, Cornatzer WE, Duerre JA (1980) S-Adenosylmethionine and S-adenosylhomocystein metabolism in isolated rat liver. Effects of L-methionine, L-homocystein, and adenosine. J Biol Chem 255:10822–10827

Chapter 3

Linkage of Methionine Dependence and Other Features of Malignancy

Robert M. Hoffman and Richard W. Erbe

Abstract

Cancer cells have an elevated methionine (MET) requirement compared to normal cells and are termed MET dependent. Cancer cells were isolated in MET-restricted (MR) medium that reverted from MET dependence to MET independence. Increased MET biosynthesis was not a prerequisite for reversion to MET independence, indicating that MET dependence was not due to reduced endogenous MET synthesis. MET-independent revertants of cancer cells concomitantly reverted for some of the other properties associated with malignancy: Of the 13 MET-independent revertants isolated 5 showed increased anchorage dependence as reflected by reduced cloning efficiencies in methylcellulose; 8 showed an increased serum requirement for optimal growth; 8 showed decreased cell density in medium containing high serum; and 3 altered their cell morphology significantly. Eight of the 13 revertants have increased chromosome numbers. Thus, by selecting for MET independence, it is possible to obtain heterogeneous reduced-malignancy revertants, indicating further a relationship between altered MET metabolism and other fundamental properties of oncogenic transformation.

Key words Methionine dependence, Methionine synthase, Cancer cells, Revertants, Methionine independence, Chromosomes, Anchorage dependence, Serum dependence, Cell morphology, Transmethylation

1 Introduction

An excess requirement for methionine (MET), termed MET dependence, is a general metabolic defect in cancer [1]. High levels of endogenous MET biosynthesis were previously observed in cancer cells that, unlike normal cells, were unable to grow in MET-restricted (MR) medium suggesting high MET usage by cancer cells [2]. In this chapter, we review results demonstrating that cancer cells can revert spontaneously from MET dependence to MET independence. We show that increased MET biosynthesis was not a prerequisite to regaining the ability to grow in MR medium. These data are consistent with our hypothesis [2] that the original defect in the transformed and malignant cells is not decreased MET biosynthesis, but increased MET usage [3]. MET

Robert M. Hoffman (ed.), *Methionine Dependence of Cancer and Aging: Methods and Protocols*, Methods in Molecular Biology, vol. 1866, https://doi.org/10.1007/978-1-4939-8796-2_3, © Springer Science+Business Media, LLC, part of Springer Nature 2019

overuse by cancer cells was demonstrated by their excess transmethylation reactions [4] and by the very bright signal of cancers imaged by [^{11}C]MET PET imaging [5]. The excessive use of MET by cancer cells is termed the "Hoffman effect" [6] analogous to the observation by Warburg of excess glucose use by cancer cells ("Warburg effect") [7].

Because MET dependence is found only in cancer cells, we previously determined whether MET-independent revertants could become normal with respect to other properties associated with oncogenic transformation, and we found that is indeed the case [8].

2 Materials

1. Doubly cloned MET-dependent human simian virus (SV40)-transformed lines, W18VA2 and SV80, and rat mammary carcinoma line, W-256, and other cancer cells [3].
2. Eagle's minimum essential medium (MEM) with 10% dialyzed fetal calf serum, without methionine (MET) and with 0.1 mM L-homocysteine (HCY) thiolactone, 0.1 mM folic acid 1.5 μM hydroxocobalamin (OH-Cbl), designated MET^-HCY^+ medium.
3. MEM with 10% dialyzed fetal calf serum, 0.1 mM MET, 0.1 mM folic acid, and 1.56 μM OH-Cbl, designated MET^+HCY^- medium [3].
4. Semisolid medium consisting of Eagle's MEM with 10% undialyzed fetal calf serum and 1.3% methylcellulose over a bed of agar.
5. Coulter counter for counting cells.
6. KCl.
7. Methanol/acetic acid.
8. Giemsa stain.
9. Phase-contrast photomicroscope.

3 Methods

1. Doubly clone MET-dependent W18VA2 and W-256 or other MET-dependent cancer cells in MET^+HCY^- medium.
2. Determine that all lines are free of mycoplasma using polymerase chain reactions (PCR) [3].
3. Inoculate parental transformed and malignant cells in 100 mm dishes with 10 mL MET^-HCY^+ medium and refeed for about 1 month.

4. Isolate focal areas of rare cancer cells growing in $MET^{-}HCY^{+}$ medium with cloning cylinders.
5. Further clone and characterize these new sublines with regard to the ability to grow in $MET^{-}HCY^{+}$ medium [3].
6. Measure 5-methyltetrahydropteroyl-glutamate:L-homocysteine *S*-methyltransferase (EC 2.1.1.13) (MET synthetase) in the parental and revertant cells as described previously [9], except equilibrate and elute the Dowex AG 1-X8 columns used to separate MET from 5-methyltetrahydrofolate (5-methyl-H_4-PteGlu) with 40 mM phosphate buffer pH 7.4 instead of water.
7. Measure 5,10-methylene-H_4 PteGlu reductase: (EC 11.1.68) as described previously [10].
8. Measure the uptake of [5-^{14}C] methyl-H_4PteGlu as described previously [2].
9. Conduct cell proliferation studies as described earlier [2] except that 60 mm petri dishes containing 4 mL of medium are used with an initial inoculum of 1.8×10^5 cells per dish.
10. Count cells with a Coulter counter [3].
11. Measure protein concentration by the method of Lowry et al. [11].
12. Isolate MET-independent revertants from doubly-cloned sublines of MET-dependent cancer cells.
13. Isolate MET-independent revertants R4, and R5a and R5b from doubly-cloned sublines of SV40-transformed human line SV80, termed sublines P4 and P5, respectively.
14. Assay anchorage dependence of the revertants by the ability of cells to form colonies in semisolid medium consisting of Eagle's MEM with 10% undialyzed fetal calf serum and 1.3% methylcellulose over a bed of agar.
15. Count only those colonies visible with a magnifying glass.
16. Refeed plates with liquid medium every 2 weeks [8].
17. Count chromosomes on preparations from logarithmic-phase cells swollen by treatment with 75 mM KC1, fixed with methanol/acetic acid, and stained with Giemsa [8].
18. Detect T-antigen in cells by immunofluorescence [12].
19. Determine serum dependence by the ability of cells to grow in minimal essential medium containing 1% fetal calf serum (undialyzed).
20. Compare cell densities during growth in Eagle's MEM medium containing 10% fetal calf serum [8].
21. Determine morphological features of cells by phase-contrast photomicroscopy [8].

4 Results

4.1 MET-Independent Revertants Regain the Ability to Grow in MR Medium

When parental MET-dependent cancer cell lines were inoculated in $MET^{-}HCY^{+}$ (MR) medium, most of the cells eventually died and detached from the surface despite weekly or twice-weekly feedings. However, after 2–4 weeks, focal areas of cells appeared which continued to grow in MR medium. These MET-independent revertant cells were cloned. The apparent reversion frequency of the W18VA2 line was approximately $1–2 \times 10^{-4}$. After many generations of growth in MET-containing medium, the revertants maintained their ability to grow in MR medium [3].

Revertants W18VA22AR1 and SV80R1 (Fig. 1) grew as well in MR medium as in MET-containing medium. This was in contrast to the parental lines which grew only transiently in MR medium and then ceased growth and eventually died. The revertants grew almost as well as their parental lines in MET-containing medium [3] (*see* **Notes 1** and **2**).

4.2 MET Synthase in MET-Dependent Cells and MET-Independent Revertants

Revertant SV80R1 contained parental levels of MET synthase under all experimental conditions tested, indicating that increased MET synthetase activity is not essential for reversion [3].

Further evidence that increased MET biosynthesis is not a prerequisite for reversion was from MET synthesis in intact cells, measured by the uptake of label from [5-^{14}C] methyl-H_4 PteGlu as

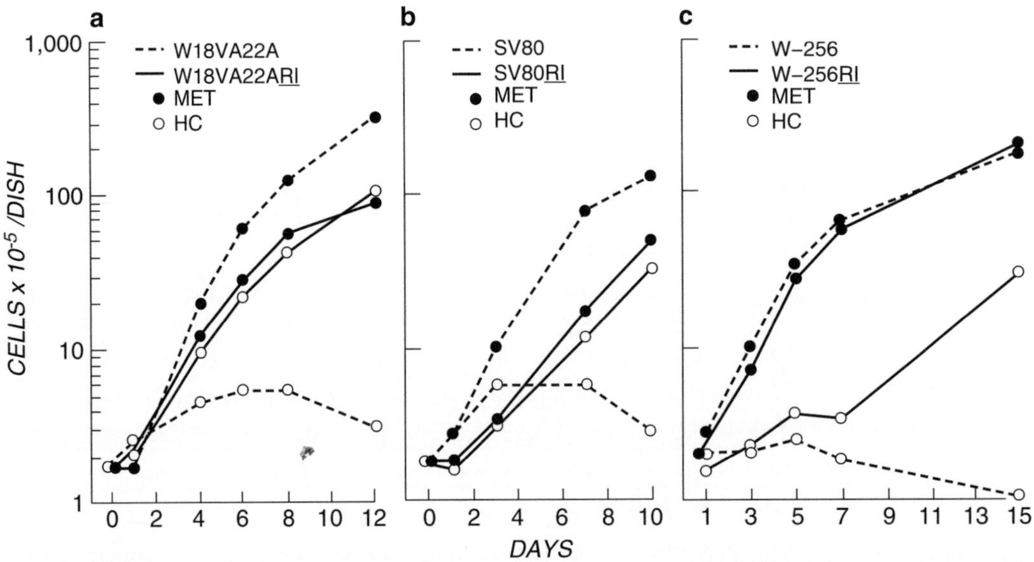

Fig. 1 Growth of parental malignant and transformed methionine (MET) auxotrophs and their MET-independent revertants in $MET^{-}HCY^{+}$ (open circle) and MET^{+} medium (filled circle). (**a**) W18VA22A and W18VA22AR1; (**b**) SV80 and SV80R1; (**c**) W-256 and W-256R1 [3]

described previously [2] (*see* **Note 1**): for example, three revertants did not take up more label than their parents [3].

The activity in cell extracts of 5,10-methylene-H_4PteGlu reductase, the enzyme catalyzing the synthesis of 5-methyl-H_4PteGlu, the methyl donor in MET biosynthesis, was similar in methionine-independent revertant SV80R2 and its parent indicating that increased activity of this enzyme is also not essential for reversion (*see* **Note 2**) [3].

4.3 Transmethylation Rates in MET-Dependent Cells and MET-Independent Revertants

In another study, revertant MET-independent cell lines had much lower basal transmethylation rates than their MET-dependent (parental cancer) cell lines. These results further indicate that the major determination of the MET dependence of cancer cells is an increase in the rate of transmethylation reactions, resulting in increased demand for MET by cancer cells [13].

4.4 Properties of Malignancy in MET-Dependent Revertants

Phase-contrast photomicrographs of a human MET-dependent, SV 40-transformed parent line, P1, and a MET-independent revertant, R1, were observed. The parental cells were stellate and contained pseudopods. The revertant cells were more pleomorphic, bipolar, and aligned more parallel, and not as stellate as their parent. The revertant cells are also larger than the parental cells and contain fewer pseudopods. The morphological differences between MET-dependent rat parent P2 and MET-independent rat revertants R2a and R2b were more pronounced (Fig. 2). The revertant cells are more bipolar, larger, and parallel than the parental cells [8].

The ability to grow well in medium containing 1% serum is characteristic of cancer cells. MET-independent revertants grew more slowly than their respective parents in 1% serum. The growth of revertant R3B was greatly reduced such that its growth was comparable to normal diploid human fibroblast MF316 under these conditions [8].

The ability to grow in a semisolid medium such as methylcellulose is characteristic of cancer cells and correlates with tumorigenicity [14]. Growth in semisolid medium indicates reduced anchorage dependence. Human revertants R1, R3b, R5a, and R5b showed a marked decrease in colony-forming efficiencies in methylcellulose and thus were considerably more normal with regard to this property. Although revertant R4 formed colonies in methylcellulose, the colonies were minute compared to those formed by the parental line, suggesting that R4 has partially reverted for this property [8].

Revertants R2, R3d, R4, R5a, and R5b and rat R2b and $R2b_2$ have reverted significantly toward normal with regard to arresting growth when confluent [8].

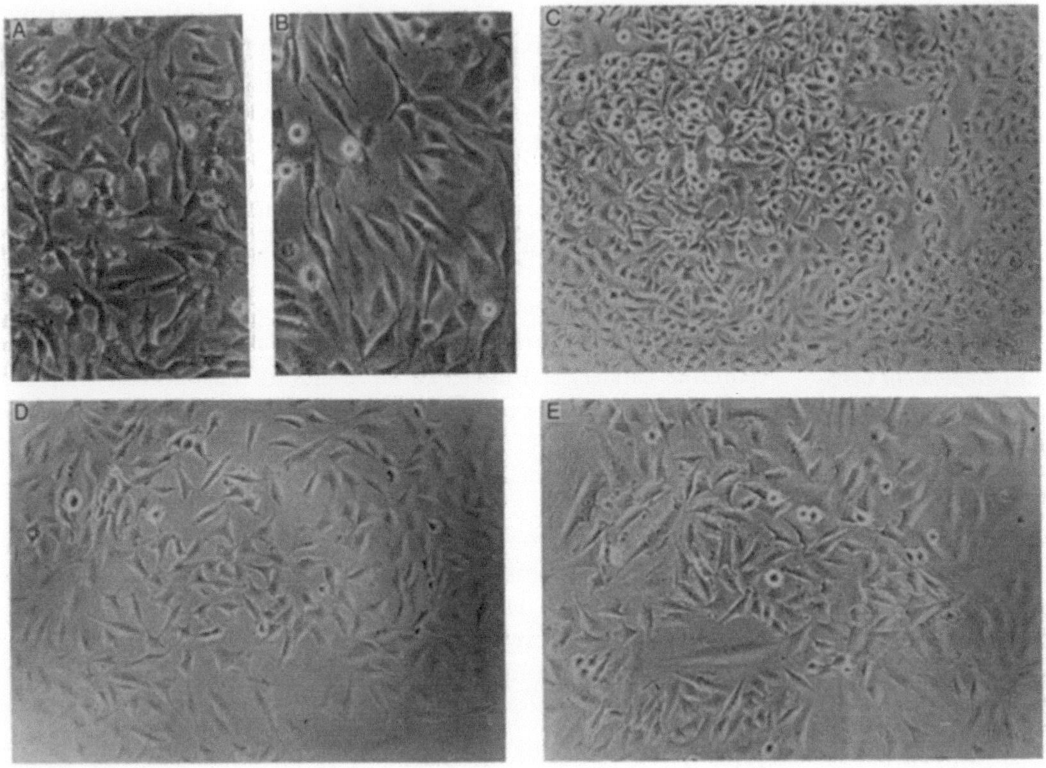

Fig. 2 Growth of cells in MET-containing medium (phase contrast, ×140). (**a**) Human parent MET auxotroph P1. (**b**) Human MET-independent revertant R1. (**c**) Rat parent MET auxotroph P2. (**d**) Rat MET-independent revertant R2a. (**e**) Rat MET-independent revertant $R2b_1$ [8]

4.5 Chromosome Content of MET-Independent Revertants

Seven out of nine revertants of SV40-transformed human cells that we have selected for MET independence also contain substantially greater numbers of chromosomes. For comparison, 20–50 metaphases from each cell line were counted. The chromosome distributions of revertants R1, R3a, and R4 are entirely distinct from those of the corresponding parental lines (Fig. 3) [8].

4.6 T Antigen in MET-Dependent Revertants

The parental human transformed lines contain SV40-specific tumor antigen (T antigen) which was detected by immunofluorescence assay. The SV40 T antigen is a virus-coded nuclear antigen [12] and was thought to be necessary for the maintenance of transformation [15]. However, studies by others of revertant cells [16], and of hybrids between mouse 3T3 cells and SV40-transformed human W18VA2 cells [17], have shown that T antigen is not sufficient to maintain the transformed state [18]. In our studies, the immunofluorescence assay (kindly performed by T. Rakusanova and P. Black) showed all revertant lines tested to contain T antigen, with lines R4 and R3b showing an immunofluorescence intermediate to that of the parents and the normal diploid fibroblast

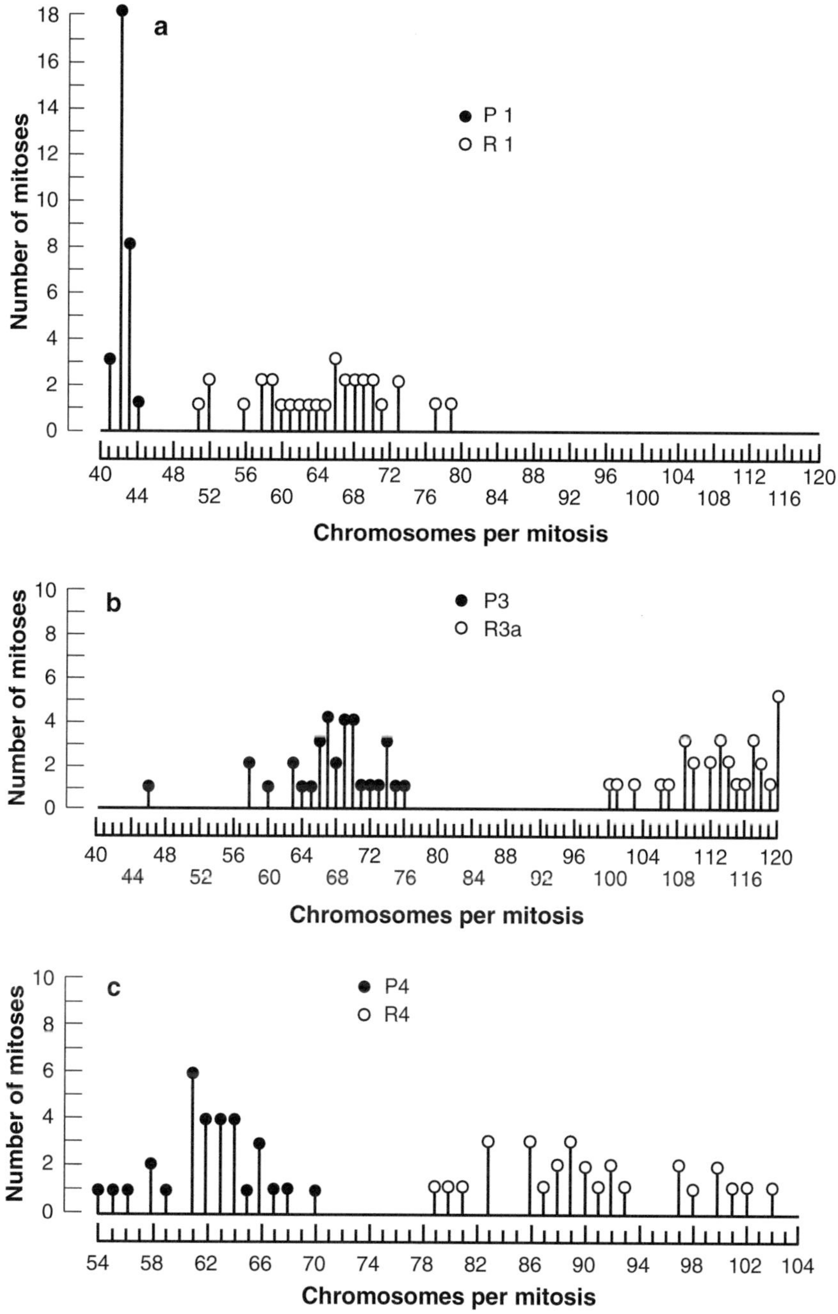

Fig. 3 Distribution of chromosome counts. (**a**) Human parent MET auxotroph P1 (filled circle) and MET-independent revertant R1 (open circle). (**b**) Human parent MET auxotroph P3 (filled circle) and MET-independent revertant R3a (open circle). (**c**) Human parent MET auxotroph P4 (filled circle) and MET-independent revertant R4 (open circle). Chromosome counts were done on preparations from logarithmic-phase cells swollen with 75 mM KCl, fixed with methanol/acetic acid, and stained with Giemsa [8]

Table 1
Summary of the properties of revertants [8]

Revertant subline	Morphological appearance	Serum dependence	Anchorage dependence	Cell density	Change in chromosome number[a]	T antigen[b]
Human						
R1	R	R	R	T	+23	+
R2	T	R	T	R	+33	+
R3a	T	R	T	T	+34	+
R3b	T	R	R	R	+16	I
R3c	T	T	T	T	-10	ND
R3d	T	R	T	R	+30	ND
R4	T	R	R	R	+28	I
R5a	T	R	R	R	+13	+
R5b	T	ND	R	R	−6	ND
Rat						
R1	T	T	T	T	−3	
R2a	R	T	T	T	+1	
$R2b_1$	R	T	T	R	+32	
$R2b_2$	T	R	T	R	ND	

R reversion toward normal, *T* properties associated with malignant transformation, *ND* not determined
[a]Difference between the mean values of parent and revertant
[b]+, Levels similar to those of fully transformed lines; I, intermediate levels as measured by immunofluorescence. T antigen in R5a was measured by immunoprecipitation, sodium dodecyl sulfate gel electrophoresis, and subsequent autoradiography [15]

MCF316. Thus, all revertants tested had at least a partially functional SV40 virus genome which was insufficient to maintain the full malignant phenotype [8].

Table 1 shows a summary of the properties of the revertants.

5 Conclusion

By the simple process of selecting for MET independence, it is possible to obtain sublines of cancer cells that have reverted toward normal with regard to various properties associated with transformation. It is possible that both the reversion to MET independence and the reduction in properties associated with oncogenic transformation are related to the ploidy changes found in most of the revertants, which possibly cause a change in the balance of chromosomes involved in the expression and suppression of malignant characteristics [19]. In any event, these results further indicate a relationship between altered MET metabolism and oncogenic transformation [8] (*see* **Note 3**).

Vanhamme and Szpirer [20, 21] showed that MET dependence can be acquired by normal cells by transfection of an activated H ras-1 oncogene. The H-ras-1-transformed cells then spontaneously reverted to MET independence at a high frequency. The reversion frequency was increased up to 400-fold by treatment of the H-ras-1-transformed cells with 5-azacytidine, which is a demethylating agent. 5-Aacytidine may have limited the aberrant transmethylation process associated with MET dependence, thereby increasing the rate of reversion from MET dependence to MET independence [20, 21] (*see* **Note 4**).

6 Notes

1. Of particular importance are MET-independent revertants SV80R1 and SV80R2 which have regained MET independence without increases in any of the three measures of MET biosynthesis. Thus, these results indicate that rates of MET synthesis do not necessarily distinguish normal MET-independent cells from MET-dependent cancer cells [3].
2. Since revertant lines SV80R1 and SV80R2 appear unaltered with regard to MET biosynthesis, they may have regained MET independence by correcting the defect that originally produced the MET dependence, possibly increased and aberrant transmethylation, which may be fundamental to carcinogenesis [3].
3. Under conditions of MET restriction, MET-dependent cancer cells can give rise to rare MET-independent revertants and in contrast to rare chemotherapy-resistant cells which arise and become more malignant [22], the MET-independent revertants become more normal. This is an important point for cancer therapy which targets MET.
4. The *ras* oncogene can also convert normal cells to MET dependence. The fact that 5-azacytidine, a DNA methylation inhibitor, causes high a rate of MET-independent reversion further suggests that the phenomena of excess and aberrant transmethylation is associated with MET dependence.

References

1. Hoffman RM (2015) Development of recombinant methioninase to target the general cancer-specific metabolic defect of methionine dependence: a 40-year odyssey. Expert Opin Biol Ther 15:21–31
2. Hoffman RM, Erbe RW (1976) High in vivo rates of methionine biosynthesis in transformed human and malignant rat cells auxotrophic for methionine. Proc Natl Acad Sci U S A 73:1523–1527

3. Hoffman RM, Jacobsen SJ, Erbe RW (1978) Reversion to methionine independence by malignant rat and SV40-transformed human fibroblasts. Biochem Biophys Res Commun 82:228–234
4. Stern PH, Hoffman RM (1984) Elevated overall rates of transmethylation in cell lines from diverse human tumors. In Vitro 20:663–670
5. Xu W, Gao L, Shao A, Zheng J, Zhang J (2017) The performance of 11C-methionine PET in the differential diagnosis of glioma recurrence. Oncotarget 8:91030–91039
6. Murakami T, Li S, Han Q, Tan Y, Kiyuna T, Igarashi K, Kawaguchi K, Hwang HK, Miyaki K, Singh AS, Hiroshima Y, Lwin TM, DeLong JC, Chishima T, Tanaka K, Bouvet M, Endo I, Eilber FC, Hoffman RM (2017) Recombinant methioninase effectively targets a Ewing's sarcoma in a patient-derived orthotopic xenograft (PDOX) nude-mouse model. Oncotarget 8:35630–35638
7. Warburg O (1956) On the origin of cancer cells. Science 123:309–314
8. Hoffman RM, Jacobsen SJ, Erbe RW (1979) Reversion to methionine independence in simian virus 40-transformed human and malignant rat fibroblasts is associated with altered ploidy and altered properties of transformation. Proc Natl Acad Sci U S A 76:1313–1317
9. Kamely D, Littlefield JW, Erbe RW (1973) Regulation of 5-methyltetrahydrofolate: homocysteine methyltransferase activity by methionine, vitamin B12, and folate in cultured baby hamster kidney cells. Proc Natl Acad Sci USA 70:2585–2589
10. Rosenblatt DS, Erbe RW (1973) Reciprocal changes in the levels of functionally related folate enzymes during the culture cycle in human fibroblasts. Biochem Biophys Res Commun 54:1627–1633
11. Lowry OH, Rosebrough NJ, Farr AL, Randall RJ (1951) Protein measurement with the Folin phenol reagent. J Biol Chem 193:265–275
12. Black PH, Rowe WP, Turner HC, Huebner RJ (1963) A specific complement-fixing antigen present in SV40 tumor and transformed cells. Proc Natl Acad Sci U S A 50:1148–1156
13. Judde JG, Ellis M, Frost P (1989) Biochemical analysis of the role of transmethylation in the methionine dependence of tumor cells. Cancer Res 49:4859–4865
14. Freedman VH, Shin SI (1974) Cellular tumorigenicity in nude mice: correlation with cell growth in semi-solid medium. Cell 3:355–359
15. Osborn M, Weber K (1975) Simian virus 40 gene A function and maintenance of transformation. J Virol 15:636–644
16. Pollack R, Wolman S, Vogel A (1970) Reversion of virus-transformed cell lines: hyperploidy accompanies retention of viral genes. Nature 228(5275):938
17. Weiss MC (1970) Further studies on loss of T-antigen from somatic hybrids between mouse cells and SV40-transformed human cells. Proc Natl Acad Sci U S A 66(1):79–86
18. Bloomfield M, Duesberg P (2015) Karyotype alteration generates the neoplastic phenotypes of SV40-infected human and rodent cells. Mol Cytogenet 8:79
19. Yamamoto T, Rabinowitz Z, Sachs L (1973) Identification of the chromosomes that control malignancy. Nat New Biol 243:247–250
20. Vanhamme L, Szpirer C (1989) Spontaneous and 5-azacytidine-induced revertants of methionine-dependent tumor-derived and H-ras-1-transformed cells. Exp Cell Res 181:159–168
21. Vanhamme L, Szpirer C (1987) Methionine metabolism defect in cells transfected with an activated HRAS1 oncogene. Exp Cell Res 169:120–126
22. St. Croix B, Flørenes VA, Rak JW, Flanagan M, Bhattacharya N, Slingerland JM, Kerbel RS (1996) Impact of the cyclin-dependent kinase inhibitor p27Kip1 on resistance of tumor cells to anticancer agents. Nat Med 2:1204–1210

Chapter 4

Isolation and Characterization of Methionine-Independent Clones from Methionine-Dependent Cancer Cells

Stacey L. Borrego, Da-Wei Lin, and Peter Kaiser

Abstract

Unlike normal cells, transformed cells are unable to grow when methionine in the growth media is restricted. Reversion to methionine independence is a rare event in transformed and malignant cells. Methionine-independent revertants provide an excellent system to identify metabolic signatures and molecular characteristics associated with methionine dependency of transformed cells. Revertants maintain the genetic background and general growth behavior of the parental cell line, except that they proliferate under methionine restriction such as in methionine-free media supplemented with homocysteine. Here we describe a general approach to generate methionine-independent revertants using the example of the triple-negative breast cancer cell line MDA-MB-468. To validate and characterize reversion we describe assays to evaluate cell proliferation and anchorage-independent growth in soft agar.

Key words Methionine, Methionine restriction, Methionine restriction resistance, Methionine independence, Homocysteine, Anchorage independence

1 Introduction

Methionine metabolism is an essential metabolic pathway in mammals. Early studies of metabolism identified a strict metabolic requirement for the amino acid methionine in transformed, malignant cells known as the "methionine dependency of cancer." When cultured in growth media where methionine has been replaced with its metabolic precursor homocysteine, malignant cells are unable to proliferate and undergo a distinct cell cycle arrest in G_1 or G_2/M [1–9]. In contrast, proliferation of non-transformed, methionine-independent cells is mostly unaffected by the metabolite replacement [10]. Reversion of transformed, methionine-dependent cells to a non-transformed methionine-independent state is a rare event, occurring approximately once in every 10,000 cells. Unlike their transformed counterparts, methionine-independent revertants can

Robert M. Hoffman (ed.), *Methionine Dependence of Cancer and Aging: Methods and Protocols*, Methods in Molecular Biology, vol. 1866, https://doi.org/10.1007/978-1-4939-8796-2_4,

proliferate in homocysteine media indefinitely and exhibit normal-like cell properties including anchorage dependence [11, 12].

Derivation of methionine-independent revertants from methionine-dependent transformed cells was originally presented by Hoffman and colleagues in 1978 using SV40-transformed human cell lines and rat breast carcinoma fibroblast cells [11, 12]. Here we describe a step-by-step procedure to isolate clonal methionine-independent cell lines derived from methionine-dependent cancer cells by prolonged culturing in homocysteine medium (*see* Subheading 3.1). We have applied this strategy to the triple-negative breast cancer cell line MDA-MB-468 and this approach is applicable to other methionine-dependent cancer cell lines. The methionine-independent revertants have similar proliferation rates in methionine-supplemented growth media as the parental cell line, continue proliferating in homocysteine media, and have lost their tumorigenic hallmark for anchorage-independent growth [5, 8].

To validate the spontaneous reversion of these clones, we describe methods for assessment of cell proliferation using the luminescent-based viability assay CellTiter-Glo® (Promega) (*see* Subheading 3.2), and anchorage independence using soft agar (*see* Subheading 3.3). The CellTiter-Glo® assay quantifies the amount of ATP from metabolically active cells, which is proportional to the number of cells in the culture. Since transformed, methionine-dependent cells are unable to proliferate in methionine-restricted homocysteine-containing growth media, measuring proliferation rates in this medium is the first step to evaluate revertant cell lines [5, 10, 13]. We and others have observed that reversion to methionine independence is typically accompanied by the loss of tumorigenic characteristics [11, 13]. While only xenograft assays can provide definitive information about the tumorigenic potential of revertant cell lines, a relatively simple evaluation of anchorage-independent growth can be informative about tumorigenic properties without animal experiments. Anchorage-independence is a well-known signature of malignant cells and soft agar assays are a stringent method for transformation detection [14]. When suspended in soft agar, malignant cell growth is unaffected and colonies form in the agar layer, whereas non-transformed cells require attachment to a solid surface and do not proliferate. Anchorage independence assays are thus simple and effective methods to compare tumorigenic potential of methionine-independent revertants from the transformed parental cell line.

Using a system of methionine-dependent and -independent cell pairs is ideal to identify unique metabolic signatures linking methionine dependence and tumorigenicity.

2 Materials

2.1 Deriving Methionine Independent Revertants from Methionine-Dependent Transformed cells

All procedures should be performed in a cell culture hood using sterile techniques and conditions. The method described uses the triple-negative breast cancer cell line MDA-MB-468 and its specific growth conditions to generate methionine-independent revertants.

2.1.1 Cell Culturing Materials

1. Methionine growth medium: Dulbecco's modified Eagle's medium with high glucose supplemented with 10% dialyzed fetal bovine serum (dFBS), 1.5 μM cyanocobalamin (vitamin B12), 4 mM L-glutamine, 100 μM L-cysteine, and 100 μM methionine (*see* **Note 1**). Filter with a 0.22 μm membrane and store at 4 °C. Warm to 37 °C before use.
2. Homocysteine growth medium: Dulbecco's modified Eagle's medium with high glucose supplemented with 10% dialyzed FBS (dFBS), 1.5 μM cyanocobalamin (vitamin B_{12}), 4 mM L-glutamine, 100 μM L-cysteine, and 370 μM DL-homocysteine (*see* **Note 2**). Filter with a 0.22 μm membrane and store at 4 °C. Warm to 37 °C before use.
3. Phosphate-buffered saline (PBS): 137 mM NaCl, 2.7 mM KCl, 10 mM Na_2HPO_4, 1.8 mM KH_2PO_4, pH 7.4. In a 1 L graduated cylinder or glass beaker with a stir bar, add 800 mL distilled water and stir at medium speed. Weigh 8 g NaCl, 0.2 g KCl, 1.44 g Na_2HPO_4, and 0.24 g KH_2PO_4 and add to stirring water. After all salts have dissolved adjust the pH to 7.4 with HCl. Add distilled water to a total volume of 1 L. Autoclave and store at room temperature.
4. Cell culture grade trypsin.
5. 150 mm, 24-well, 6-well, and 100 mm cell culture plates.
6. 200 μL Micropipettor with sterile tips.

2.2 Luminescent Measurement of Cell Viability

The majority of transformed, malignant cell lines are methionine dependent and cannot proliferate when cultured in methionine-free homocysteine-containing media. In comparison, non-transformed and primary cells can utilize homocysteine and continue to proliferate when methionine is not available in the growth media. To determine if a cell line is methionine independent, we routinely use the luminescent cell viability assay CellTiter-Glo® (Promega), which provides a quick readout for cell proliferation (*see* **Note 3**).

2.2.1 Materials

1. Methionine growth media (described in Subheading 2.1, **item 1**).
2. Homocysteine growth media (described in Subheading 2.1, **item 2**).

3. PBS (described in Subheading 2.1, **item 3**).
4. Cell culture-grade trypsin.
5. 96-Well white plates with clear plastic bottom.
6. CellTiter-Glo® luminescent viability assay (Promega): Reconstitute reagent per the manufacturer's instructions. Aliquot 10 mL in 15 mL conical tubes. Store at −20 °C.
7. Luminometer plate reader.

2.3 Assessment of Anchorage Independence with Soft Agar

All procedures should be prepared in sterile conditions using sterile reagents, media, and glassware. The following protocol provides instructions for preparing ten 0.35% soft agar assays in 35 mm dishes.

2.3.1 Base Agar

1. 1% w/v Low-temperature gelling agar: Prepare a minimum of 10 mL 1% low-temperature gelling agar in sterile water. In a sterilized glass bottle with a stir bar, warm 10 mL sterile water to 37 °C. With the stir bar at medium speed, add 100 mg low-temperature gelling agar to warm water and stir until completely dissolved. Keep agar in a 40 °C water bath for immediate use (*see* **Note 4**).
2. 2× Methionine growth medium: 1× methionine growth medium is described in Subheading 2.1, **item 1**. Prepare 10 mL growth medium with twice the amount of additives, including FBS and antibiotics (*see* **Note 5**). Warm to 40 °C in a water bath.
3. 35 mm Sterile Petri dishes (*see* **Note 6**).

2.3.2 Top Agar Layer with Cell Suspension

1. 0.7% w/v Low-temperature gelling agar: Prepare a minimum of 10 mL 0.7% low-temperature gelling agar in sterile water. In a sterilized glass bottle with a stir bar, warm 10 mL sterile water to 40 °C. With the stir bar on medium speed, add 70 mg low-temperature gelling agar to warm water and stir until completely dissolved. Keep agar in a 40 °C water bath for immediate use (*see* **Note 7**).
2. 1× Methionine growth medium for preparation of cell suspension (*see* **Note 5**).
3. 2× Methionine growth medium: 1× methionine growth medium is described in Subheading 2.1, **item 1**. Prepare 10 mL growth medium with twice the amount of additives including FBS and antibiotics (*see* **Note 5**). Warm to 40 °C in a water bath.
4. PBS (described in Subheading 2.1, **item 3**).
5. Hemocytometer to prepare cell suspension.
6. Cell culture-grade trypsin for adherent cells.

7. Serum-containing growth medium to collect cells after trypsin-induced cell dissociation.
8. Cell suspension of 6667 cells per 1 mL in 2× growth medium (*see* **Notes 8–10**).

2.3.3 Assay Maintenance

1. 1× methionine growth medium warmed to 37 °C (described in Subheading 2.1, **item 1**, *see* **Note 5**).

2.3.4 Staining Colonies

1. 0.005% crystal violet solution prepared in 50% ethanol.
2. PBS.

3 Methods

3.1 Deriving Methionine-Independent Revertants from Methionine-Dependent Transformed Cells

1. Culture cells in a 150 mm cell culture plate in methionine growth medium until they reach 80% confluency.
2. Remove and discard methionine growth medium and add 10 mL pre-warmed (37 °C) PBS to the plate to wash the cell monolayer. Swirl plate to remove all traces of methionine and aspirate PBS wash.
3. Perform a second 10 mL PBS wash and aspirate to discard.
4. Add 20 mL pre-warmed methionine-free homocysteine-containing growth medium to the cell culture plate and return cells to humidified incubator at 37 °C.
5. In the first week, replace the medium every day to remove detached cells. Aspirate the current growth medium and wash once with 10 mL pre-warmed PBS. Replenish the cells with 20 mL pre-warmed homocysteine medium.
6. In the second week, replace the medium every 2 days to remove detached cells and replenish media components.
7. Use a microscope to identify areas of growing cells.
8. Continue to culture cell colonies until they are large enough to be visualized without a microscope.
9. Once the colonies can be visualized without a microscope cells can be isolated and transferred to a 24-well plate.
10. Prepare a 24-well plate for cell transfer by filling wells with 500 μL pre-warmed homocysteine growth medium.
11. Remove and discard growth medium of cell-culture plates containing cell colonies.
12. Wash once with 10 mL PBS and aspirate to discard.
13. Add 10 mL pre-warmed homocysteine growth medium to cell culture plates to prevent cell dehydration during colony isolation.

14. To collect a single colony, hold the plate at a 45-degree angle to clear the medium from the region of interest.
15. Using a micropipettor with a sterile tip gently touch the tip to the cell colony and lift (*see* **Note 11**).
16. Transfer colony to a 24-well plate and gently resuspend to mix (*see* **Note 12**).
17. Place cells in a humidified incubator at 37 °C and allow selected clones to grow.
18. When cells have grown to about 80% confluency, use standard subculturing methods to dissociate cells from 24-well plates and replate in 6-well plates (*see* **Note 9**).
19. At this point, cells can be switched back to methionine growth medium or maintained in methionine-free homocysteine-containing medium for further selection (*see* **Note 5**).
20. Continue to culture cells and expand clonal cell lines as necessary.

3.2 Luminescent Measurement of Cell Viability

This assay is performed over the course of several days. Each 96-well plate is collected for each time point. We typically perform this assay over 6 days, collecting time points at 0, 2, 4, and 6 days, and thus we require four identically-seeded 96-well plates. To ensure data quality, we seed at least four wells per treatment for each time point.

1. From cultured cells, prepare a cell suspension to be seeded into 96-well white plates with a clear plastic bottom (*see* **Note 9**).
2. Seed 2000–10,000 cells per well in each 96-well plate (*see* **Note 13**). Allow the cells to attach to the plate for at least 16 h before proceeding.
3. Wash the cells twice with 200 μL PBS per well and aspirate all residual liquid from each well (*see* **Note 14**).
4. Add 100 μL of either methionine or homocysteine growth medium and return all plates to the cell culture incubator at 37 °C except for the day 0 plate—see below (*see* **Note 15**).
5. To collect each time point, remove the plate from the cell culture incubator and place directly in a −80 °C freezer (*see* **Note 16**).
6. Thaw an adequate amount (100 μL/well) of CellTiter-Glo® reagent for 1 h at room temperature.
7. Remove samples from −80 °C and immediately add 100 μL/well of CellTiter-Glo® (*see* **Notes 17** and **18**).
8. Allow the plate to reach room temperature before proceeding to a luminometer plate reader. The reaction is stable for 1 h (*see* **Note 19**) (Fig. 1).

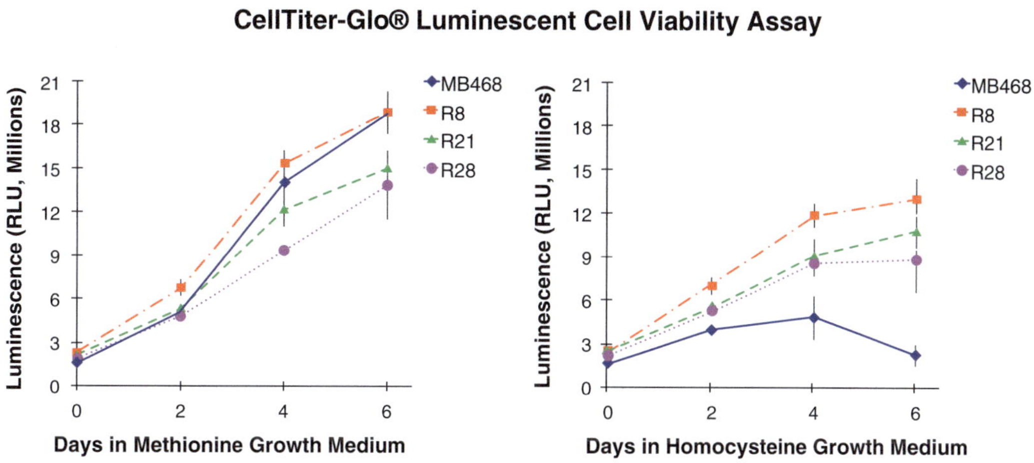

Fig. 1 MDA-MB-468 cancer cells and the methionine-independent revertant clones MDA-MB-468res-R8, -21, and -R28 were cultured in either methionine or homocysteine growth medium. Samples were collected at 0, 2, 4, and 6 days and treated with CellTiter-Glo®. Unlike the methionine-independent revertants, the cancer cell line MDA-MB-468 cannot proliferate in methionine-free homocysteine-containing growth media

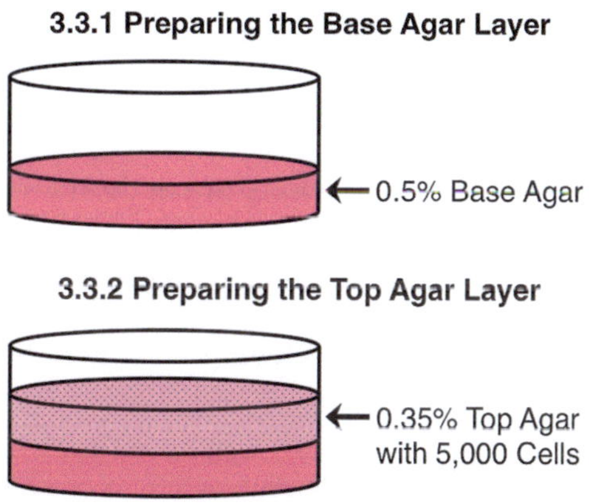

Fig. 2 Soft agar assays are a stringent method for cell-transformation detection. Each assay comprises two layers, a lower 0.5% agar base layer (described in Subheading 3.3.1) and an upper 0.35% agar top layer containing the cells of interest (described in Subheading 3.3.2)

3.3 Assessment of Anchorage Independence with Soft Agar (Fig. 2)

3.3.1 Preparing the Base Agar Layer

1. 0.5% agar base: In 50 mL conical tube, gently combine 10 mL 1% agar and 10 mL 2× complete growth medium until fully mixed while preventing bubbles in the solution. This will prepare 20 mL of 0.5% agar.
2. Add 1.5 mL 0.5% agar base to each 35 mm Petri dish. Gently swirl to ensure that the bottom of each dish is completely covered. The remaining 0.5% agar can be discarded.
3. Set dishes aside for a minimum of 30 min at room temperature to allow agar to solidify (*see* **Note 20**).

3.3.2 Preparing the Top Agar Layer

1. If the dishes with the base layer are prepared ahead of time, remove from 4 °C and allow to equilibrate to room temperature for at least 30 min.
2. Prepare dishes with base agar appropriately for samples and positive and negative controls (*see* **Note 21**).
3. For blank assays in triplicate, mix 2.25 mL 0.7% agar with 2.25 mL 2× growth medium in 15 mL conical tubes. Gently mix to avoid the introduction of bubbles. Pipette 1.5 mL onto the top of three dishes containing a base layer.
4. For cell suspension assays in triplicate, add 2.25 mL 0.7% agar to 15 mL conical tubes containing 2.25 mL cell suspension in 2× growth medium. Gently mix to avoid the introduction of bubbles and damage to cells. Pipette 1.5 mL into three dishes with base layer.
5. Place dishes at 4 °C for 30 min to solidify (*see* **Note 22**).
6. Incubate dishes at 37 °C in humidified incubator for 10–30 days.

3.3.3 Assay Maintenance

1. Add 0.75 mL of 1× growth medium to plates one or two times per week to prevent the agar from dehydrating.
2. Ensure the incubator's humidity by maintaining water levels if necessary. A lack of humidity will cause the agar to dehydrate resulting in cell death.

3.3.4 Staining Colonies

1. Aspirate any remaining medium from the dish without disturbing the agar by holding the dish at a 45-degree angle allowing the medium to collect on the side of the dish.
2. Add 0.5 mL of 0.005% crystal violet for a minimum of 1 h. Gently agitate dishes with a rocker on a low setting at room temperature (*see* **Note 23**).
3. Aspirate the crystal violet solution from the dishes without disturbing the agar.
4. Quickly add 0.5 mL 1× PBS to the dish, swirl, and aspirate. Do not leave the dish in PBS; the agar will soften and become too difficult to handle (*see* **Note 24**).
5. Count colonies using a dissecting microscope or scan (Fig. 3) (*see* **Note 25**).

4 Notes

1. The medium described is the recommended culturing condition for MDA-MB-468 cells; this should be modified for the cell line of interest. Dialyzed fetal bovine serum (dFBS) must be used to eliminate FBS as a source for methionine and other

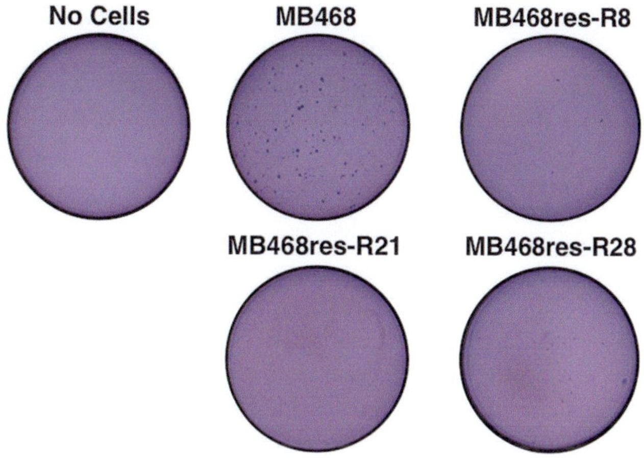

Fig. 3 Methionine-independent revertant clones MDA-MB-468res-R8, -R21, and -28 form fewer and smaller clones in soft agar compared to the parental MDA-MB-468 cell line. Control plate does not contain cells

amino acids. Our DMEM of choice is high glucose without glutamine, cysteine, methionine, or homocysteine and thus these components must be supplemented.

2. Homocysteine can be readily oxidized and must be stored at −20 °C. We prepare homocysteine medium in small portions of 100 mL and discard any excess medium after 1 week. For our experiments we use DL-homocysteine; however, L-homocysteine is commercially available. If L-homocysteine is used the final concentration should be 185 μM.
3. A number of alternative assays such as MTT (3-(4, 5-dimethylthiazol-2-yl)-2, 5-diphenyltetrazolium bromide) or sulforhodamine B can also be used [15, 16].
4. It is best to use the prepared soft agar immediately but it can be stored at room temperature and melted again for future use. Properly seal glass bottles to prevent water evaporation, which increases agar density. When agar is reheated, maintain in a water bath for 30 min to lower the temperature before use.
5. For standard culturing and anchorage independence assays it is unnecessary to use dFBS in the growth medium because methionine dependence is not being assessed. Generally dFBS is more expensive and we only use it prior to and during experiments in which cells cultured in methionine and homocysteine growth medium are being compared.
6. Assays can be prepared in 6-well plates instead of 35 mm Petri dishes. However, we have found that assays in 6-well plates evaporate at different rates depending on the location of the well in the plate and thus we recommend using individual dishes for each assay.

7. Certain cell types are sensitive to the percentage of top agar; determine if 0.3 or 0.4% agar is best for the cell type of interest. In our assays for MDA-MB-468 cells we choose to use a final concentration of 0.35% agar.
8. The number of cells used per assay needs to be optimized. We found that 5000 cells per assay is optimal for MDA-MB-468 cells.
9. We use trypsin to release the adherent cells from the cell-culturing surface. First, aspirate current medium and wash cells with pre-warmed PBS to remove all traces of serum. Aspirate PBS, add pre-warmed trypsin to cover the cell monolayer, and swirl the plate to ensure that trypsin is evenly distributed. We use 0.5% trypsin and generally need to incubate our cells for 10 min at 37 °C; however, trypsin percentage and incubation times will vary depending on trypsin potency, cell type, and cell density and therefore incubation time should be monitored and kept to a minimum. Collect cells by adding serum-containing growth medium and gently pipette up and down to break up any cell clumps. Transfer cell suspensions to 15 mL conical tubes and centrifuge (300 × *g*, 5 min, room temperature). Aspirate the supernatant and resuspend pellets thoroughly in 1× methionine growth medium.
10. Cell suspensions should be prepared as normally done during subculturing or as described in **Note 9**. After centrifugation, aspirate the supernatant and resuspend pellets thoroughly in 1× methionine growth medium to prepare for cell counting. Count the resuspended cells using a hemocytometer. For three assays using 5000 cells per assay we need 2.25 mL of 15,000 cells (5000 cells/0.75 mL or 6667 cells/mL). Transfer the equivalent of 15,000 cells to a new 15 mL conical tube. Centrifuge, aspirate supernatant, and resuspend cell pellets in 2.25 mL 2× methionine growth medium. Adjust accordingly for quantity of assays and cell number.
11. If the cells do not lift off the plate easily you can gently slide the pipette tip from one side of the colony to the other. This may cause cell damage and should not be used as a first option. Alternatively, cloning cylinders can be used to harvest cells using trypsin-induced dissociation.
12. It is fine if the colony does not completely break up into a single-cell suspension; the cells will still adhere and grow in the 24-well plate. Trypsin will be used in a later step to disrupt the colony and produce a single-cell suspension during replating.
13. Plating number depends on cell size. For example, MDA-MB-468 cells are smaller than MDA-MB-231 and thus we use 8000 cells/well of MDA-MB-468 and 3000 cells/well of MDA-MB-231.

14. It is crucial to remove all of the residual methionine from the growth media and PBS washes before treating with methionine-free homocysteine-containing media.
15. To compare proliferation rates of each cell line throughout the time course, each plate should have the same cell line treated in both methionine and homocysteine growth media.
16. These samples can be stored in −80 °C for up to 1 month.
17. When using an electric multichannel pipette, always use 5 mL more CellTiter-Glo® then calculated to ensure that the bottom of the reagent reservoir is covered. Unused reagent can be recycled and stored at −20 °C.
18. A significant reduction in luciferase signal occurs when the reagent is added to cells kept at room temperature for an extended period before adding the CellTiter-Glo® reagent.
19. The luciferase in the CellTiter-Glo® reagent mixture utilizes ATP from sample cells to produce luminescent signals as a cell-viability-per-cell-number readout. If the experimental procedure severely affects ATP production it will be inadequate to use CellTiter-Glo® to measure cell viability.
20. These plates can be stored for up to 1 week at 4 °C. Stack plates, wrap in foil, and store upside down. For best results, prepare the base layer 1–2 days in advance before adding the top layer.
21. We recommend plating each cell line in replicates of no less than three. Including a positive control and an assay without cells is recommended. Positive controls should be an anchorage-independent tumorigenic cell line; we have used the triple-negative breast cancer cell line MDA-MB-468. An assay with top and base layers without cells is helpful for a background control and also monitors any contamination.
22. Placing the assays at 4 °C will ensure that the agar is fully solidified before incubating at 37 °C and will not harm the cells. In our experience, if the agar does not completely solidify at room temperature before placing in the incubator, the agar will remain in a semisolid state and the assay will be difficult to work with for quantification.
23. An alternative for colony-staining is nitro-blue tetrazolium chloride.
24. When staining the cells it is important not to disturb the agar. Having been placed at room temperature, treated with crystal violet, and washed with PBS all make the agar soft and easily damaged or aspirated into a vacuum, if touched.
25. Methionine dependence can also be assessed by sensitivity to methioninase [17].

References

1. Chello PL, Bertino JR (1973) Dependence of 5 methyltetrahydrofolate utilization by L5178Y murine leukemia cells in vitro on the presence of hydroxycobalamin and transcobalamin II. Cancer Res 33:1898–1904
2. Halpern BC, Clark BR, Hardy DN et al (1974) The effect of replacement of methionine by homocystine on survival of malignant and normal adult mammalian cells in culture. Proc Natl Acad Sci U S A 71:1133–1136. https://doi.org/10.1073/pnas.71.4.1133
3. Hoffman RM, Erbe RW (1976) High in vivo rates of methionine biosynthesis in transformed human and malignant rat cells auxotrophic for methionine. Proc Natl Acad Sci U S A 73:1523–1527. https://doi.org/10.1073/pnas.73.5.1523
4. Stern PH, Wallace CD, Hoffman RM (1984) Altered methionine metabolism occurs in all members of a set of diverse human tumor cell lines. J Cell Physiol 119:29–34
5. Booher K, Lin DW, Borrego SL, Kaiser P (2012) Downregulation of Cdc6 and pre-replication complexes in response to methionine stress in breast cancer cells. Cell Cycle 11:4414–4423
6. Lin DW, Chung BP, Kaiser P (2013) S-adenosylmethionine limitation induces p38 mitogen-activated protein kinase and triggers cell cycle arrest in G1. J Cell Sci 127:50–59
7. Hoffman RM, Jacobsen SJ (1980) Reversible growth arrest in simian virus 40-transformed human fibroblasts. Proc Natl Acad Sci U S A 77:7306–7310
8. Sugimura T, Birnbaum SM, Winitz M et al (1959) Quantitative nutritional studies with water-soluble, chemically defined diets. VIII. The forced feeding of diets each lacking in one essential amino acid. Arch Biochem Biophys 81:448–455
9. Hoffman RM (2015) Development of recombinant methioninase to target the general cancer-specific metabolic defect of methionine dependence: a 40-year odyssey. Expert Opin Biol Ther 15:21–31
10. Mecham JO, Rowitch D, Wallace CD et al (1983) The metabolic defect of methionine dependence occurs frequently in human tumor cell lines. Biochem Biophys Res Commun 117:429–434. https://doi.org/10.1016/0006-291X(83)91218-4
11. Hoffman RM, Jacobsen SJ, Erbe RW (1979) Reversion to methionine independence in simian virus 40-transformed human and malignant rat fibroblasts is associated with altered ploidy and altered properties of transformation. Proc Natl Acad Sci U S A 76:1313–1317
12. Hoffman RM, Jacobsen SJ, Erbe RW (1978) Reversion to methionine independence by malignant rat and SV40-transformed human fibroblasts. Biochem Biophys Res Commun 82:228–234. https://doi.org/10.1016/0006-291X(78)90600-9
13. Borrego SL, Fahrmann J, Datta R et al (2016) Metabolic changes associated with methionine stress sensitivity in MDA-MB-468 breast cancer cells. Cancer Metab 4:9. https://doi.org/10.1186/s40170-016-0148-6
14. Mori S, Chang JT, Andrechek ER et al (2010) An anchorage-independent cell growth signature identifies tumors with metastic potential. Oncogene 28:2796–2805. https://doi.org/10.1038/onc.2009.139.An
15. Mosmann T (1983) Rapid colorimetric assay for cellular growth and survival: application to proliferation and cytotoxicity assays. J Immunol Methods 65:55–63. https://doi.org/10.1016/0022-1759(83)90303-4
16. Skehan P, Storeng R, Scudiero D et al (1990) New colorimetric cytotoxicity assay for anticancer-drug screening. J Natl Cancer Inst 82:1107–1112
17. Tan Y, Xu M, Hoffman RM (2010) Broad selective efficacy of recombinant methioninase and polyethylene glycol-modified recombinant methioninase on cancer cells *in vitro*. Anticancer Res 30:1041–1046

Chapter 5

Tumor-Specific S/G_2-Phase Cell Cycle Arrest of Cancer Cells by Methionine Restriction

Robert M. Hoffman and Shuya Yano

Abstract

Cancer cells require elevated amounts of methionine (MET) and arrest their growth under conditions of MET restriction (MR). This phenomenon is termed MET dependence. Fluorescence-activated cell sorting (FACS) first indicated that the MET-dependent SV40-transformed cancer cells were arrested in the S and G_2 phases of the cell cycle when under MR. This is in contrast to a G_1-phase accumulation of cells, which occurs only in MET-supplemented medium at very high cell densities and which is similar to the G_1 cell-cycle block which occurs in cultures of normal fibroblasts at high density. When the human PC-3 prostate carcinoma cell line was cultured in MET-free, homocysteine-containing (MET^-HCY^+) medium, there was an extreme increment in DNA content without cell division indicating that the cells were blocked in S phase. Recombinant methioninase (rMETase) treatment of cancer cells also selectively trapped cancer cells in S/G_2: The cell cycle phase of the cancer cells was visualized with the fluorescence ubiquitination cell cycle indicator (FUCCI). At the time of rMETase-induced S/G_2-phase trap, identified by the cancer cells' green fluorescence by FUCCI imaging, the cancer cells were administered S-phase-dependent chemotherapy drugs, which interact with DNA or block DNA synthesis such as doxorubicin, cisplatin, or 5-fluorouracil (5-FU) and which were highly effective in killing the cancer cells. In contrast, treatment of cancer cells with drugs in the presence of MET, only led to the majority of the cancer cell population being blocked in G_0/G_1 phase, identified by the cancer cells becoming red fluorescent in the FUCCI system. The G_0/G_1 blocked cells were resistant to the chemotherapy. MR has the potential for highly effective cell-cycle-based treatment strategy for cancer in the clinic.

Key words Cancer cells, Methionine dependence, Methionine restriction, Cell cycle, Arrest, S/G_2 phase, chemotherapy

1 Introduction

Cancer cells are unable to proliferate when methionine (MET) is restricted. This phenomenon is termed MET dependence [1]. Normal cells can grow well when MET is restricted [2, 3].

To understand the biochemical basis of the MET-dependent phenotype, it was important to know the effects of MET restriction (MR) on the cancer cell cycle [3].

Robert M. Hoffman (ed.), *Methionine Dependence of Cancer and Aging: Methods and Protocols*, Methods in Molecular Biology, vol. 1866, https://doi.org/10.1007/978-1-4939-8796-2_5,

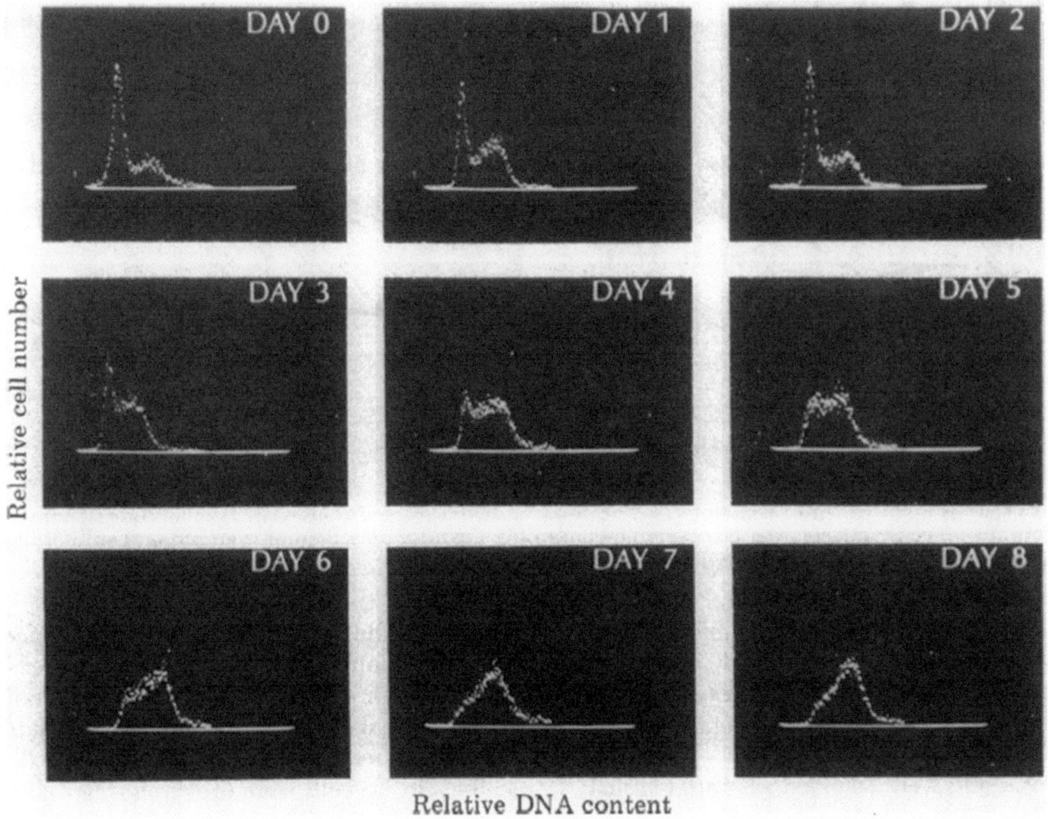

Fig. 1 Fluorescence-activated cell sorting (FACS) to determine cell-cycle position in SV40-trasnformed human line P5 (subclone of SV80). Days indicate time of incubation in MET-restricted medium [3]

Fluorescence-activated cell sorting (FACS) demonstrated that the SV40-transformed human cancer cells were arrested in the S and G_2 phases of the cell cycle upon MR (Fig. 1). This is in contrast to a G_1-phase accumulation of cells, which occurs only in MET-supplemented medium at very high densities and which is similar to the G_1 block seen in cultures of normal fibroblasts at high density (Fig. 2) [3].

When the human PC-3 prostate carcinoma cell line was cultured under MR, there was a large increment in DNA content without cell division indicating an S-phase arrest (Fig. 3) [4].

We also demonstrated that the Yoshida tumor growing in nude mice can be induced by an MR diet to an S/G_2 cell-cycle block [5].

The S/G_2 trap that cancer cells enter upon MR was exploited for selective chemotherapy in vitro. In cultures that were initiated with equal amounts of cancer cells and human diploid fibroblasts, MR culture medium and doxorubicin (DOX), an S-phase drug, followed by MET repletion with vincristine, an anti-mitosis drug, were totally effective at selectively eliminating a MET-dependent human sarcoma and three MET-dependent human carcinomas

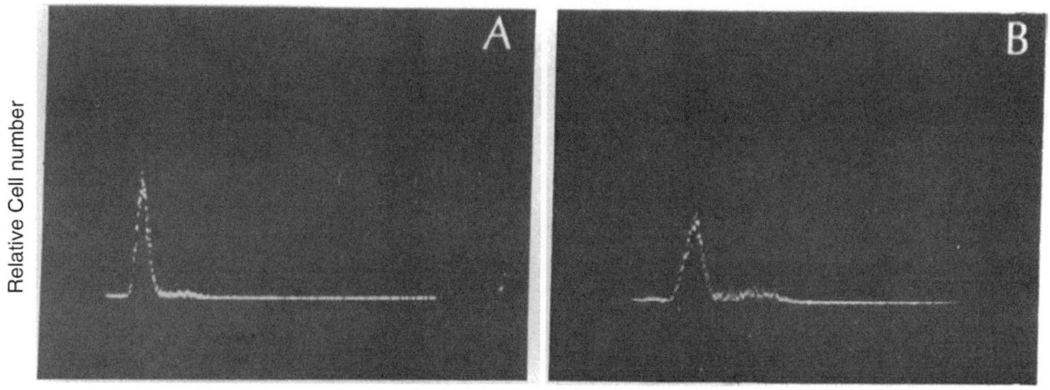

Fig. 2 FACS to determine cell cycle position. (**a**) Confluent culture of diploid human embryonic fibroblast line AF2. (**b**) Dense culture of SV40-transformed human line P1 (subclone of W18VA2) in MET-containing medium [3]

from the co-culture. This chemotherapeutic procedure used was not toxic to normal cells growing alongside the cancer cells. The chemotherapy procedure was ineffective when conducted totally in MET-containing medium [6, 7].

2 Materials

1. Human SV40-transformed cell lines W18VA2 and SV80 [8] or other cancer cells.
2. Yoshida sarcoma cells.
3. MKN45 human stomach cancer cells.
4. Penicillin.
5. Streptomycin.
6. L-Glutamine.
7. Eagle's minimal essential medium (lacking MET and choline chloride) with nonessential amino acids (GIBCO).
8. Fetal bovine serum (Irvine Scientific, Santa Ana, CA).
9. Glucose.
10. Sodium pyruvate.
11. Ferric nitrate.
12. Folic acid.
13. Hydroxycobalamin.
14. NaCl.
15. L-MET or DL-homocysteine thiolactone (HCY).
16. Corning roller bottles (490 cm^2).
17. DNase.

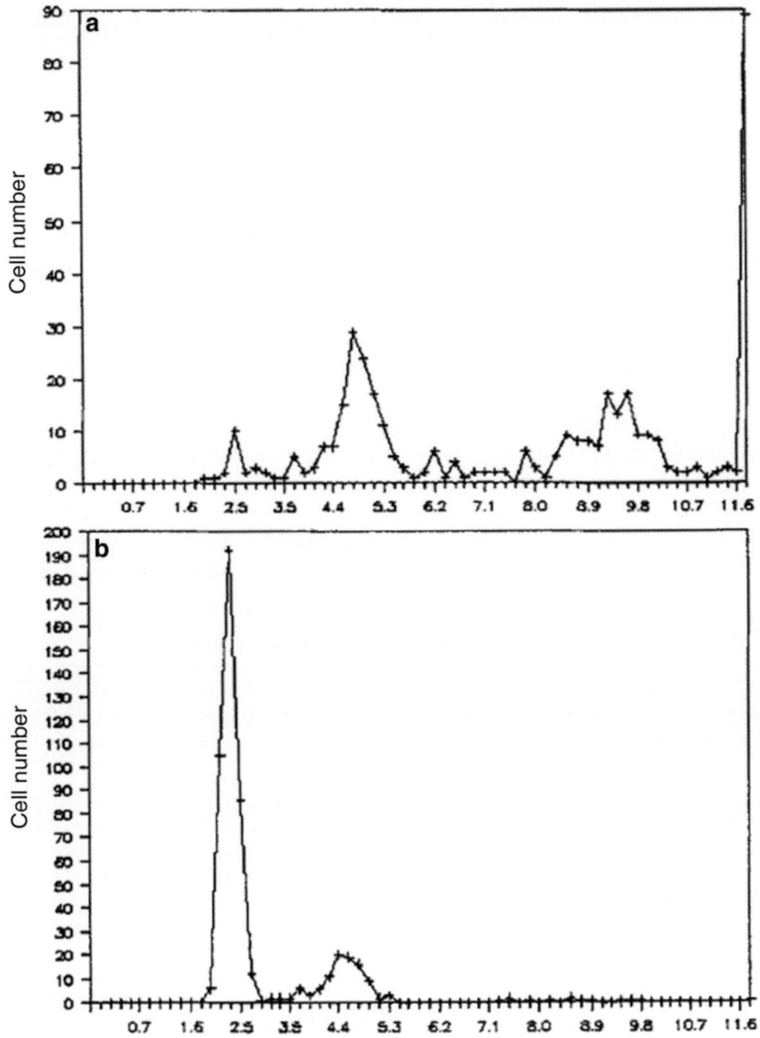

Fig. 3 DNA content of PC-3 cells cultured for 14 days in MR medium (**a**) or in MET-containing medium (**b**). Cells were fixed with Fix-Rite and stained by the Feulgen method. The DNA content of the nucleus of each cells was measured by determined integrated optical density with a Cambridge Instrument Quantimet-520 image analysis system [4]

18. Soybean trypsin inhibitor.
19. Formaldehyde.
20. HCl.
21. Acriflavine.
22. Coulter counter.
23. Giemsa stain.

24. Four- to 5-week-old outbred *nu/nu* nude mice (AntiCancer Inc., San Diego, CA).
25. Defined mouse diets with and without MET (Teklad, Madison, WI).
26. Hydrochloric acid.
27. Cambridge Instruments Quantimet-520 or equivalent to measure DNA content.
28. Recombinant L-methionine α-deamino-γ- mercaptomethane lyase (recombinant methioninase, rMETase) [EC 4.4.1.11] from *Pseudomonas putida*, previously cloned in *Escherichia coli* (AntiCancer Inc., San Diego, CA).
29. FUCCI (fluorescence ubiquitination cell cycle indicator) (MBL, Nagoya, Japan).
30. Confocal laser scanning microscope (FV1000; Olympus, Tokyo, Japan).

3 Methods

3.1 Culture Conditions and Preparation for Cell Sorting

1. Grow cells in Corning roller bottles (490 cm^2) in MET-containing MEM medium with or without DL-homocysteine (HCY).
2. After incubation, rinse cells twice with phosphate-buffered saline (PBS) and detach from the plastic with trypsin at room temperature.
3. Enumerate cells in a Coulter counter.
4. Treat cells with DNase and soybean trypsin inhibitor and fix in formaldehyde as described [9].
5. Fix cells for at least 24 h and hydrolyze in 4 M HCl for varying periods of time (20 min at room temperature is standard procedure).
6. Immediately following hydrolysis, stain the cells with acriflavine for 5 min and wash with acid alcohol as described [9].
7. Resuspend the cells in water and analyze at a wavelength of 488 nm with a fluorescence-activated cell sorter (FACS) [9].
8. Use Giemsa stain to quantitate cell growth and cloning efficiency [3].

3.2 Mice

1. Use 4- to 5-week-old outbred *nu/nu* nude mice [5, 7].
2. Inject cancer cells (1×10^7) in the nude mice previously grown in Eagle's minimum essential medium with 10% fetal calf serum at the axillary and inguinal sites [5].

3.3 Diets

1. Use defined MR or normal diets.
2. Feed the mice in one group a MET-containing diet and feed the mice in the other group an MR diet.
3. Give mice in each group equal measured amounts of either diet.
4. Start the defined diets on day 2 after the injection of cancer cells in the nude mice.
5. House the mice on the MR diets separately from mice on the normal diets [5].
6. Measure the lengths of the major and minor axes of tumors with calipers.
7. Evaluate the growth of the tumors every 3 days [5].

3.4 DNA Staining

1. Incubate the slides containing 3–5 μm histological sections of the tumors from animals on either diet, in preheated 1 N hydrochloric acid at 60° for 20 rain.
2. Rinse the slides with distilled water 6 times to remove excess acid and stain with Schiff's reagent for 20 min at room temperature.
3. Treat with two successive changes of freshly prepared sulfurous acid rinse and wash in running tap water for 5 min.
4. After dehydration, cover slides for DNA analysis [5].

3.5 Determination of Cell Cycle Position by DNA-Content Measurement

1. Use a Cambridge Instruments Quantimet-520 system or equivalent to determine the DNA content of cell nuclei by measuring integrated absorbance of each cell [10].
2. Measure 500 cells per slide.
3. The integrated absorbance is directly proportional to DNA content.
4. Determine the G_1 reference peak in the tissues of the control animals as the first major peak in the histogram [5].

3.6 Imaging of FUCCI-Expressing Cancer Cells

1. Acquire time-lapse images of HeLa and MCF-7 cells stably transfected with FUCCI vectors using a confocal laser scanning microscope [11–13].

4 Results

In MR medium, cancer cells accumulated in the late-S/G_2 phases of the cell cycle as determined by fluorescence-activated cell sorting (FACS) (Fig. 1). By day 7 the G_1 peak had disappeared, leaving a large asymmetric peak phase at G_2/M (Fig. 1). This G_2/M peak probably contained a significant fraction of cells in S and G_2 phases [3].

In contrast to their behavior in MR medium, most of the MET-dependent cancer cells accumulated in G_1 phase when cultures were grown to high density in MET-containing medium. Figure 2 compares dense cancer cells with confluent normal diploid human cells in MET-containing medium [3] (*see* **Note 2**).

At the beginning of the incubation period in MR medium, approximately 50% of the cancer cells were in G_1, 30–35% in S, and 10–15% in G_2; by the end of the incubation period in MET-containing medium, approximately 10–15% of the cells were in G_1, 30–35% in S, and 50% in G_2 (Fig. 1). For cancer cells in MET-containing medium, approximately 50% of the cells were in G_1, 30–35% in S, and 15–20% in G_2 (Fig. 2) (*see* **Note 1**) [3].

When the human PC-3 prostate carcinoma cell line was cultured under MR, there was a large increment in DNA content without cell division indicating an S-phase block (Fig. 3) [4].

4.1 DNA Content Measurement by Image Analysis of Cells from Tumors Growing in Nude Mice on $MET^{+}HCY^{-}$ and MR Diets

Cell cycle analysis demonstrated that cells from the tumors grown in mice on the MR diet had a much greater DNA content than the cells from the tumors grown in mice on the MET-containing diet. These results thus indicate that an S/G_2 block occurred in the Yoshida sarcoma grown in nude mice on the MR diet (*see* **Note 1**) [5].

4.2 Recombinant Methionine (rMETase) Trap of Cancer Cells in S/G_2 Visualized by FUCCI Imaging

rMETase trapped HeLa-FUCCI cells in S/G_2 phase before cell division (Fig. 4). rMETase continued to trap HeLa-FUCCI cells in S/G_2 phase over time without entry into mitosis (Fig. 4) [14]. The ability of rMETase to induce the S/G_2-phase cell-cycle trap on the cancer cells was dose dependent (Fig. 5).

We subsequently demonstrated that using rMETase to deplete MET and thereby trap cancer cells in S/G_2, and FUCCI imaging to detect the onset of the cell-cycle block by color-coded imaging, chemotherapy could become effective on the S/G_2-trapped cancer cells (Fig. 6) [7].

4.3 rMETase Induces Mitotic Catastrophe After Late S/G_2 Trap Visualized by FUCCI Imaging

HeLa-FUCCI cells were treated with rMETase for more than 80 h. HeLa-FUCCI cells trapped in late S/G_2 phase did not divide and their nuclei turned red, after which they died (Fig. 7). These results showed that MET was indispensable for cell division, and therefore rMETase induced mitotic catastrophe [14–17].

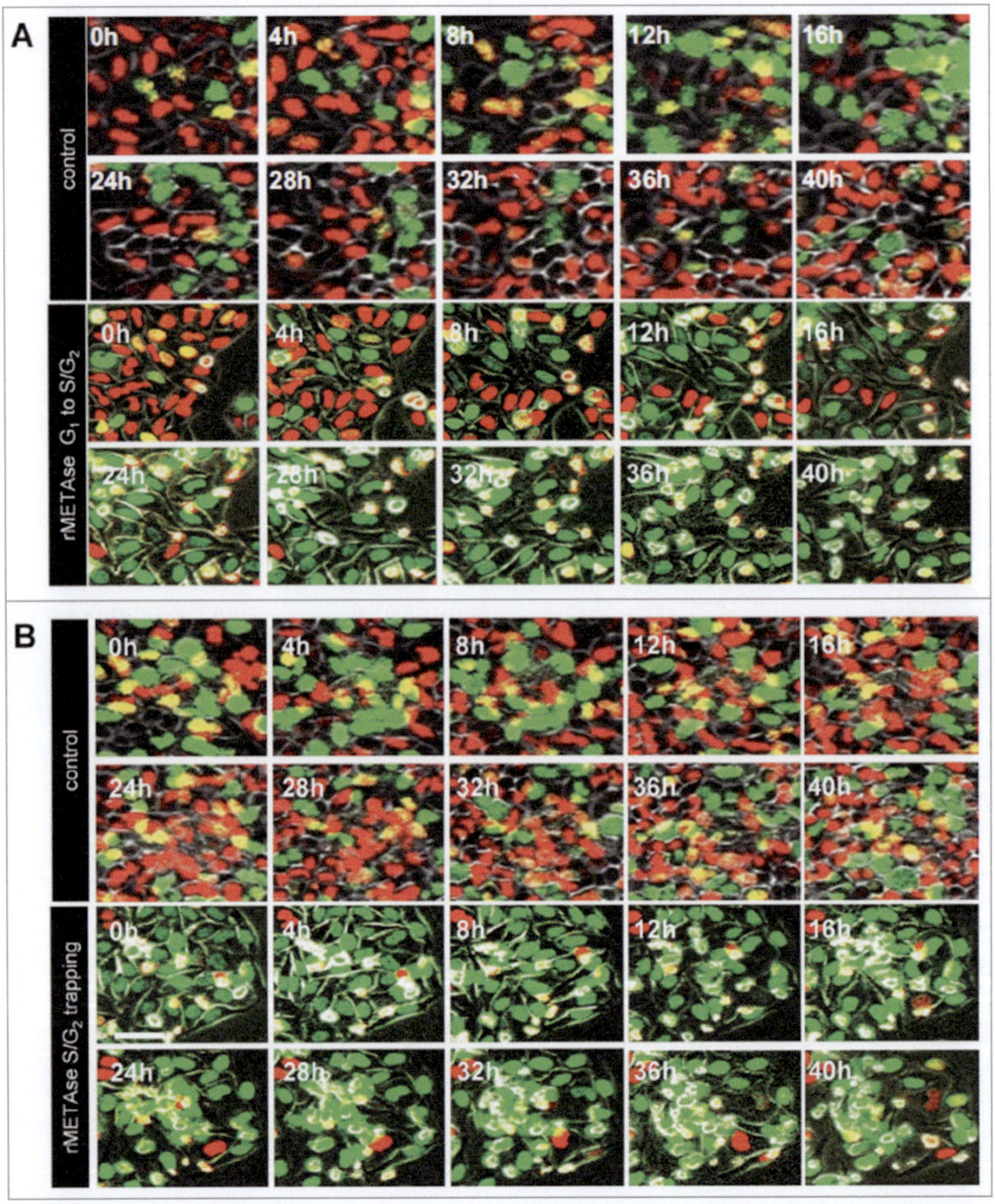

Fig. 4 rMETase traps cancer cells in S/G_2 phase. Time-course imaging of HeLa-FUCCI cells treated with rMETase. After seeding on 35 mm glass dishes and culture overnight, HeLa-FUCCI cells were treated with rMETase at a dose of 1.0 unit/mL. (**a**) Kinetics of rMETase trapping of cells in S/G_2. (**b**) Maintenance of rMETase trap in S/G_2 over time. All images were acquired with the FV1000 confocal microscope (Olympus, Tokyo, Japan). The cells in G_0/G_1, S, or G_2/M phases appear red, yellow, or green, respectively [14]

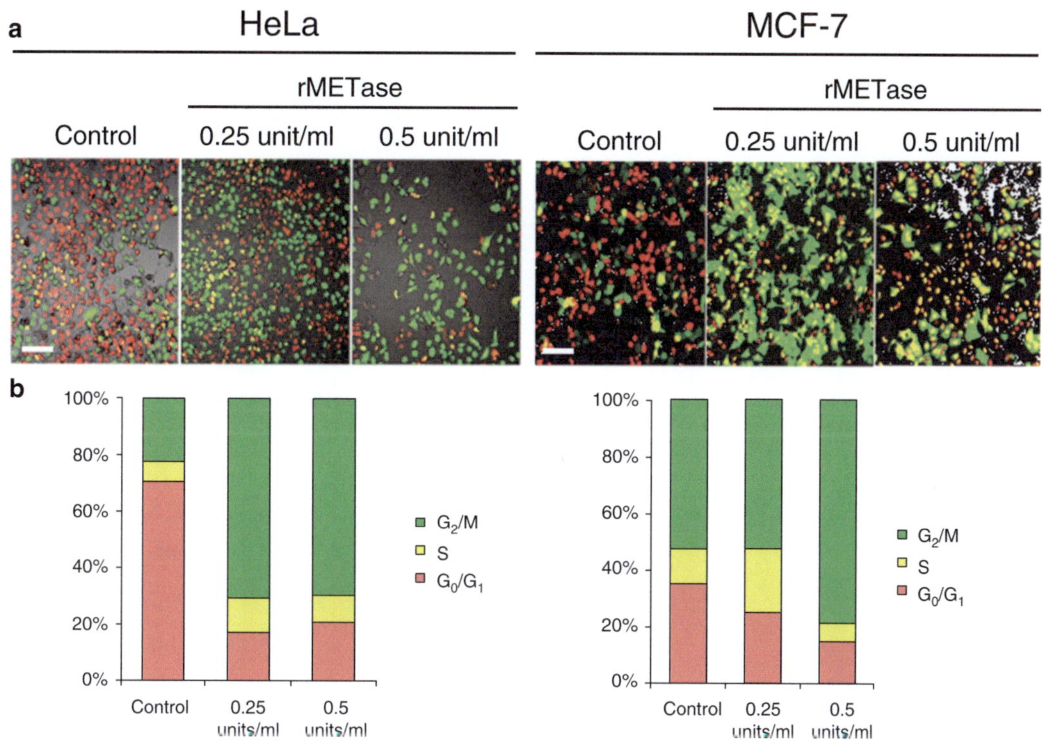

Fig. 5 rMETase traps cancer cells in S/G_2 phase. After seeding on 35 mm glass dishes and culture overnight, HeLa cells and MCF-7 cells were treated with rMETase, at the indicated doses, for 48 h. (**a**) Representative images of control or rMETase-treated cells. (**b**) Histogram shows the percentages of cells in G_1 (red), early S (yellow), or late S/G_2/M (green). Cells at each cell-cycle phase were quantitatively assessed by counting the number of cells with each color. $N = 5$ experiments were analyzed. Scale bars: 50 μm [7]

5 Notes

1. After incubation in MR medium, cancer cells could resume growth in MET-containing medium in mass culture but rapidly lost the ability to clone in MET [3].
2. The SV40-transformed cells in $MET^{+}HCY^{-}$ medium become dense and slowed their growth; they accumulate in G_1 phase almost to the extent that normal human diploid fibroblasts do at confluence [3].

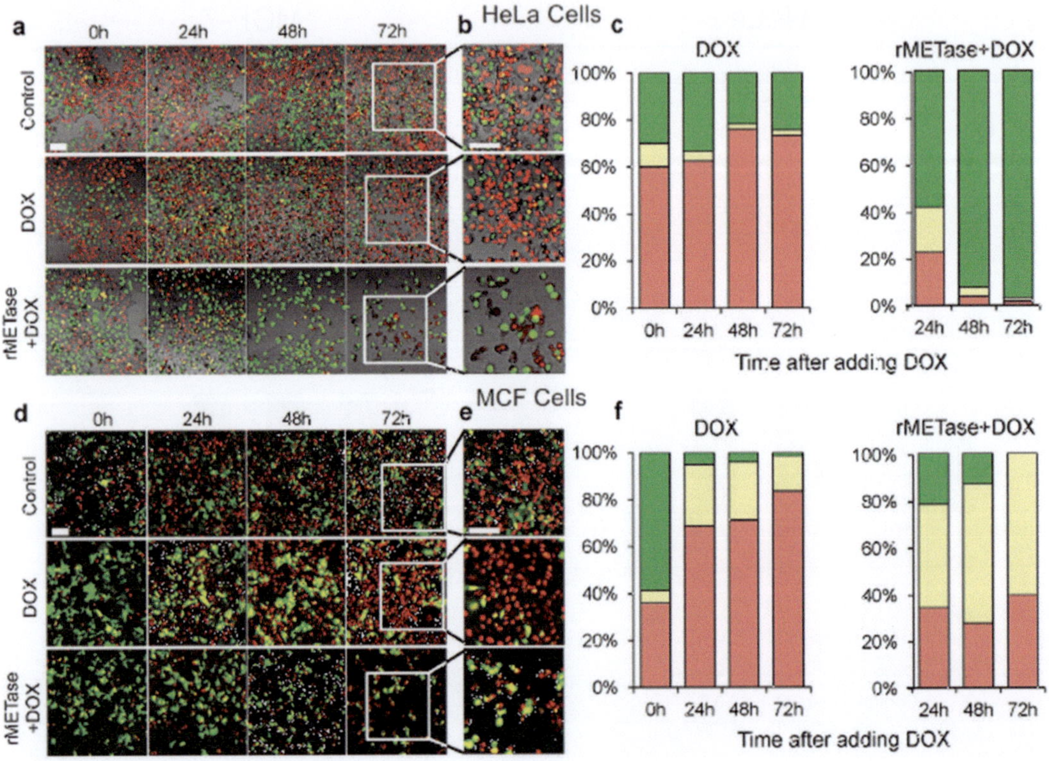

Fig. 6 FUCCI cell-cycle analysis during chemotherapy with and without rMETase. After overnight culture, HeLa cells (**a–c**) and MCF-7 cells (**d–f**) were treated with 0.25 unit/mL rMETase for 48 h and then were treated with 0.5 μg/mL doxorubicin (DOX) (HeLa cells) or 2.5 μg/mL DOX (MCF-7) for 72 h. For conventional chemotherapy, after culture for 48 h, HeLa cells (**a–c**) and MCF-7 cells (**d–f**) were treated with 0.5 μg/mL DOX (HeLa cells) or 2.5 μg/mL DOX (MCF-7) for 72 h. (**a**, **b**, **d**, **e**) Representative images acquired with the FV-1000 are shown. (**c**, **f**). Histograms show the percentages of cells G_1(red), early S (yellow), or late $S/G_2/M$ (green). Cells at each cell-cycle phase were quantitatively assessed by counting the number of cells with each color. $N = 5$ experiments were analyzed. Scale bars: 50 μm [7]

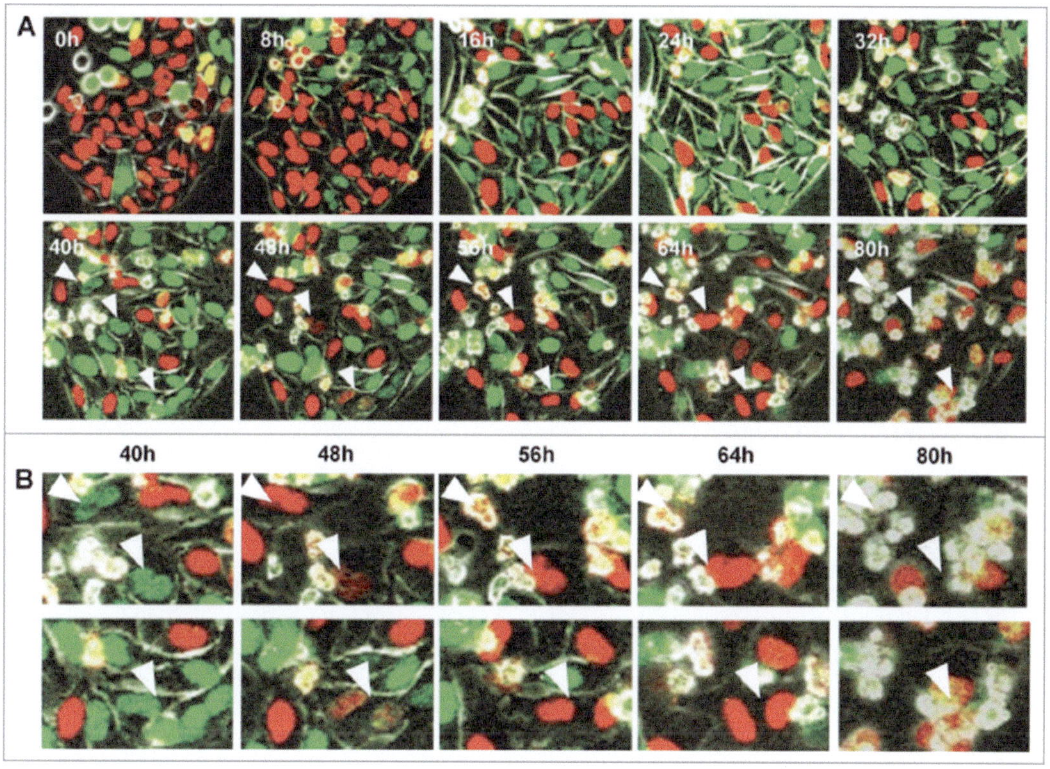

Fig. 7 Prolonged administration of rMETase-induced mitotic catastrophe after late-S/G$_2$-phase blocking. (**a**) Time-lapse imaging of HeLa-FUCCI cells treated with rMETase. After seeding on 35 mm glass dishes and culture overnight, HeLa-FUCCI cells were treated with rMETase at a dose of 1.0 unit/mL for 80 h. All images were acquired with the FV1000 confocal microscope (Olympus, Tokyo, Japan). The cells in G$_0$/G$_1$, S, or G$_2$/M phases appear red, yellow, or green, respectively. (**b**) High-magnificent images of A. Arrowheads refer to a cell dying from mitotic catastrophe [14]

References

1. Hoffman RM (2015) Development of recombinant methioninase to target the general cancer-specific metabolic defect of methionine dependence: a 40-year odyssey. Expert Opin Biol Ther 15:21–31
2. Kamely D, Littlefield JW, Erbe R (1973) Regulation of 5-methyltetrahydrofolate: homocysteine methyltransferase activity by methionine, vitamin B12, and folate in cultured baby hamster kidney cells. Proc Natl Acad Sci U S A 70:2585–2589
3. Hoffman RM, Jacobsen SJ (1980) Reversible growth arrest in simian virus 40-transformed human fibroblasts. Proc Natl Acad Sci U S A 77:7306–7310
4. Guo HY, Herrera H, Hoffman RM (1993) Unchecked DNA synthesis and blocked cell division induced by methionine deprivation in a human prostate cancer cell line. In Vitro Cell Dev Biol 29A:359–361
5. Guo H, Lishko V, Herrera H, Groce A, Kubota T, Hoffman RM (1993) Therapeutic tumor-specific cell-cycle block induced by methionine starvation in vivo. Cancer Res 53:5676–5679
6. Stern PH, Hoffman RM (1986) Enhanced in vitro selective toxicity of chemotherapeutic agents for human cancer cells based on a metabolic defect. J Natl Cancer Inst 76:629–639
7. Yano S, Li S, Han Q, Tan Y, Bouvet M, Fujiwara T, Hoffman RM (2014) Selective methioninase-induced trap of cancer cells in S/G$_2$ phase visualized by FUCCI imaging

confers chemosensitivity. Oncotarget 5:8729–8736

8. Hoffman RM, Jacobsen SJ, Erbe RW (1979) Reversion to methionine independence in simian virus 40-transformed human and malignant rat fibroblasts is associated with altered ploidy and altered properties of transformation. Proc Natl Acad Sci U S A 76:1313–1317

9. Kraemer PM, Deaven LL, Crissman HA, Van Dilla MA (1972) In: Du-Praw EJ (ed) Advances in cell and molecular biology, vol 2. Academic Press, New York, pp 47–108

10. Guo HY, Herrera H, Groce A, Hoffman RM (1993) Expression of the biochemical defect of methionine dependence in fresh patient tumors in primary histoculture. Cancer Res 53:2479–2483

11. Yano S, Zhang Y, Miwa S, Tome Y, Hiroshima Y, Uehara F, Yamamoto M, Suetsugu A, Kishimoto H, Tazawa H, Zhao M, Bouvet M, Fujiwara T, Hoffman RM (2014) Spatial-temporal FUCCI imaging of each cell in a tumor demonstrates locational dependence of cell cycle dynamics and chemoresponsiveness. Cell Cycle 13:2110–2119

12. Yano S, Miwa S, Mii S, Hiroshima Y, Uehara F, Yamamoto M, Kishimoto H, Tazawa H, Bouvet M, Fujiwara T, Hoffman RM (2014) Invading cancer cells are predominantly in G_0/G_1 resulting in chemoresistance demonstrated by real-time FUCCI imaging. Cell Cycle 13:953–960

13. Yano S, Tazawa H, Hashimoto Y, Shirakawa Y, Kuroda S, Nishizaki M, Kishimoto H, Uno F, Nagasaka T, Urata Y, Kagawa S, Hoffman RM, Fujiwara T (2013) A genetically engineered oncolytic adenovirus decoys and lethally traps quiescent cancer stem-like cells into $S/G_2/M$ phases. Clin Cancer Res 19:6495–6505

14. Yano S, Takehara K, Zhao M, Tan Y, Han Q, Li S, Bouvet M, Fujiwara T, Hoffman RM (2016) Tumor-specific cell-cycle decoy by *Salmonella typhimurium* A1-R combined with tumor-selective cell-cycle trap by methioninase overcome tumor intrinsic chemoresistance as visualized by FUCCI imaging. Cell Cycle 15:1715–1723

15. Castedo M, Perfettini JL, Roumier T, Andreau K, Medema R, Kroemer G (2004) Cell death by mitotic catastrophe: a molecular definition. Oncogene 23:2825–2837

16. Chow JPH, Poon RYC (2010) Mitotic catastrophe. In: Enders G (ed) Cell cycle deregulation in cancer. Springer, New York, pp 79–96

17. Vakifahmetoglu H, Olsson M, Zhivotovsky B (2008) Death through a tragedy: mitotic catastrophe. Cell Death Differ 15:1153–1162

Chapter 6

Preclinical Breast Cancer Models to Investigate Metabolic Priming by Methionine Restriction

Elena Strekalova, Dmitry Malin, Harisha Rajanala, and Vincent L. Cryns

Abstract

We have developed a novel therapeutic paradigm ("metabolic priming") for cancer whereby restriction of the essential amino acid methionine activates a number of cell-stress-response pathways that can be selectively targeted to enhance the therapeutic impact of methionine restriction. One example of metabolic priming is the combination of methionine restriction with proapoptotic TRAIL receptor-2 (TRAIL-R2) agonists. Methionine restriction enhances the cell surface expression of TRAIL-R2 selectively in transformed breast epithelial cells and renders them more susceptible to cell death induction by TRAIL-R2 agonists in cellular and murine models of breast cancer. This methods review focuses on preclinical models of breast cancer to investigate metabolic priming by methionine restriction. Multiple cell-based methods are detailed to measure cell viability, cell survival, caspase activity, apoptosis, and matrix detachment-induced cell death (anoikis). In addition, we describe an orthotopic model of metastatic breast cancer that utilizes mCherry-fluorescently-labeled human breast cancer cells. This model captures the entire metastatic cascade from the mammary gland to the lung and mimics key features of the human disease. These breast-cancer models can be readily adapted to other tumor types. Overall, we provide a stepwise, translationally-relevant approach to study metabolic priming in the context of cancer.

Key words Methionine, Metabolism, TRAIL, Breast cancer, Metastasis, Apoptosis, Therapeutics, Murine models

1 Introduction

Depletion of the essential amino acid methionine has been demonstrated to initiate apoptosis and inhibit cell-cycle progression in a broad range of cancer cell lines and primary cancer cells [1–4]. These cellular effects of methionine restriction (MR) lead to suppression of tumor growth in many murine models of cancer [5, 6]. Although clinical trials of dietary MR in patients with advanced solid tumors have demonstrated the safety of prolonged dietary MR for up to 39 weeks, these studies have failed to demonstrate significant clinical activity of MR alone or in combination with cytotoxic agents [7–9]. We postulated that a more detailed understanding of the cellular stress response to MR would enable

Robert M. Hoffman (ed.), *Methionine Dependence of Cancer and Aging: Methods and Protocols*, Methods in Molecular Biology, vol. 1866, https://doi.org/10.1007/978-1-4939-8796-2_6, © Springer Science+Business Media, LLC, part of Springer Nature 2019

us to utilize MR to expose targetable vulnerabilities in cancer cells and enhance the therapeutic efficacy of MR by specifically targeting these pathways. Viewed from this context, we envision MR as a novel paradigm to metabolically prime tumor cells to respond to cancer drugs that target stress-response pathways induced by MR.

As proof of principle, we observed that MR robustly enhances the cell-surface expression of the proapoptotic TNF-related apoptosis-inducing ligand (TRAIL) receptor 2 (TRAIL-R2/DR5) in clinically-aggressive triple-negative breast cancer cells (TNBC), which lack expression of the estrogen receptor (ER), progesterone receptor (PR), and human epidermal growth factor receptor 2 (HER2) [10]. The pro-apoptotic TRAIL receptor pathway has been extensively studied as a potential cancer therapy because soluble recombinant TRAIL ligand and agonistic antibodies targeting pro-apoptotic TRAIL receptors (TRAIL-R1 and TRAIL-R2) have demonstrated robust tumor-selective activity in preclinical models with little toxicity [11]. However, these agents have not demonstrated efficacy in clinical trials in patients with advanced malignancies [12–15].

We postulated that MR would prime TNBC cells to respond to TRAIL-R2 agonists by enhancing the cell surface expression of its molecular target, TRAIL-R2. To this end, we observed that preincubating a panel of human TNBC cells in methionine-free medium selectively sensitized them to the agonistic TRAIL-R2 monoclonal antibody lexatumumab but had little effect on their sensitivity to diverse cytotoxic agents [10]. Intriguingly, untransformed human breast epithelial cells failed to upregulate cell surface of expression of TRAIL-R2 in response to MR and were largely resistant to the combination of MR and lexatumumab, underscoring the potential tumor selectivity of our metabolic priming approach. We also tested this approach in an orthotopic model of TNBC that recapitulates many features of the human disease, including triple-negative receptor expression and extensive visceral metastases including the lungs [10, 16]. In this metastatic murine model, a 3-week administration of a methionine-free diet alone or lexatumumab alone modestly inhibited primary tumor growth, but neither agent suppressed lung metastases [10]. However, the combination of MR and lexatumumab was more effective at inhibiting primary tumor growth than either intervention alone and resulted in significant suppression of lung metastases. These antitumor effects of MR were accompanied by enhanced expression of TRAIL-R2 expression in mammary tumors and modest weight loss [10]. Overall, these findings underscore the potential utility of MR to metabolically prime cancer cells to pro-apoptotic TRAIL-R2 agonists by augmenting cell-surface expression of their molecular target.

In this methods review, we focus on cellular models of breast cancer to investigate the effects of MR on cell viability, apoptosis, and caspase activation as well as murine breast-cancer models to examine the antitumor effects of MR in vivo. Although the focus is clinically aggressive TNBC models and the TRAIL receptor pathway, these methods could be readily adapted to incorporate diverse tumor types and other molecular vulnerabilities induced by MR. As noted previously, our strategy utilizes MR to metabolically prime tumors to respond to rationally-selected cancer drugs based on exposed molecular liabilities rather than envisioning MR as a stand-alone therapy. Our goal is to provide a detailed description of relevant preclinical breast cancer models to facilitate investigation in this exciting field.

2 Materials

2.1 Cell Lines

1. Human TNBC cell lines: MDA-MB-231 and MDA-MB-468 cells are available from ATCC (*see* **Note 1**) while GILM2 TNBC cells are described elsewhere [17].
2. Human breast epithelial cell lines: Human MCF-10A breast epithelial cells stably expressing oncogenic RasV12 or empty vector (*see* **Note 2**) are described previously [18].
3. For in vivo experiments, MDA MB 468 cells stably expressing mCherry fluorescent protein (468-mCherry) are utilized to enable fluorescence imaging of tumors [10].

2.2 Cell Culture Reagents

1. MDA-MB-231 TNBC cells: Maintain in DMEM/F12 medium supplemented with 10% FBS and 100 units/mL penicillin/streptomycin (Thermo Fisher Scientific). Culture MDA-MB-468 and MDA-MB-468-mCherry cells in DMEM with 10% FBS and 100 units/mL penicillin/streptomycin (Thermo Fisher Scientific). Grow GILM2 cells in DMEM/F12 supplemented with 10% FBS, insulin/transferrin/sodium selenite mix, and 100 units/mL penicillin/streptomycin (Thermo Fisher Scientific). Culture MCF-10A stably expressing RasV12 or empty vector in DMEM/F12 medium supplemented with 5% horse serum (Thermo Fisher Scientific), 20 ng/mL EGF (Sigma-Aldrich), 10 μg/mL insulin (Sigma-Aldrich), 100 ng/mL cholera toxin (Sigma-Aldrich), 0.5 mg/mL hydrocortisone (Sigma-Aldrich), and 100 units/mL penicillin/streptomycin.
2. For MR experiments, supplement RPMI-1640 medium without methionine (Thermo Fisher Scientific) but containing other nutrients and FBS (MR medium, *see* **Note 3**) to closely match the original media for each cell line (complete media).

2.3 Cell Viability Reagents

1. Measure cell viability using a colorimetric MTS assay (CellTiter 96 Aqueous One Solution Cell Proliferation Assay, Promega).
2. Stain surviving cells with crystal violet (Sigma-Aldrich, *see* **Note 4**).

2.4 Apoptosis Reagents

1. Score apoptotic cells by flow cytometry-based annexin V labeling (Annexin-PE Apoptosis Detection Kit, BD Bioscience).
2. Measure caspase-3/7 activity in cell lysates using a luminescence assay (Caspase-Glo 3/7, Promega).
3. Purchase HPLC-purified doxorubicin (DOX) from Sigma-Aldrich.
4. Obtain agonistic monoclonal antibodies against TRAIL-R1 (mapatumumab) or TRAIL-R2 (lexatumumab) from Human Genome Sciences.

2.5 Anoikis Reagents

1. Grow TNBC cells in adherent culture as in Subheading 2.2 or in suspension on Corning Costar Ultra-Low Attachment Plates (Thermo Fisher Scientific) in medium supplemented with 1% methylcellulose (Sigma-Aldrich) to prevent cell aggregation.

2.6 TRAIL Receptor Expression Reagents

1. Synthesize total RNA to cDNA using the iScript cDNA Synthesis Kit (Bio-Rad).
2. Purchase oligonucleotide primers from Integrated DNA Technologies.
3. Use fluorescein isothiocyanate (FITC)-conjugated monoclonal antibodies (mAbs) against TRAIL-R1 (Abcam, ab59047), TRAIL-R2 (Abcam, ab53319), and control IgG (Abcam, ab37356) for cell-surface detection of TRAIL receptor expression.

2.7 Mice and Murine Model Reagents

Establish a fluorescence orthotopic model of metastatic TNBC using mCherry-labeled human MDA-MB-468 cells in female NOD SCID IL-2 receptor γ chain knockout (NSG) mice (Jackson Laboratory) [10] (*see* **Notes 5** and **6**). Whenever possible, use pharmacologic grade drugs and reagents.

1. Purchase female 4–5-week-old NSG mice (*see* **Note 7**) from Jackson Laboratories.
2. Control diet: 15% Protein diet (Envigo/Teklad TD.01084).
3. MR diet: Isocaloric 15% protein methionine-free (0% methionine, Envigo/Teklad TD.140119).
4. Image mCherry-fluorescent metastases at autopsy using a Leica MZ10F fluorescence stereomicroscope.

3 Methods

3.1 MTS Cell-Viability Assay

1. Trypsinize actively-growing TNBC cells and count viable cells by trypan blue exclusion using a hemocytometer. Plate 3–5 × 10^3 cells in each well of a 96-well plate (triplicate wells). Allow the cells to adhere overnight (*see* **Notes 8** and **9**).
2. Wash cells with PBS and add control or MR media for 72 h.
3. Add DOX (0–3.4 μM) or agonistic TRAIL receptor mAbs (0–4 μg/mL) for an additional 48 h.
4. Measure cell viability using the CellTiter 96 Aqueous One Solution Cell Proliferation Assay (Promega). Add 20 μL MTS reagent to each well of the 96-well plate. Measure absorbance at 490 nm in triplicate wells 1 h later using a microplate reader. Cell viability is expressed as the percentage of viable cells relative to control cells (*see* **Notes 10** and **11**).

3.2 Crystal-Violet Cell-Survival Assay

1. Plate cells (3 × 10^5 cells/well) on 6-well plates. Allow cells to adhere overnight.
2. Wash cells with PBS and add complete or MR media for 48 h.
3. Add DOX (0–3.4 μM) or TRAIL receptor mAbs (0–4 μg/mL) for an additional 24–48 h.
4. Fix surviving cells, stain with crystal violet solution (40% ethanol, 60% PBS, and 0.5% crystal violet), and count (*see* **Note 12**).
5. Present representative images and quantitation of multiple experiments (Fig. 1).

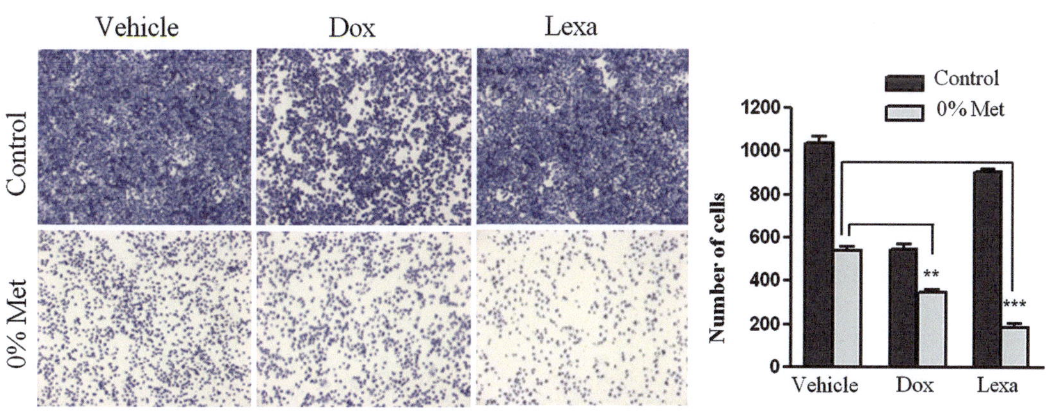

Fig. 1 Crystal violet survival assay of MDA-MB-468 TNBC cells grown in control media or methionine-free medium for 24 h and then treated with vehicle, doxorubicin (DOX) (3.4 μM) or the TRAIL-R2 agonist lexatumumab (4 μg/mL) for an additional 48 h. Representative images (left panel) and quantitative analysis of three independent experiments (right panel). $^{**}P < 0.01$, $^{***}P < 0.001$. Reproduced from [10] with permission from the American Association for Cancer Research

3.3 Annexin V Labeling

1. Grow TNBC cells (3×10^5 cells/well) in 6-well plates in complete or MR media for 48 h.
2. Add DOX (0–3.4 mM) or TRAIL receptor mAb (0–2 μg/mL) for an additional 6 h.
3. Collect supernatant. Trypsinize cells and collect by gentle centrifugation for 5 min at $314 \times g$ in a tabletop centrifuge.
4. Determine annexin V labeling using the Annexin-PE Apoptosis Detection Kit (BD Bioscience). Wash cells in PBS and resuspend at 1×10^6 cells/mL in 1× Annexin V Binding Buffer (10 mM Hepes/NaOH (pH 7.4), 0.14 M NaCl, 2.5 mM $CaCl_2$).
5. Place 100 μL of resuspended cells in a 5 mL conical tube wrapped in aluminum foil to exclude light. Add 5 μL of PE Annexin V and DAPI (1 μg/mL) and incubate at RT for 15 min.
6. Analyze cells in a flow cytometer (LSRII, BD Biosciences). Annexin V-PE-positive cells are detected using a blue laser (Ex 496 nm/Em 578 nm), while DAPI-positive cells are counted using a violet laser (Ex 358 nm/Em 460 nm).
7. Present flow cytometry data using annexin V labeling on the *x*-axis and DAPI staining on the *y*-axis (Fig. 2, *see* **Note 13**).

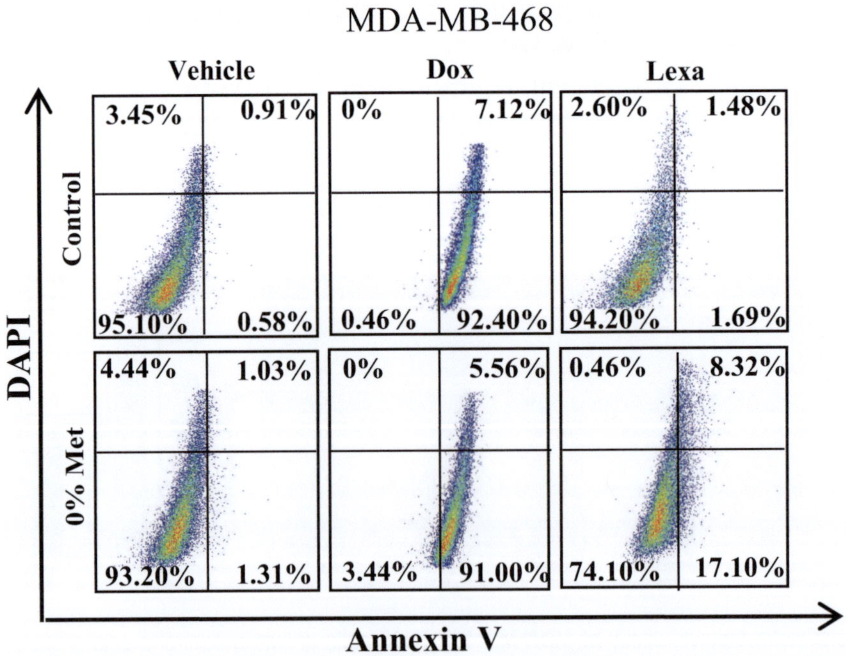

Fig. 2 Annexin V flow cytometry analysis of MDA-MB-468 TNBC cells grown in control medium or methionine-free medium for 48 h and then treated with vehicle, DOX (3.4 μM), or the TRAIL-R2 agonist lexatumumab (2 μg/mL) for an additional 6 h. The percentage of TNBC cells in each quadrant is indicated. Reproduced from [10] with permission from the American Association for Cancer Research

3.4 Caspase-3/7 Activity Assay

1. Seed TNBC cells (2.5×10^3 cells/well) on black-welled 96-well plates overnight. Allow to adhere overnight.
2. Wash cells in PBS and add 100 μL complete or MR medium for 48 h.
3. Add DOX (0–3.4 μM) or TRAIL receptor mAb (0–2 μg/mL) for an additional 16–24 h.
4. Measure caspase-3/7 activity using the Caspase-Glo 3/7 kit (Promega). Add 100 μL of Caspase GLO reagent with added Hoechst dye (10 μM) and incubate for 1 h at room temperature. Detect caspase activity by measuring luminescence using a multimode microplate reader (Synergy H1, BioTek).
5. In order to normalize the signal to cell number, remove media from the plate, and wash cells once with PBS. Visualize nuclei by Hoechst staining and measure fluorescence (Ex 361 nm/ Em 497 nm) using the same microplate reader.

3.5 Anoikis Assay

1. Seed 1.0×10^4 cells/well in 96-well Corning Costar Ultra-Low attachment plates in complete or MR medium supplemented with 1% methylcellulose (Sigma-Aldrich) for 48 h.
2. Add vehicle, DOX (0–3.4 μM), or agonistic TRAIL receptor mAb (0–2 μg/mL) for an additional 24 h.
3. Measure cell viability with the MTS assay in 96-well plates as described in Subheading 3.1.
4. Use the annexin V (Subheading 3.3) and caspase-3/7 (Subheading 3.4) assays and TNBC cells grown on Ultra Low attachment plates to assess the impact of matrix detachment on apoptosis and caspase activation, respectively.

3.6 TRAIL Receptor Expression

3.6.1 RT-PCR

1. Grow TNBC cells (3×10^5 cells/well) in 6-well plates in complete or MR medium for 48 h.
2. Isolate total RNA using SpinSmart™ Total RNA Mini Purification Kit (Denville Scientific) and then synthesize cDNA from total RNA using the iScript cDNA Synthesis Kit (Bio-Rad) following the manufacturers' protocols.
3. Amplify cDNAs PCR using the iQ SYBR Green Supermix (Bio-Rad) and detect with CFX96 Real-Time PCR Detection System (Bio-Rad). Use the following primer pairs: TRAIL-R1 (forward 5-CAGAGGGATGGTCAAGGTCAAGG-3, reverse 5-CCACAACCTGAGCCGATGC-3), TRAIL-R2 (forward 5-CGCTGCACCAGGTGTGATT-3, reverse 5-GTGCCTTC TTCGCACTGACA-3), glyceraldehyde-3-phosphate dehydrogenase (GAPDH) used to normalize gene expression. Primers for GAPDH are forward 5-GAAGGTGAAGGTCGGAGTC-3, and reverse 5-GAAGATGGTGATGGGATTTC-3. Amplify 50–400 ng cDNA in a 25 μL reaction volume containing a

SYBR Green Supermix (Bio-Rad). Use cycling conditions at 95 °C for 5 min, followed by a 40-cycle amplification at 95 °C for 15 s, and 59 °C for 45 s. Perform experiments two times. Each sample is analyzed in triplicate.

4. Represent real-time PCR results as Ct values (the threshold PCR cycle for detecting the PCR product). Normalize RNA expression in each sample with GAPDH expression in each experiment.

3.6.2 Flow Cytometry

1. Culture TNBC cells (3×10^5 cells/well) in 6-well plates in complete or MR medium for 72 h.
2. Trypsinize and collect cells by gentle centrifugation for 5 min at $314 \times g$ in a tabletop centrifuge.
3. Wash cells with PBS and incubate with FITC-conjugated mAbs against TRAIL-R1, TRAIL-R2, or control IgG in ice-cold PBS containing 2.5% BSA for 45 min in the dark.
4. Wash cells three times with cold PBS containing 2.5% BSA and resuspend in PBS containing DAPI (1 μg/mL).
5. Analyze cells using a LSRII flow cytometer. FITC-positive cells are detected using a blue laser (Ex 495 nm/Em 519 nm). Detect DAPI-positive cells with a violet laser (Ex 358 nm/Em 460 nm) and exclude nonviable cells from the analysis.

3.7 Fluorescence Orthotopic Models of Metastatic Breast Cancer

1. Allow female 4–5-week-old NSG mice to recover from the stress of transportation for up to 1 week in the vivarium. Maintain NSG mice in appropriate barrier facilities as warranted by their immunocompromised nature.
2. Resuspend 2×10^6 MDA-MB-468-mCherry TNBC cells in 100% Matrigel (BD Bioscience).
3. Anesthetize mice using 2.5–5% vaporized isoflurane via a nose cone and then inject TNBC cells into the lactiferous ducts of the fourth mammary gland bilaterally using a 27-gauge needle (*see* **Note 14**).
4. Measure tumors weekly with vernier calipers and calculate tumor volume using the formula: tumor volume $(\text{mm}^3) = (\text{length} \times \text{width}^2) \times \pi/6$ [19]. Weigh mice weekly.
5. Randomize mice to treatment groups when mean tumor volume is 100–150 mm^3 (typically 2–3 weeks depending on the tumor model). Include four treatment groups: control diet + vehicle, MR diet + vehicle, control diet + TRAIL receptor agonist, and MR diet + TRAIL receptor agonist (*see* **Note 15**). Administer agonistic TRAIL receptor mAbs 10 mg/kg twice weekly by intraperitoneal injection using a 27-gauge needle.

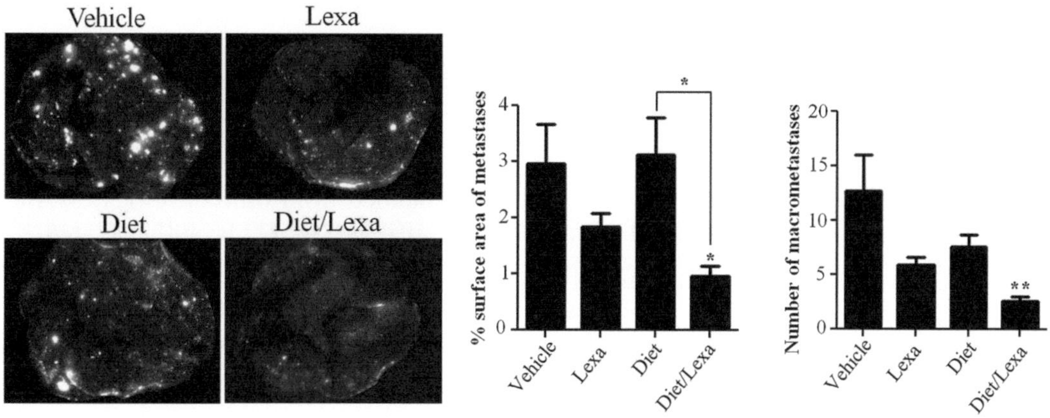

Fig. 3 MDA-MB-468-mCherry lung metastases in female NSG mice treated with vehicle, lexatumumab (10 mg/kg *i.p.* twice weekly for 3 weeks), methionine-free diet for 3 weeks, or methionine-free diet plus lexatumumab. Representative fluorescence ex vivo images of lungs (left) and quantitation of percentage of lung surface area occupied by metastases and number of macrometastases (at least 0.1 mm). $*P < 0.05$, $**P < 0.01$. Reproduced from [10] with permission from the American Association for Cancer Research

6. Monitor mice daily on therapy (*see* **Note 16**). Weigh mice and measure tumor volumes weekly.
7. Euthanize mice in 3 weeks or sooner if mice develop tumors >1.5 cm in any dimension or show signs of distress. Perform terminal intracardiac puncture under deep isoflurane anesthesia to obtain blood for complete blood count, electrolytes, liver function, and kidney function tests.
8. Dissect euthanized mice and remove lungs as a single intact organ.
9. Image lungs ex vivo by fluorescence microscopy and capture images with a digital camera.
10. Quantitate metastatic tumor burden using NIH Image J software to analyze digital images for the number of fluorescent metastases per lung and % surface area of lung occupied by metastases (Fig. 3).
11. Score the number of lung metastases by routine hematoxylin and eosin (H&E) staining of formalin-fixed paraffin-embedded (FFPE) sections of lung tissue. Perform H&E staining of FFPE sections of liver, brain, and kidney to assess systemic toxicity. Briefly, incubate deparaffinized and dehydrated sections (10 μm) with hematoxylin for 3 min, wash with tap water and then with deionized water, incubate with eosin for 1 min, and then wash with 100% ethanol.

4 Notes

1. Early-passage cell lines should be used for experiments and tested periodically for mycoplasma contamination using commercially available kits (e.g., Universal Mycoplasma Detection Kit, ATCC). Cell lines obtained from other investigators and from ATCC more than 1 year ago should be authenticated.
2. MCF-10A cells stably expressing oncogenic Ras or empty vector serve as isogenic models of transformed or untransformed breast epithelial cells [18], respectively, to evaluate the tumor selectivity of therapies.
3. Serum contains modest concentrations of methionine (approximately 3 μM or 0.3 μM for 10% FBS). For dose–response experiments at lower methionine concentrations, dialyzed FBS and methionine-free media should be used. Recent findings suggest that fasting methionine levels in healthy human subjects range from 3 to 30 μM [20].
4. Multiple assays are used to assess cell viability (MTS and crystal violet) and apoptosis (annexin V and caspase activation) to validate findings.
5. The use of fluorescently-labeled human TNBC cells facilitates imaging of primary and metastatic tumors [10, 19, 21]. In addition, fluorescently-labeled circulating cancer cells can be directly isolated from blood in tumor-bearing mice [22].
6. The orthotopic model of metastatic TNBC in this chapter captures the entire metastatic cascade from primary tumor to lung metastases and faithfully recapitulates the human disease with regard to triple-negative status and lung metastases. This is a major advantage over many other metastatic models, such as tail-vein injection, which only model the later stages of metastasis (extravasation and organ colonization) [23, 24].
7. The use of NSG mice, which lack B cells, T cells, and NK cells, rather than athymic nude mice, which lack only T cells, enhances the metastatic potential of orthotopic mammary tumors [25]. However, they may also be less hardy than athymic nude mice and require reductions in dosing of toxic agents such as chemotherapy drugs.
8. MTS assay experiments are performed in triplicate wells to minimize variability due to plating differences. The use of multichannel pipettes (e.g., eight channels) enhances speed and fidelity of cell plating, particularly for large experiments.
9. We typically use 100 μL of medium/well in 96-well plates to provide adequate "cushion" to prevent dislodging cells during media manipulations.

10. Statistical significance of intergroup differences is assessed by ANOVA with appropriate post-tests using GraphPad Prism software. Cell model experiments are performed at least three times.
11. MTS cell-viability results can be normalized to control cells and expressed as fold differences if desired.
12. Crystal-violet cell-survival assays can also be performed with a drug/media "washout" period. Treated cells are returned to control medium for several days to assess the long-term impact of transient MR and/or drug treatment.
13. For annexin V labeling experiments, treated cells are scored in each quadrant of the flow cytometry analysis (Fig. 2). Viable cells are double negative for annexin V and PE (left lower quadrant). Early apoptotic cells are positive for annexin V because they have externalized phosphatidylserine and negative for DAPI because they have intact plasma membranes preventing DAPI staining of nuclei (right lower quadrant). Late apoptotic/necrotic cells are double positive for annexin V and DAPI (right upper quadrant). Cellular/nuclear debris are annexin V negative and DAPI positive (left upper quadrant). We prefer to show flow cytometry results directly because they contain all these data.
14. Intraductal injection of breast cancer cells, in comparison to the standard mammary fat pad injection, facilitates metastasis in murine models [26].
15. We typically use ten mice per group (each with two primary mammary tumors) to evaluate the therapeutic impact of treatments on primary and metastatic tumor burden.
16. Our metabolic priming approach combines short-term (days to few weeks) complete MR (methionine-free diet) in combination with TRAIL receptor agonists. Mice lose weight on a methionine-free diet (approximately 2 g over 3 weeks [10]) but can tolerate this diet for at least 5 weeks.

Acknowledgments

We are indebted to Robin Humphreys for providing agonistic TRAIL receptor mAbs. This work was supported by grants from the V Foundation for Cancer Research, Breast Cancer Research Foundation, Avon Breast Cancer Crusade, UW Carbone Cancer Center pilot funding, and the Wisconsin Partnership Program.

References

1. Guo HY, Herrera H, Groce A, Hoffman RM (1993) Expression of the biochemical defect of methionine dependence in fresh patient tumors in primary histoculture. Cancer Res 53:2479–2483
2. Kreis W, Baker A, Ryan V, Bertasso A (1980) Effect of nutritional and enzymatic methionine deprivation upon human normal and malignant cells in tissue culture. Cancer Res 40:634–641
3. Lu S, Hoestje SM, Choo EM, Epner DE (2002) Methionine restriction induces apoptosis of prostate cancer cells via the c-Jun N-terminal kinase-mediated signaling pathway. Cancer Lett 179:51–58
4. Mecham JO, Rowitch D, Wallace CD, Stern PH, Hoffman RM (1983) The metabolic defect of methionine dependence occurs frequently in human tumor cell lines. Biochem Biophys Res Commun 117:429–434
5. Hoshiya Y, Guo H, Kubota T, Inada T, Asanuma F, Yamada Y et al (1995) Human tumors are methionine dependent in vivo. Anticancer Res 15:717–718
6. Sugimura T, Birnbaum SM, Winitz M, Greenstein JP (1959) Quantitative nutritional studies with water-soluble, chemically defined diets. VII. Nitrogen balance in normal and tumor-bearing rats following forced feeding. Arch Biochem Biophys 81:439–447
7. Durando X, Thivat E, Farges MC, Cellarier E, D'Incan M, Demidem A et al (2008) Optimal methionine-free diet duration for nitrourea treatment: a phase I clinical trial. Nutr Cancer 60:23–30
8. Epner DE, Morrow S, Wilcox M, Houghton JL (2002) Nutrient intake and nutritional indexes in adults with metastatic cancer on a phase I clinical trial of dietary methionine restriction. Nutr Cancer 42:158–166
9. Thivat E, Farges MC, Bacin F, D'Incan M, Mouret-Reynier MA, Cellarier E et al (2009) Phase II trial of the association of a methionine-free diet with cystemustine therapy in melanoma and glioma. Anticancer Res 29:5235–5240
10. Strekalova E, Malin D, Good DM, Cryns VL (2015) Methionine deprivation induces a targetable vulnerability in triple-negative breast cancer cells by enhancing TRAIL receptor-2-expression. Clin Cancer Res 21:2780–2791
11. Nair P, Lu M, Petersen S, Ashkenazi A (2014) Apoptosis initiation through the cell-extrinsic pathway. Methods Enzymol 544:99–128
12. Camidge DR, Herbst RS, Gordon MS, Eckhardt SG, Kurzrock R, Durbin B et al (2010) A phase I safety and pharmacokinetic study of the death receptor 5 agonistic antibody PRO95780 in patients with advanced malignancies. Clin Cancer Res 16:1256–1263
13. Herbst RS, Eckhardt SG, Kurzrock R, Ebbinghaus S, O'Dwyer PJ, Gordon MS et al (2010) Phase I dose-escalation study of recombinant human Apo2L/TRAIL, a dual proapoptotic receptor agonist, in patients with advanced cancer. J Clin Oncol 28:2839–2846
14. Herbst RS, Kurzrock R, Hong DS, Valdivieso M, Hsu CP, Goyal L et al (2010) A first-in-human study of conatumumab in adult patients with advanced solid tumors. Clin Cancer Res 16:5883–5891
15. Trarbach T, Moehler M, Heinemann V, Kohne CH, Przyborek M, Schulz C et al (2010) Phase II trial of mapatumumab, a fully human agonistic monoclonal antibody that targets and activates the tumour necrosis factor apoptosis-inducing ligand receptor-1 (TRAIL-R1), in patients with refractory colorectal cancer. Br J Cancer 102:506–512
16. Toft DJ, Cryns VL (2011) Minireview: basal-like breast cancer: from molecular profiles to targeted therapies. Mol Endocrinol 25:199–211
17. Lev DC, Kiriakova G, Price JE (2003) Selection of more aggressive variants of the gI101A human breast cancer cell line: a model for analyzing the metastatic phenotype of breast cancer. Clin Exp Metastasis 20:515–523
18. Moyano JV, Evans JR, Chen F, Lu M, Werner ME, Yehiely F et al (2006) αB-crystallin is a novel oncoprotein that predicts poor clinical outcome in breast cancer. J Clin Invest 116:261–270
19. Malin D, Chen F, Schiller C, Koblinski J, Cryns VL (2011) Enhanced metastasis suppression by targeting TRAIL receptor 2 in a murine model of triple-negative breast cancer. Clin Cancer Res 17:5005–5015
20. Mentch SJ, Mehrmohamadi M, Huang L, Liu X, Gupta D, Mattocks D et al (2015) Histone methylation dynamics and gene regulation occur through the sensing of one-carbon metabolism. Cell Metab 22:861–873
21. Malin D, Strekalova E, Petrovic V, Deal AM, Al Ahmad A, Adamo B et al (2014) αB-crystallin: a novel regulator of breast cancer metastasis to the brain. Clin Cancer Res 20:56–67
22. Halo TL, McMahon KM, Angeloni NL, Xu Y, Wang W, Chinen AB et al (2014) NanoFlares

for the detection, isolation, and culture of live tumor cells from human blood. Proc Natl Acad Sci U S A 111:17104–17109

23. Fu X, Le P, Hoffman RM (1993) A metastatic orthotopic-transplant nude-mouse model of human patient breast cancer. Anticancer Res 13(4):901–904
24. Li X, Wang J, Yang M, Baranov E, Jinag P, Sun F, Moussa AR, Hoffman RM (2002) Optically imageable metastatic model of human breast cancer. Clin Exp Metastasis 19(4):347–350
25. Puchalapalli M, Zeng X, Mu L, Anderson A, Hix Glickman L, Zhang M et al (2016) NSG mice provide a better spontaneous model of breast cancer metastasis than athymic (nude) mice. PLoS One 11:e0163521
26. Harrell JC, Dye WW, Allred DC, Jedlicka P, Spoelstra NS, Sartorius CA et al (2006) Estrogen receptor positive breast cancer metastasis: altered hormonal sensitivity and tumor aggressiveness in lymphatic vessels and lymph nodes. Cancer Res 66:9308–9315

Chapter 7

Efficacy of Methionine-Restricted Diets on Cancers In Vivo

Robert M. Hoffman, Yasunori Hoshiya, and Weiyan Guo

Abstract

Methionine (MET) dependence is the elevated requirement of cancer cells for MET. Cancer cells are arrested when MET is restricted in late S/G_2 phase of the cell cycle. MET dependence may be the only known general metabolic defect in cancer. This chapter reviews the in vivo efficacy of dietary MET restriction (MR) to arrest human-cancer cell-line tumors and mouse tumors in nude mice. Human cancer xenografts in nude mice, when fed a MET-free diet, had greatly inhibited tumor growth. The body weight of mice on the MET-free diet was found to be maintainable by once-per-week administration of MET. These results suggested that MET dependence can be an important target for human cancer treatment. Yoshida sarcoma in nude mice on a MET-depleted diet regressed. MET depletion resulted in the extended survival of the tumor-bearing mice. These experiments are a prelude to further clinical studies of the efficacy of MR diets on cancer patients.

Key words Methionine dependence, Human cancer, Sarcoma, Cell lines, Yoshida sarcoma, Nude mice, Methionine-free diet, Tumor growth inhibition

1 Introduction

Methionine (MET) dependence is the inability of cancer cells to grow under MET restriction (MR) [1]. MET dependence has been observed in cancer cells but not in normal cells [2]. MET dependence is probably due at least in part to excess MET utilization for aberrant methylation reactions in tumor cells [3]. Under the condition of MR, MET-dependent cells, unlike normal cells, can not divide and arrest in the late S/G_2 phase of the cell cycle [4, 5].

We have reported that many human malignant cell lines and fresh human cancers originating from all organs were MET dependent in vitro [6, 7]. Rodent tumors, in particular the Yoshida sarcoma, have been found to be MET dependent in vivo [7–10]. MET dependence also occurs in human cancer in vivo as observed in a study of human tumor xenografts in nude mice fed a MET-free diet [5, 11].

Robert M. Hoffman (ed.), *Methionine Dependence of Cancer and Aging: Methods and Protocols*, Methods in Molecular Biology, vol. 1866, https://doi.org/10.1007/978-1-4939-8796-2_7,

2 Materials

1. Four–six-week-old male and female BALB/C *nu/nu* nude mice [5, 11].
2. Human breast (R-27), colon (Co-4, COLO-205), and lung (H-460, H-522) cancer cell lines: R-27 was established as a cultured cell line from a tamoxifen-resistant variant of MCF-7 in 1981 by Nawara [12] and was established in nude mice in Keio University [13, 14]. Co-4 was established in the Pathology Division of the Japanese National Cancer Center Research Institute (Tokyo, Japan). COLO-205, H-460, and H-522 were kindly supplied by Dr. Jacqueline Plowman of the US National Cancer Institute [11]. The Yoshida sarcoma is described in reference [5].
3. Hanks' balanced salt solution.
4. TD 930020 (MET-containing diet) and TD 92077 (MET-free diet) (TEKLAD, Madison, WI).

3 Methods

3.1 Mice

1. Use 4- to 5-week-old outbred *nu+/nu* + mice [5].
2. Inject cancer cells (1×10^7) in nude mice previously grown in Eagle's minimum essential medium with 10% fetal calf serum in each mouse at the axillary and inguinal sites [5].

3.2 Transplantation

1. Resect tumors aseptically in the exponential growth phase in nude mice.
2. Cut away necrotic tissues and cut the remaining viable tumor tissue into fragments about 3–4 mm in diameter and place in Hanks' balanced salt solution.
3. Subcutaneously transplant the tumor fragments to either side of the backs of nude mice.
4. Subcutaneously transplant female mice with the R-27 human breast cancer xenograft.
5. Administer one-time dose of 17-β-estradiol dipropionate at 5 mg/kg intramuscularly to the female nude mice [11].
6. Inject a suspension of Yoshida sarcoma and other cancer cell lines (1×10^7 cells) previously grown in Eagle's minimum essential medium with 10% fetal calf serum in each mouse at the axillary and inguinal site.

3.3 Diets

1. Divide mice into two groups of four to five.
2. Feed mice in the control group with the MET-containing diet every day.

3. Feed mice in the treatment group with the MR diet every day.
4. Feed mice in the treatment group bearing human breast tumor R-27 the MR diet for six consecutive days each week and with the MET-containing diet 1 day each week. Feed mice equal amounts on each day [5, 11].

3.4 Tumor Measurement

1. Measure the length and width of the tumors with sliding calipers three times a week.
2. Measure the body weight of the mice at the same time.
3. Estimate the tumor weight according to the following formula: Tumor weight (mg) = length (mm) × [width (mm)]^2/2.

3.5 DNA Staining

1. Make slides containing histological 3 μm sections of tumors and normal colon and liver tissue taken immediately after death of animals.
2. Incubate slides in preheated 1 N hydrochloric acid at 60 °C for 20 min.
3. Rinse the slides with distilled water six times to remove excess acid.
4. Stain with Schiff's reagent for 20 min at room temperature, treat with two successive changes of freshly prepared sulfurous acid rinse, and wash in running tap water for 5 min.
5. After dehydration, coverslip slides for DNA analysis [5].

3.6 Cell-Cycle Position Determination by DNA Measurement

1. Use a Cambridge Instruments Quantimet-520 system or equivalent to determine the DNA content of cell nuclei by measuring integrated absorbance of each cell [7].
2. Measure 500 cells per slide.
3. Integrated absorbance is directly proportional to DNA content.
4. Determine the G1 reference peak in the tissues of the control animals as the first major peak in the histogram [5].

3.7 Statistical Analysis

1. Evaluate the antitumor effect of the MR diet by the T/C ratio (%), where T is the actual tumor weight of the treated group and C is the actual tumor weight of the control group.
2. Perform statistical analysis of the data with the Student's *t*-test [11].

4 Results

The growth of human tumors was inhibited in nude mice fed the MR diet with statistical significance for COLO-205, H-460, and Co-4. Lung cancer H-522 and colon cancer COLO-205 seemed to

Table 1
Effect of dietary MET depletion on the growth of human tumor xenografts in nude mice [11]

Human tumor xenograft	T/C of tumor weight (%)	*P*-value
H-522	31.4	0.001
Colo-205	33.6	0.041
R-27	43.6	0.067 (N.S.)
H-460	55.0	0.004
Co-4	55.1	0.005

Tumors were transplanted subcutaneously and measured as described in the Methods. Tumor weights were compared at the end of the experiment in mice on the MET-containing and MR diets. Tumors were grown for 14–39 days [11]

be the most MET dependent with T/C values of approximately 30% (Table 1) [11].

For the R-27 tumor-bearing mice, the weekly schedule of 6 days on the MET-restricted diet and 1 day on the MET-containing diet reduced the body weight loss to only 10.2% over the 33-day treatment period. The T/C ratio was 43.6% for this tumor [11].

When the ratios of tumor inhibition to body weight loss due to the MR diet were determined, the MR diet had a strong selective effect against the tumors. Using this value, lung tumor H-522 and breast tumor R-27 were most MET dependent with ratios under 50% [11] (*see* **Notes 1** and **2**).

4.1 Yoshida Sarcoma Growth In Vivo in Nude Mice on Methionine-Containing and MR Diets

The Yoshida tumor grew very rapidly in nude mice on the MET-containing diet after s.c. injection of 10^7 cells in the axillary and inguinal sites of the mouse. These animals were all dead by day 12 (Fig. 1). In contrast, in the mice on the MR diet, the tumors grew with a lag, and then rapidly, and then started to regress, with a subsequent 81% reduction from the peak ($P < 0.05$, paired Student's *t*-test) (Table 2). In two subsequent experiments containing 12 mice, the tumors initially grew and then regressed on average more than 50% on the MR diet ($P < 0.05$), thereby repeating the initial result [5] (*see* **Note 3**).

4.2 Cell Cycle Analysis of Tumors Growing in Nude Mice on Methionine-Containing and Methionine-Free Diets

Cell cycle analysis demonstrated that cells from the tumors grown in mice on the MR diet had a much greater DNA content than the cells from the tumors grown in mice on the methionine-containing diet, indicating a cell cycle arrest in the S/G_2 phase [5, 7].

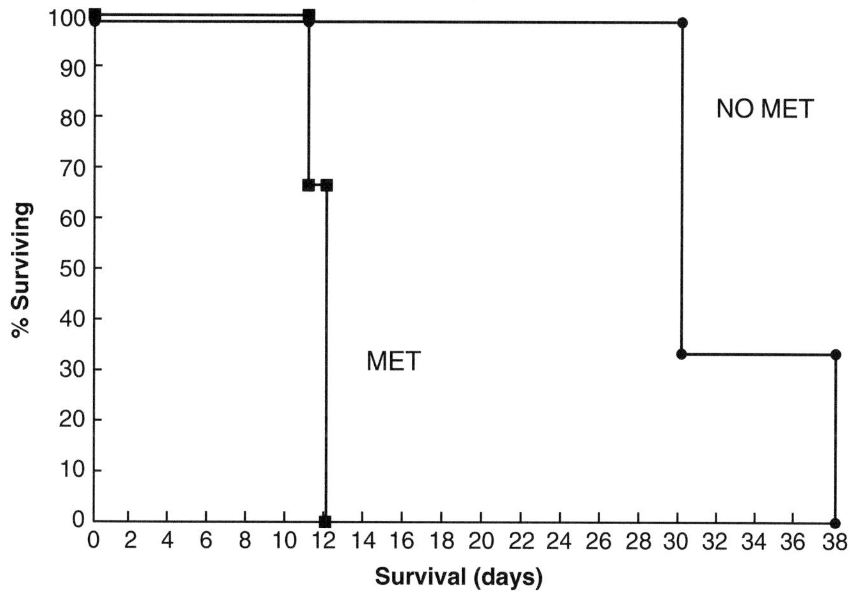

Fig. 1 Representative survival curve of three nude mice bearing the Yoshida sarcoma on the methionine-containing diet and three nude mice on the MR diet. Note that the animals on the MR diets survived much longer ($P < 0.05$, paired Student's *t*-test) [5]

Table 2
Regression of the total estimated tumor weight of the Yoshida sarcoma on an MR diet [5]

Mouse site	Peak estimated tumor wt (mg)	Postregression estimated tumor wt (mg)
A	1353.7	18.7
I	181.1	27.0
A	870.4	281.0
I	207.7	80.0
A	1053.0	252.0
I	273.6	70.3
Av. for all values	$656.6 \pm 205.2^{a, b}$	$121.5 \pm 47.0^{a, b}$

A axillary site, *I* inguinal site
[a]Mean ± SE
[b]$P < 0.05$, paired Student's *t* test
Tumors were grown in nude mice and weights were estimated as described [5]

4.3 Body Weights of Yoshida Sarcoma-Bearing Animals on MET-Containing and Met-Restricted Diet

There was no significant difference ($P > 0.05$, paired Student's t test) between the mean carcass weight of the mice on the two diets (taken on day 10, before any mice died). Mouse body weight on the MR diet was relatively constant for a long period, even during the time of tumor regression, indicating that tumor regression was not just a function of total body weight loss. The mice also maintained a normal performance status as determined by their ambulatory ability for approximately 30 days on the MR diet, suggesting minimal relative toxicity (data not shown) [5] (*see* **Note 4**).

4.4 Survival of Nude Mice with Yoshida Sarcoma on MET-Containing and MR Diets

The nude mice bearing the Yoshida tumor on the MET-containing diet were all dead by day 12. In contrast, the Yoshida tumor-bearing mice on the MR diet were all alive at day 30, with the last animal dying at day 38. There was a significant difference between the mean survival time of the two groups, at $P < 0.05$ by paired Student's t-test [5] (*see* **Note 5**).

5 Notes

1. Since normal cells can synthesize MET from homocysteine (HCY), the MR diet was also depleted of HCY and choline to allow extensive depletion of MET in the mouse blood.
2. The results presented here demonstrate that MET dependence actually occurs in human tumors in vivo and suggest that MET dependence is a potential selective target for human cancer treatment [11].
3. The initial growth of the tumor on the MR diet could be due to cellular and extracellular MET stores. The extended administration of the MR diet seemed to be a key factor in demonstrating that tumor regression could occur. Apparently tumor regression allowed the animals to have extended survival on the MR diet [5].
4. It should be noted that during the period of tumor regression the carcass weight of the animals stayed relatively constant, demonstrating that weight loss was not a factor in the tumor regression. The maintenance of constant weight and the animals' high performance status during prolonged periods of MR indicated that MR diets may be relatively nontoxic in the period investigated [5].
5. The results of the studies reviewed in this chapter were used to design clinical trials for cancer patients on MR diets. (Please see chapter 9 in the present volume).

References

1. Hoffman RM (2015) Development of recombinant methioninase to target the general cancer-specific metabolic defect of methionine dependence: a 40-year odyssey. Expert Opin Biol Ther 15:21–31
2. Hoffman RM (1984) Altered methionine metabolism, DNA methylation and oncogene expression in carcinogenesis: a review and synthesis. Biochim Biophys Acta 738:49–87
3. Stern PH, Hoffman RM (1984) Elevated overall rates of transmethylation in cell lines from diverse human tumors. In Vitro 20:663–670
4. Hoffman RM, Jacobsen SJ (1980) Reversible growth arrest in simian virus 40-transformed human fibroblasts. Proc Natl Acad Sci U S A 77:7306–7310
5. Guo HY, Lishko VK, Herrera H, Groce A, Kubota T, Hoffman RM (1993) Therapeutic

tumor-specific cell cycle block induced by methionine starvation in vivo. Cancer Res 53:5676–5679

6. Mecham JO, Rowitch D, Wallace CD, Stern PH, Hoffman RM (1983) The metabolic defect of methionine dependence occurs frequently in human tumor cell lines. Biochem Biophys Res Commun 117:429–434
7. Guo HY, Herrera H, Groce A, Hoffman RM (1993) Expression of the biochemical defect of methionine dependence in fresh patient tumors in primary histoculture. Cancer Res 53:2479–2483
8. Goseki N, Yamazaki S, Endo M (1992) Antitumor effect of methionine-depleting total parenteral nutrition with doxorubicin administration on Yoshida sarcoma-bearing rats. Cancer 69:1865–1872
9. Breillout F, Hadida F, Echinard-Darin P, Lascaux V, Poupon M-F (1987) Decreased rat rhabdomyosarcoma pulmonary metastases in response to a low methionine diet. Anticancer Res 7:861–867
10. Breillout F, Antoine E, Poupon M-F (1990) Methionine dependency of malignant tumors: a possible approach for therapy. J Natl Cancer Inst 82:1628–1632
11. Hoshiya Y, Guo H, Kubota T, Inada T, Asanuma F, Yamada Y, Koh J, Kitajima M, Hoffman RM (1995) Human tumors are methionine dependent in vivo. Anticancer Res 15:717–718
12. Nawara H, Bronzert D, Lippman ME (1981) Isolation and characterization of a tamoxifen-resistant cell line derived from MCF-7 human breast cancer cells. J Biol Chem 256:5016–5021
13. Kubota T, Kubouchi K, Koh J, Enomoto K, Ishibiki K, Abe O (1983) Human breast carcinoma (MCF-7) serially transplanted into nude mice. Jpn J Surg 13:381–384
14. Fukutomi T, Kubota T, Ikeda T, Isobe Y, Kikuyama S, Shimada A, Nakamura A, Nishiumi T, Enomoto K, Ishibiki K, Abe O (1986) Experimental combined hormone therapy on human breast carcinomas serially transplanted into nude mice. Jpn J Cancer Res 77:92–97

Chapter 8

Dietary Methionine Restriction-Based Cancer Chemotherapy in Rodents

Robert M. Hoffman and Peter H. Stern

Abstract

The elevated methionine (MET) requirement for the growth of tumors, first observed by Sugimura in 1959, termed MET dependence, is a potentially highly effective therapeutic target. Proof of this principle is that when MET restriction (MR) was initially established in co-cultures of cancer and normal cells, MET dependence could be exploited to selectively kill cancer cells without killing co-cultured normal cells. MET-dependent cells become reversibly blocked in the late S/G_2 phase of the cell cycle under MR enabling selective and effective S-phase chemotherapy against these blocked cancer cells. Subsequent MET repletion with an anti-mitotic drug was totally effective at selectively eliminating the MET-dependent cancer cells enabling the normal MET-dependent cells to take over the culture. We have also observed that the MET analog ethionine (ETH) is synergistic with MR in arresting the growth of the Yoshida sarcoma both in vitro and eliminating metastasis when transplanted to nude mice. MR increased the efficacy of cisplatinum (CDDP) against the MX-1 human breast carcinoma cell line when grown in nude mice. MR increased 5-fluorouracil (5-FU) efficacy on a human gastric cancer xenograft, SC-1-NU, in nude mice. MET-restricted total parenteral nutrition (MR TPN) was effective in Yoshida sarcoma-bearing rats. MR TPN with doxorubicin (DOX) and vincristine (VCR) resulted in significant tumor suppression and prolonged survival of Yoshida-sarcoma-bearing rats. These results were the basis of subsequent studies that used methioninase to effect MR for effective cancer therapy.

Key words Cancer, Methionine dependence, Methionine restriction, Diet, Cell cycle, Chemotherapy, S/G_2 phase, Cell cycle arrest, Total parenteral nutrition (TPN)

1 Introduction

Methionine (MET) dependence, the elevated requirement for MET, is a phenomenon found only in cancer [1–3]. MET dependence is defined as the inability or greatly reduced ability of cancer cells to grow when the MET is restricted (MR). A broad range of human tumors tested in our and other laboratories, including carcinomas, sarcomas, and neurologic tumors, were found to be

Robert M. Hoffman (ed.), *Methionine Dependence of Cancer and Aging: Methods and Protocols*, Methods in Molecular Biology, vol. 1866, https://doi.org/10.1007/978-1-4939-8796-2_8, © Springer Science+Business Media, LLC, part of Springer Nature 2019

absolutely MET dependent in that they were totally unable to grow in MET-restricted medium [4]. Thus it is possible that MET dependence is a general metabolic defect in cancer. Normal cells grow quite well under MET restriction [5].

When MET-dependent cancer cells were placed in MR medium, the cancer cells arrested in the late S/G_2 phase of the cell cycle over a period of 9 days, thus synchronizing them for immediate entry into mitosis when MET was repleted [6]. We took advantage of this cell-cycle block of MET-dependent cancer cells incubated in MET-restricted medium to selectively eliminate MET-dependent cancer cells from a mixed population with normal MET-independent cells by the use of the cell cycle-dependent drugs doxorubicin (DOX) and vincristine (VCR) [7].

Brillout et al. [8, 9] found for MET-dependent tumors that a MR diet lowered the metastatic potential of tumors without significant effects on local tumor growth in rats. Goseki et al. [10] observed that a MR total parenteral nutrition (TPN) mixture for rats bearing the Yoshida sarcoma slowed tumor growth and extended the survival of the rats, especially with the use of DOX. Yoshida et al. [11] observed that administration of MET-depleted TPN slowed growth of the AH 109A ascites hepatoma in rats [12].

We have demonstrated that the Yoshida tumor growing in nude mice on a MR diet has a late S/G_2 cell-cycle block, indicating that a tumor-selective cell-cycle block can indeed be achieved in vivo [13]. We also observed that the Yoshida tumor in nude mice can actually regress with prolonged dietary MR, resulting in an extended survival period of the mice [13].

In an attempt to completely arrest the Yoshida sarcoma growing in nude mice, we have administered the combination of a MET-depleted diet and the methionine analog ethionine (ETH) which acts as a competitive inhibitor for MET-utilizing enzymes [12].

Sequential administration of MR TPN, (DOX), a drug acting on the late S/G_2-phase cells, and VCR, an anti-mitotic drug, was highly effective against the Yoshida sarcoma in rats. MET-restricted TPN potentiated the efficacy of 5-FU in a clinical trial of gastric cancer [14].

2 Materials

1. Cancer cell lines: Human gastric cancer xenograft, SC-1-NU [15]. HOS-1A, a clone of the human MET-dependent osteogenic sarcoma HOS [8]; HOS-1A-R3, a partially MET-independent revertant derived from HOS-1A [16]; PC-3-1C, a clone of the human MET-dependent prostate carcinoma PC-3 [17]; A2182-5D, a clone of the

MET-dependent lung-cancer A2182 [4]; MCF-7, a human MET-dependent breast-cancer cell line [4]; human breast-cancer xenograft MX-1 and Yoshida sarcoma cells.

2. Normal cell strain FS-3, a normal diploid fibroblast cell strain derived from human foreskin.
3. Eagle's minimum essential medium.
4. Fetal bovine serum.
5. L-Methionine (L-MET).
6. L-Homocysteine thiolactone (L-HCY).
7. Folic acid.
8. Hydroxocobalamin.
9. 6-Well cluster plates.
10. Doxorubicin (DOX).
11. Vincristine (VCR).
12. Cisplatinum (CDDP).
13. 5-Fluorouracil (5-FU).
14. Methanol.
15. Giemsa's stain.
16. Athymic *nu/nu* mice.
17. MET-containing diet (Teklad, Madison, WI [16]).
18. MET-depleted diet (Teklad).
19. Formalin.
20. Paraffin.
21. Hematoxylin and eosin (H&E).
22. Phosphate-buffered saline (PBS).
23. Hanks' balanced salt solution [19].
24. Male Donryu rats (Shizuoka Laboratory Animal Center, Shizuoka, Japan).
25. Microinfusion pump.
26. [^{3}H]thymidine [14].
27. AO-90 total parenteral infusion [14].
28. Pan-Amin S total parenteral infusion [14].

3 Methods

3.1 Co-culture with MET-Dependent Cancer Cells and MET-Independent Cells to Demonstrate that MR and Cell-Cycle-Dependent Chemotherapy Can Selectively Eliminate the Cancer Cells

1. Grow cells in Eagle's minimum essential medium containing 10% fetal bovine serum and supplemented with either 100 μM L-MET or 100 μM L-HCY thiolactone and 100 μM folic acid and 1.5 μM hydroxocobalamin (MR medium), selective conditions that distinguish MET-dependent cells from MET-independent cells [1–4, 6, 20].
2. Seed cells in 6-well cluster plates in $MET^{+}HCY^{-}$ medium.
3. After 24-h incubation, divide groups in the following manner: Maintain one control group for each cancer cell type in $MET^{+}HCY^{-}$ medium. Maintain another control group in $MET^{-}HCY^{+}$ medium for 10 days and then place in $MET^{+}HCY^{-}$ medium. Place a third group in $MET^{+}HCY^{-}$ medium containing DOX for 10 days and then switch to drug-free $MET^{+}HCY^{-}$ medium. Place a fourth group in $MET^{+}HCY^{-}$ medium. Incubate co-cultures in $MET^{-}HCY^{+}$ medium with DOX for 10 days before switching to drug-free $MET^{+}HCY^{-}$ medium. Incubate groups 5 and 6 in $MET^{+}HCY^{-}$ and $MET^{-}HCY^{+}$ medium, respectively, for 10 days; treat with $MET^{+}HCY^{-}$ medium containing VCR for 24 h; and then place in drug-free $MET^{+}HCY^{-}$ medium for the remainder of the experiment. Incubate groups 7 and 8 in $MET^{+}HCY^{-}$ and $MET^{-}HCY^{+}$ medium, respectively, containing DOX. After 10 days, treat for 24 h with $MET^{+}HCY^{-}$ medium containing VCR and then place in drug-free $MET^{+}HCY^{-}$ medium for the duration of the experiment.
4. Conduct the experiment for a total of 31 days.
5. Replace the medium at 3- to 4-day intervals.
6. Take photomicrographs of the cells at various time periods.
7. After the experiment are completed, fix the cells in methanol, stain with Giemsa, and photograph again [7].

3.2 Demonstrate that MR Potentiates Ethionine (ETH) Chemotherapy

1. Seed Yoshida sarcoma cell line in vitro at 10^3 cells/mL.
2. Culture the cells in MEM Earle's media with 10% fetal calf serum containing MET at 5 μm, 10 μm, and 100 μm, and ETH at concentrations of 5 μm, 50 μm, 100 μm, 500 μm, and 1000 μm in various combinations.
3. Count cells every day.
4. Randomly divide 5-week-old nude mice into four groups. Each group should consist of three mice.
5. Inject Yoshida sarcoma cells (8×10^3) in suspension in an axillary site in each nude mouse.

6. Feed group 1 mice a defined MET-containing diet. Feed group 2 mice a defined MR diet. Feed group 3 mice the defined MET-containing diet and administer ETH ip twice daily at 25 mg/kg. Treat group 4 mice with 25 mg/kg ETH as above on the MR diet.
7. Measure tumor size with a caliper each day.
8. Determine tumor size by the length of the longest axis times the length of the shortest axis.
9. Measure body weight each day.
10. After the mice die, fix the liver, lung, kidney, and colon of the mice in 10% formalin.
11. Dehydrate the tissues, embed in paraffin, and section at 5 μm.
12. Stain the slides with hematoxylin and eosin (H&E) and analyze for metastasis by light microscopy [12].

3.3 Demonstrate that MR Potentiates CDDP and 5-FU

1. Subcutaneously transplant MX-1 human breast cancer on the backs of nude mice under ether anesthesia.
2. Feed mice in the control and CDDP-only groups the MET-containing diet every day. Feed mice in the MR group and MR/CDDP group the MR diet for six consecutive days each week.
3. Treat mice in the CDDP-only group and MR/CDDP group with CDDP intraperitoneally at a dose of 1 mg/kg on the fourth day after MR for three consecutive weeks.
4. Estimate the tumor weight according to the following formula:

$$\text{Tumor weight (mg)} = \text{length (mm)} \times [\text{width (mm)}]^2/2$$

5. Resect the tumors and freeze in liquid nitrogen as quickly as possible.
6. Assess the intra-tumor concentration of total platinum in the samples by flameless atomic absorption spectrophotometry [21].
7. Subcutaneously transplant nude mice with SC-l-NU stomach cancer.
8. Treat mice with 5-FU intraperitoneally at a dose of 30 mg/kg/week for 4 weeks on the fourth day after the initiation of the MR diet.
9. In the 5-FU-alone group, administer 5-FU at the same time and the same dose as the MR group, but in the MET-containing diet.
10. Evaluate antitumor efficacy by the T/C ratio (%), where T is the tumor weight of the treated group and C is the tumor weight of the control group at the time of sacrifice [15].

3.4 Determine Efficacy of MR TPN on Mitosis of Yoshida Sarcoma in Rats

1. Transplant ascites-type Yoshida sarcoma (5×10^6) cells. i.p. in 7-week-old male Donryu rats, weighing approximately 200 g.
2. Cannulate each rat in the vena cava soon after transplantation (day 0).
3. During the TPN period, the rats should receive no solid food except the freely-fed group.
4. To analyze the effect of MET-depleted TPN on the cell cycle of cancer cells, use the autoradiographic analytical method of labeled mitosis, using [^{3}H]thymidine.
5. Give one group of rats TPN with AO-90 (MR TPN) for 7 days and administer i.p. pulse injection of 500 mCi/kg [^{3}H]thymidine on day 5.
6. Give another group of rats TPN with Pan-Amin S (MET-containing TPN) for 7 days. Administer [^{3}H]thymidine to each rat in the same dose and manner as the AO-90 group.
7. Give another group of rats AO-90 regimen for 4 days, and then change TPN to Pan-Amin S regimen from the time of i.p. administration of 500 mCi/kg [^{3}H]thymidine.
8. Give another group of rats TPN for 4 days with AO-90 regimen, and then change to Pan-Amin S regimen. 16 h before the changeover, administer [^{3}H]thymidine.
9. Give another group of rats TPN for 6 days without any amino acid, and then administer [^{3}H]thymidine on day 5.
10. Give another group of rats solid food and water ad libitum for 7 days, and then administer [^{3}H]thymidine to each rat.
11. Use a microinfusion pump for constant administration of each TPN solution.
12. After i.p. administration of [^{3}H]thymidine, obtain 0.05 mL ascites fluid from each rat every 1–2 h for 60–72 h [14].

3.5 Determine Efficacy of MR TPN with DOX and VCR Administration on the Yoshida-Sarcoma-Bearing Rats

1. Transplant Yoshida sarcoma cells (1×10^4) into adipose tissue on the back (day 0) of 48 7-week-old male Donryu rats.
2. Cannulate 32 rats in the vena cava immediately after tumor transplantation (on day 0) and start TPN immediately after tumor transplantation (day 0).
3. Divide rats into two groups, AO-90 (MR TPN) and Pan-Amin S (MET-containing TPN) and maintain TPN for 8 days.
4. Do not feed the rats during TPN.
5. Subdivide the rats in both groups according to DOX and VCR administrations into four groups: AO-90 + (DOX and VCR) group; AO-90 group; Pan-Amin S + (DOX and VCR) group; and Pan-Amin S group.

6. Feed the remaining 16 rats with solid food and water ad libitum (freely fed group) and divide into 2 groups according to the administration of freely fed with or without (DOX and VCR).
7. Divide the rats into six experimental groups as follows: AO-90 + (DOX and VCR) group ($n = 8$): Give rats TPN with AO-90 for 8 days, followed by TPN with Pan-Amin S for 3 days. Give each rat DOX three times (days 3, 5, and 7) at a dose of 0.5 mg/kg per one time via i.p. injection. Administer VCR at a dose of 0.05 mg/kg on days 9, 10, and 11, and at a dose of 0.1 mg/kg on days 12 and 13.
8. In the AO-90 group ($n = 8$), maintain rats in the same manner as the AO-90 + (DOX and VCR) group except for DOX and VCR.
9. In the Pan-Amin S+(DOX and VCR) group ($n = 8$), administer TPN for 11 days with Pan-Amin. Administer DOX and VCR at the same dose and manner as in the AO-90 + (DOX and VCR) group.
10. In the Pan-Amin S group ($n = 8$), maintain the rats in the same manner as in the Pan-Amin S + (DOX and VCR) group without DOX and VCR administration.
11. In the freely-fed+ (DOX and VCR) group ($n = 8$), feed the rats with solid food and water ad libitum and give each rat DOX and VCR at the same dose and manner as in the AO-90 + (DOX and VCR) group.
12. In the freely-fed group ($n = 8$), maintain rats in the same manner as in the freely-fed + (DOX and VCR) group without DOX and VCR administration.
13. During TPN, individually house rats in metabolic cages and use a microinfusion pump for constant administration of TPN solutions.
14. From day 12, feed all rats in all groups with solid food and water ad libitum during the experiments without TPN.
15. Determine the life span of each rat [14].

4 Results

4.1 MR Chemotherapy In Vitro

In co-culture experiments with MET-dependent cancer cells and MET-independent normal cells, chemotherapy in $MET^{+}HCY^{-}$ medium (groups 1, 3, 5, 7) could not prevent the proliferation of HOS-1A osteosarcoma cells. Placement of the co-culture in $MET^{-}HCY^{+}$ medium (group 2) selectively reduced the rate of cancer cell growth but did not eliminate the cancer cells. $MET^{-}HCY^{+}$ medium containing DOX (group 4) did not greatly enhance the selective killing of the cancer cells. The use of

MET^-HCY^+ medium followed by VCR in MET^+HCY^- medium (group 6) was more selective against the cancer cells but still did not completely eliminate the cancer cells. The combination chemotherapy of DOX in MET^-HCY^+ medium followed by VCR in MET^+HCY^- medium for 24 h and then drug-free MET^+HCY^- medium (group 8) was the only procedure that resulted in a culture completely free of HOS-1A cells while still allowing proliferation of the normal fibroblasts [7] (*see* **Note 1**).

4.2 Antitumor Efficacy of ETH With and Without MR In Vivo

The percent inhibition of Yoshida sarcoma growth in nude mice on the MR diet was 64% compared to control tumor-bearing animals on the MET-containing diet (Fig. 1). ETH (25 mg/kg) given to Yoshida-sarcoma-bearing nude mice on the MR diet resulted in an 87.1% inhibition rate compared to control animals. In contrast, ETH (25 mg/kg) given on the MET-containing diet had only a 7.5% inhibition rate on the growth of the Yoshida sarcoma ($p < 0.01$) [12].

The body weights of the animals on the MR diet with ETH were similar to the body weights of the animals on the MR diet only. The body weights of the animals under these two conditions

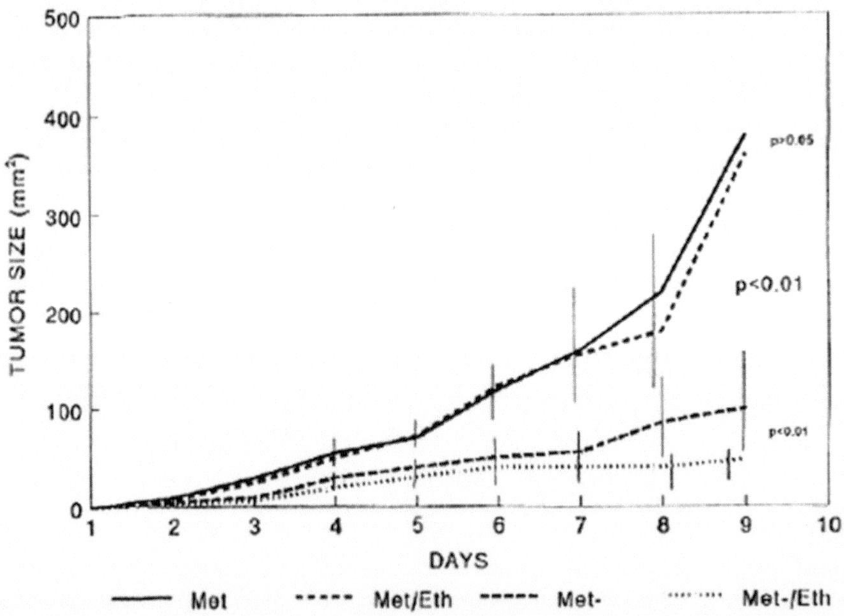

Fig. 1 Effect of ethionine administration and methionine depletion on tumor growth in nude mice. Yoshida sarcoma cells (8×10^5) in suspension were injected in an axillary site in each nude mouse. Mice were divided into four groups. Group 1 mice were given a defined MET-containing diet. Group 2 mice were fed a defined MR diet. Group 3 mice were treated with ethionine at 25 mg/kg i.p. twice a day on the MET-containing diet. Group 4 mice were treated with 25 mg/kg ethionine i.p. twice a day on the MR diet. Each group consisted of three animals. The tumor area was measured by the equation: length of the longest axis × length of the shortest axis [12]

remained essentially constant from day 4 to day 9 after an initial loss resulting in no animal deaths. Tumor growth then ceased in the animals on the MR diet receiving ETH after day 6 [12].

4.3 Anti-Metastatic Efficacy of ETH With and Without MR

No metastases were found in Yoshida-sarcoma-bearing mice treated with ETH (25 mg/kg) on the MR diet compared to the 43% on the MR diet without ETH and 75% on a MET-containing diet without ETH [12].

4.4 MR Enhanced Efficacy of CDDP and 5-FU on Human Mammary Tumors In Vivo

The treated/control MX-1 mammary tumor ratios of CDDP-only was 68.9% in the MET-containing diet. The MR diet by itself resulted in a T/C ratio of 94.4%. A T/C ratio of 31% resulted with CDDP in combination with the MR diet (Fig. 2). MR more than doubled the antitumor efficacy of CDDP with statistical significance of $p < 0.05$ [19].

The efficacy of the MR diet and 5-FU was investigated on human SC-1-NU stomach cancer in nude mice. The T/C ratio of the actual tumor weight was 63.1% in the MR group with a statistically-significant difference relative to control at $p < 0.01$ (Fig. 3) [15]. Tumor growth was strongly inhibited by the combination of MR diet and 5-FU, $p < 0.05$, compared to 5-FU treatment on the MET-containing diet [15] (*see* **Note 2**).

4.5 Efficacy of MR TPN Combined with Chemotherapy

All rats with the Yoshida sarcoma in the AO-90 MR TPN with DOX and VCR group survived more than 28 days after the initiation of the experiment. Of the rats which received no chemotherapy

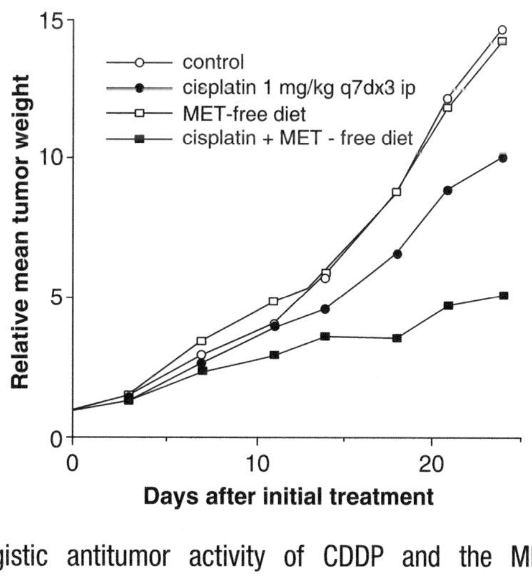

Fig. 2 Synergistic antitumor activity of CDDP and the MR diet. CDDP was administered i.p. at a dose of 1 mg/kg once a week for 3 weeks. The MR diet was given for 6 days each week with the control diet given on the seventh day [19]

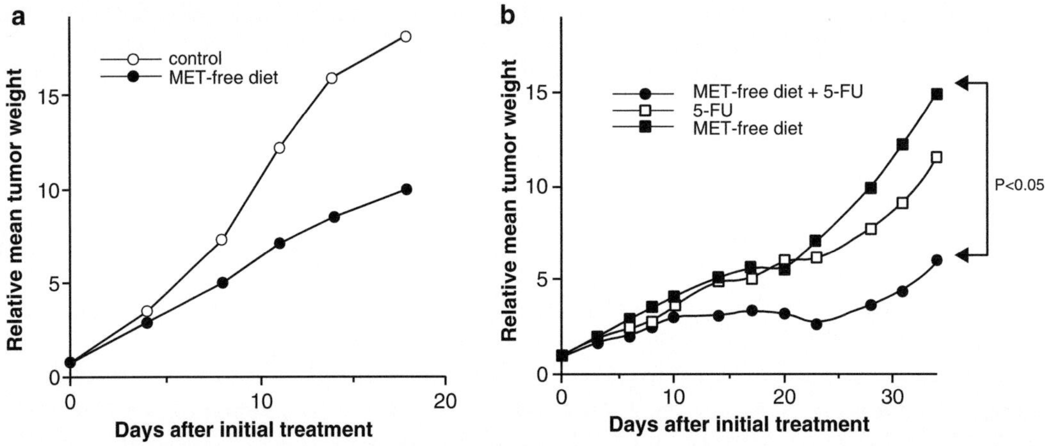

Fig. 3 MR diet modulates 5-FU efficacy on the human gastric cancer xenograft, SC-1-NU. (**a**) Shows the effect of MR-alone relative to untreated control. The MR-free diet was given for 6 days each week followed by the control diet given on the seventh day. (**b**) Shows the effect of 5-FU alone and the combination of 5-FU and the MR diet relative to the MR diet alone. Mice treated with combination therapy received intraperitoneal 5-FU at a dose of 30 mg/kg for 4 weeks on the fourth day after each initiation of MR. In the 5-FU-alone group, 5-FU was administered at the same time and same dose as the combination group [15]

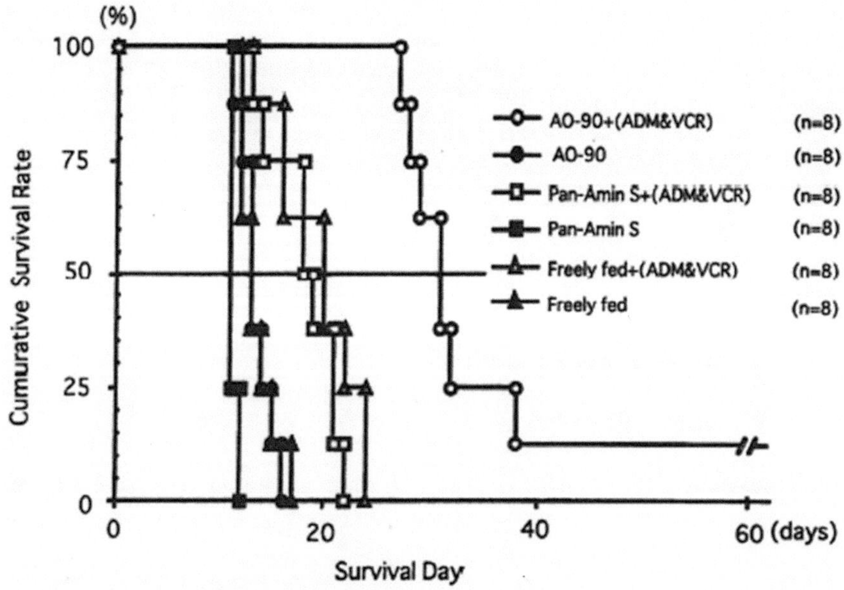

Fig. 4 Life span of the rats in six experimental groups [14]

including AO-90 MR TPN and MET Pan-Amin TPN and freely fed groups, all died within 16 days (Fig. 4). All rats which received DOX and VCR in the presence of MET died by day 22 [14] (*see* **Note 3**).

5 Notes

1. Late S/G_2-phase cell-cycle arrest caused by MR could selectively potentiate the sensitivity of the cancer cells to drugs acting on the late S/G_2-phase cells. Anti-mitotic drugs became effective after the reversal of the MR cell-cycle block in cell culture.
2. MR may act as an effective biochemical modulator for 5-FU [10, 22].
3. This was the first demonstration that sequential administration of DOX and VCR in the same animal was effective using MR. MR TPN was useful combined with not only single anticancer agents such as 5-FU [22, 23] and DOX, but also an antimitotic drug, such as VCR [14].

References

1. Hoffman RM (2015) Development of recombinant methioninase to target the general cancer-specific metabolic defect of methionine dependence: a 40 year odyssey. Expert Opin Biol Ther 15:21–31
2. Hoffman RM (1984) Altered methionine metabolism, DNA methylation and oncogene expression in carcinogenesis. Biochim Biophys Acta 738:49–87
3. Hoffman RM (1985) Altered methionine metabolism and transmethylation in cancer. Anticancer Res 5:1–30
4. Mecham JO, Rowitch D, Wallace CD, Stern PH, Hoffman RM (1983) The metabolic defect of methionine dependence occurs frequently in human tumor cell lines. Biochem Biophys Res Commun 117:429–434
5. Duvigneaud V, Dyer HM, Harmon J (1935) The growth-promoting properties of homocysteine when added to cysteine-deficient diet and the proof of structure of homocysteine. J Biol Chem 101:719–726
6. Hoffman RM, Jacobsen SJ (1980) Reversible growth arrest in simian virus 40-transformed human fibroblasts. Proc Natl Acad Sci U S A 77:7306–7310
7. Stern PH, Hoffman RM (1986) Enhanced in vitro selective toxicity of chemotherapeutic agents for human cancer cells based on a metabolic defect. J Natl Cancer Inst 76:629–639
8. Breillout F, Hadida F, Echinard-Darin P, Lascaux V, Poupon MF (1987) Decreased rat rhabdomyosarcoma pulmonary metastases in response to a low methionine diet. Anticancer Res 7:861–867
9. Breillout F, Antome E, Poupon MF (1990) Methionine dependency of malignant tumors: a possible approach for therapy. J Natl Cancer Inst 82:1628–1632
10. Goseki N, Yamazaki S, Endo M (1992) Antitumor effect of methionine-depleting total parenteral nutrition with doxorubicin administration on Yoshida sarcoma-bearing rats. Cancer 69:1865–1872
11. Yoshida S, Yamasaki K, Kaibara A, Takagi K, Noake T, Ishibashi N, Kakegawa T (1995) Effect of methionine-deprived total parenteral nutrition on tumor protein turnover in rats. Cancer 76:1275–1282
12. Guo H, Tan Y, Kubota T, Moossa AR, Hoffman RM (1996) Methionine depletion modulates the antitumor and antimetastatic efficacy of ethionine. Anticancer Res 16:2719–2723
13. Guo H, Lishko VK, Herrera H, Kubota T, Hoffman RM (1993) Therapeutic tumor-specific cell cycle block induced by methionine starvation in vivo. Cancer Res 53:5676–5679
14. Nagahama T, Goseki N, Endo M (1998) Doxorubicin and vincristine with methionine depletion contributed to survival in the Yoshida sarcoma bearing rats. Anticancer Res 18:25–32
15. Hoshiya T, Kubota T, Inada T, Kitajima M, Hoffman RM (1997) Methionine-depletion modulates the efficacy of 5-fluorouracil in human gastric cancer in nude mice. Anticancer Res 17:4371–4376
16. Hoffman RM, Jacobsen SJ, Erbe RW (1978) Reversion to methionine independence by malignant rat and SV40-transformed human

fibroblasts. Biochem Biophys Res Commun 82:228–234

17. Kaighn M, Narayan KS, Ohnuki Y, Lechner JF, Jones LW (1979) Establishment and characterization of a human prostate carcinoma cell line (PC-3). Invest Urol 17:16–25
18. Ovejera AA, Houchens DP, Barker AD (1978) Chemotherapy of human tumor xenografts in genetically athymic mice. Ann Clin Lab Sci 8:50–56
19. Hoshiya Y, Kubota T, Matsuzaki SW, Kitajima M, Hoffman RM (1996) Methionine starvation modulates the efficacy of cisplatin on human breast cancer in nude mice. Anticancer Res 16:3515–3517
20. Coalson DW, Mecham JO, Stern PH, Hoffman RM (1982) Reduced availability of endogenously synthesized methionine for S-adenosylmethionine formation in methionine-dependent cancer cells. Proc Natl Acad Sci U S A 79:4248–4251
21. Leroy AF, Wehling MI, Sponseller HL, Friauf WS, Solomon RE, Dedrick RL, Litterst CL, Gram TE, Guarino AM, Becker DA (1977) Analysis of platinum in biological materials by flameless atomic absorption spectrophotometry. Biochem Med 18:184–191
22. Goseki N, Yamazaki S, Shimojyu K, Kando F, Maruyama M, Endo M, Koike M, Takahashi H (1995) Synergistic effect of methionine-depleting total parenteral nutrition with 5-fluorouracil on human gastric cancer: a randomized, prospective clinical trial. Jpn J Cancer Res 86:484–489
23. Goseki N, Endo M, Onodera T, Kosaki G (1991) Anti-tumor effect of L-methionine-deprived total parenteral nutrition with 5-fluourouracil administration on Yoshida sarcoma-bearing rats. Ann Surg 213:83–88

Chapter 9

Clinical Studies of Methionine-Restricted Diets for Cancer Patients

Robert M. Hoffman

Abstract

Methionine (MET) restriction (MR) has been shown to arrest cancer growth and sensitizes tumors to chemotherapy. MR total parenteral nutrition (MR TPN) with a chemotherapy-containing amino acid solution ("AO-90") (lacking both MET and L-cysteine[CYS]) showed synergistic effects with 5-fluorouracil (5-FU) in tumor-bearing rats and in a Phase I clinical trial with gastrointestinal tract cancers compared to 5-FU in a MET-containing TPN. All gastric cancer patients underwent gastrectomy. Resected tumors in the AO-90 group showed significant reduction of cancer histologically, while almost no effect was seen in the control group. A Phase II clinical trial of dietary MR combined with cystemustine treatment for melanoma or glioma was carried out. Twenty-two patients (20 with metastatic melanoma and 2 with recurrent gloma) received a median of four cycles of the combination of a 1-day MR diet with cystemustine (60 mg/m^2) every 2 weeks. This combination was well tolerated (toxicity and nutritional status). The median disease-free survival was 1.8 months and the median survival was 4.6 months, with two long-duration stabilizations. MET depletion in plasma was 40%. In another study, eight patients with a variety of metastatic solid tumors were enrolled in a Phase I clinical trial of a commercially available MR medical food. Participants remained on the experimental diet for an average of 17.3 weeks. Plasma methionine levels fell from 21.6 to 9 μm within 2 weeks, a 58% decline. The only side effect was weight loss of approximately 0.5 kg per week. A feasibility study combining dietary MR with a FOLFOX regimen in patients with metastatic colorectal cancer was carried out. The plasma MET concentration was reduced by dietary MR by 58% on the first day of the MR diet. Among the four patients evaluable for response, three experienced a partial response and one patient had disease stabilization. The results of the above-described clinical trials indicate the clinical potential of MR.

Key words Methionine restriction, Clinical trial, Cancer, Methionine (MET) dependence, Total parenteral nutrition (TPN), MET-restricted TPN, 5-Fluorouracil, 5-FU, Gastric cancer, Resection, Histological response

1 Introduction

Methionine (MET) restriction (MR) has been shown to arrest cancer growth and sensitize tumors to chemotherapy [1–23], due to an S/G_2 cell-cycle block [24–27]. In Sato lung carcinoma-bearing rats, the MET concentration in the tumor tissue was significantly

Robert M. Hoffman (ed.), *Methionine Dependence of Cancer and Aging: Methods and Protocols*, Methods in Molecular Biology, vol. 1866, https://doi.org/10.1007/978-1-4939-8796-2_9, © Springer Science+Business Media, LLC, part of Springer Nature 2019

reduced by MR total parenteral nutrition (TPN) compared to a MET-infused control group [7, 13].

A randomized prospective clinical trial demonstrated MR TPN with 5-fluorouracil (5-FU) (AO-90) had more antitumor efficacy on gastric cancer patients undergoing tumor resection compared to MET-containing TPN with 5-FU, based on histopathological examination of the resected materials [13].

Chloroethylnitrosoureas (CENUs), such as carmustine (BCNU), fotemustine, nimustine (ACNU), and cystemustine, are used with limited efficacy in metastatic malignant melanoma and in recurrent glioma [28–32].

Mouse studies have tested the combination of MR and CENUs demonstrating that MR significantly improved the therapeutic index of CENUs [8, 16, 33, 34]. The combination of MR and CENU treatment increased sensitivity to BCNU and cystemustine in human brain tumor xenografts in athymic nude mice and in B16 melanoma tumors grafted in syngeneic mice [16, 34].

The synergistic effect of the combination of MR and nitrosourea treatment in cancer patients was first determined in a Phase I clinical trial of dietary MR combined with cystemustine in patients with metastatic melanoma or recurrent glioma, in order to determine the optimal duration of the MR diet. Optimal plasma MET depletion (41%) was obtained on the first day of the diet [35]. Then in a Phase II trial a 1-day dietary MR combined with cystemustine therapy was carried out with efficacy [28].

A Phase I clinical trial consisted of dietary MR alone for adults with advanced solid tumors. All patients on the trial were maintained on an enteral diet. Enteral MR for several weeks was safe and reduced plasma MET levels [36].

Since MR can individually potentiate the different chemotherapeutic agents used in the FOLFOX regimen, a clinical trial combining dietary MR with the FOLFOX regimen in patients with metastatic colorectal cancer was carried out with efficacy [37].

2 Materials

1. The AO-90 (MR TPN) group consisted of four males and three females, aged from 55 to 78 (average 67.1), all with gastric cancer; three were stage IV and four were stage III. The control group included six males and one female, aged 49 to 75 (average 62.4); five all with gastric cancer were stage IV and 2 were stage III [13].
2. Proteamine 12X (Tanabe Pharmaceutical Co., Ltd., Tokyo).

3. Paraffin.
4. Hematoxylin and eosin.
5. Alcian blue.
6. XMET Maxamum (SHS, Liverpool, UK).
7. Hominex-2 Amino Acid-Modified Medical Food (Ross Products Division, Abbott Laboratories, Columbus, OH).
8. FOLFOX6 consisting of oxaliplatinum (100 mg/m^2), leucovorin (DL racemic mixture, 400 mg/m^2), and 5-fluorouracil (5-FU) (2400 mg/m^2) [37].
9. P680 HPLC pump, ASI-100 automated sample injector (Dionex, Voisin-Le-Bretonneux, France) with post-column ninhydrin derivatization, model PCX5200 (Pickering Laboratories, Mountain View, CA, USA), or equivalent.

3 Methods

3.1 AO-90 TPN Clinical Trial

3.1.1 Protocol for Preoperative TPN Treatment

1. Administer TPN intravenously with 5-FU at a daily dose of 500 mg/body for 24 consecutive hours (total 4.0 g/body) from 7 days before tumor resection until completion of gastrectomy.
2. Administer MR AO-90 as a sole nitrogen source with glucose, lipid, electrolytes, vitamins, and minerals.
3. Administer Proteamine 12X, an amino acid solution containing L-MET and other nutrients, to the control group [13].
4. Restrict all patients from eating in order to prevent protein intake during the TPN treatment [13].

3.1.2 Histopathological Examination of Resected Tumors

1. Cut sections approximately 5 mm wide from the center of the cancer, including adjacent gastric wall with no cancer invasion, and fix with 10% formalin.
2. Embed these sections in paraffin and slice to about 4 μm thick.
3. Perform hematoxylin and eosin (H&E) staining and Alcian blue and PAS double staining [13].
4. Conduct histological examination of cancer tissue to evaluate the therapeutic response according to the following histological criteria:

   Grade 0: No effect; almost no treatment-induced tumor degeneration or necrosis is seen.

   Grade 1: Slight effect; (a) very slight effect; degeneration or necrosis affects <1/3 of the cancer cells. (b) Slight effect; degeneration, necrosis, or liquefaction of 1/3–2/3 of the cancer cells.

Grade 2: Moderate effect; marked degeneration, necrosis, liquefaction, or disappearance of more than two-thirds of the cancer cells.

Grade 3: Marked effect; the entire tumor is necrotic or liquefied, has disappeared, or has been replaced by granulation tissue or fibrosis [13].

5. Use the Mann-Whitney U-tests for statistical analysis of histological response [13].

3.1.3 MR Diet Combined with Cystemustine Clinical Trial

1. Enroll patients presenting with histological proof of metastatic melanoma or recurrent high-grade glioma [28].
2. Administer patients four cycles of cystemustine every 2 weeks as conventionally used [4, 16, 17] combined with a MR diet for at least five cycles.
3. At each cycle, during the hospitalization period, feed patients a standard diet on the first day and the MR diet on the following day.
4. Administer cystemustine at noon on the day the MR diet is consumed [28].
5. Administer cystemustine *i.v.* at 60 mg/m^2, infused for 15 min in 100 mL 5% dextrose [28].
6. Mix the XMET Maxamum and soluble DUOCAL which contains no MET to meet the energy and nitrogen requirements of a 70 kg man with a total energy intake of 2510 kcal/day and 1 g of protein/kg body weight per day.
7. Advise the patients to eat the MR diet throughout the day [28].
8. Monitor patient compliance with the MR diet by calculating the percentage of the MR diet that was ingested, versus the MET-free diet administered (theoretical intake).
9. Weigh the patients and calculate the body mass index (BMI) [weight (kg)/height (m^2)].
10. Assess disease response by CT scans or MRI after four cycles.
11. For plasma MET concentration determination, collect blood samples in heparinized tubes every day at 8 a.m. (just before the first meal) and at noon (4 h after the start of the MR diet).
12. Deproteinize all samples immediately using sulfosalicylic acid (50 mg/mL plasma).
13. After centrifugation (4 °C, 3500 rpm, 10 min), store the supernatants at −80 °C until analysis.
14. Quantify the plasma MET concentrations in the supernatant by ion-exchange chromatography using high-performance liquid chromatography with a coefficient of variation of the internal standard within and between runs of <5% [28].

3.1.4 MR Diet Alone

1. Enter patients with histological or cytological proof of metastatic cancer who were refractory to standard therapy or had a cancer with no standard therapy [36].
2. Before therapy, evaluate plasma amino acid profile, total plasma homocysteine (HCY), complete blood count, platelet count, sodium, potassium, chloride, carbon dioxide, blood urea nitrogen, creatinine, glucose, calcium, protein, albumin, phosphorus, uric acid, serum aspartate aminotransferase, serum alanine aminotransferase, bilirubin, lactate dehydrogenase, alkaline phosphatase, lipoprotein panel, prothrombin time, and partial thromboplastin time.
3. Repeat serum chemistries and blood counts every 2 weeks.
4. Repeat calcium and lipoprotein panel every 8 weeks [36].

3.1.5 Measurement of Plasma Amino Acids

1. Perform plasma amino acid analysis using a Dionix high-performance liquid chromatograph with post-column ninhydrin detection.
2. Determine total plasma HCY by electrospray tandem mass spectroscopy.
3. Measure the plasma amino acid profile and total plasma HCY levels twice per week for the first 2 weeks and every other week thereafter [36].

3.1.6 Administration of MR Diets

1. Place patients on the Hominex-2 Amino Acid-Modified Medical Food, which is approved for treatment of patients with homocystinuria. Hominex-2 contains essentially no MET.
2. Serve Hominex-2 as the primary dietary protein source for all patients [36].
3. Place the first four patients on a modular diet designed to provide 2 mg of methionine and ~25 kcal per kilogram per day, consisting of low-protein cereals, grains, and breads; fruits; vegetables; margarines and oils; and simple carbohydrates (sodas, hard candies, sugars, and drink mixes).
4. During this period, mix Hominex-2 with water and/or low-protein broth in an effort to maximize the amount of food that patients could consume [36].
5. Modify the diet so that Hominex-2 is served as the primary source of protein and energy.
6. Formulate the Hominex-2 mixtures using powdered, citrus-flavor drink mixes, protein-free bouillon, tomato juice, sucrose, and canola oil.

7. Formulate the Hominex-2 "shakes" on the basis of the energy requirements of each patient. Allow the patient 4–5 shakes per day to meet 100% of their protein requirements (0.8 g protein/kg) and ~75% of their energy requirements.
8. Use regular food to provide up to 2 mg MET/kg/day as well as the remaining energy needs [36].

3.1.7 FOLFOX Combined with MR Diet

1. Enroll patients with histologically proven adenocarcinoma of the colon or rectum [37].
2. Give patients the MR diet from 8.00 a.m. on D1 to noon on D3 and the FOLFOX chemotherapy regimen during 48 h from 12.00 a.m. on D1 to 12 a.m. on D3 [37].

4 Results

4.1 AO-90 TPN Study

None of the 14 patients showed any major complication, such as marked myelosuppression, hypoproteinemia, liver dysfunction, or anastomotic leakage, due to preoperative TPN treatment. The MR TPN increased the anti-tumor efficacy of 5-FU and other chemotherapy drugs [11–13] (*see* **Notes 1–6**).

4.2 Clinical Parameters of MR Diets

Durando et al. first demonstrated that an MR diet was able to reduce plasma MET levels 41% (after feeding) from the first day of the MET-free diet and found no effect of extending the MET-free diet period to 2, 3, or 4 days [35].

Patients consumed 78% of the MET-free diet at 2300 kcal/day. Body weight remained normal and stable. Plasma albumin levels were normal and unchanged comparing before and after treatment. Thrombocytopenia, leukopenia, and neutropenia were the main toxicities. Seventeen patients were evaluable for response after the fourth cycle using CT scans or MRI. Three patients showed a disease stabilization of 3.4-, 7-, and 29.4-month duration, respectively. Four patients died because of disease progression. One patient, not evaluated by medical imaging, was considered as having disease progression after clinical evaluation. The median time to progression of the 22 patients was 1.8 months (range: 0.4–29.4 months) and median overall survival was 4.6 months (range: 0.4–55 months) [28]. During the MET-free diet day, the plasma MET decrease was 53% after 4 h from the start of the MET-free diet from 25 μmol/L at 8 a.m. D1 to 12.5 μmol/L at 12 p.m. [28].

4.3 MR Diet Clinical Trial

4.3.1 Macronutrient Intake: Energy Intake Increased During the Clinical Trial

MET intake fell from a mean of 21 mg/kg/day to 2 mg/kg/day on the MR diet. Mean plasma MET levels decreased from 22 to 9 μM within 2 weeks, a 58% decrease. Total plasma HCY levels trended downward (Fig. 1). All patients lost 0.5 kg per week at a constant rate throughout the study. This study was the first to show that MR via an enteral diet for several weeks is safe and feasible in adults with advanced solid tumors [36].

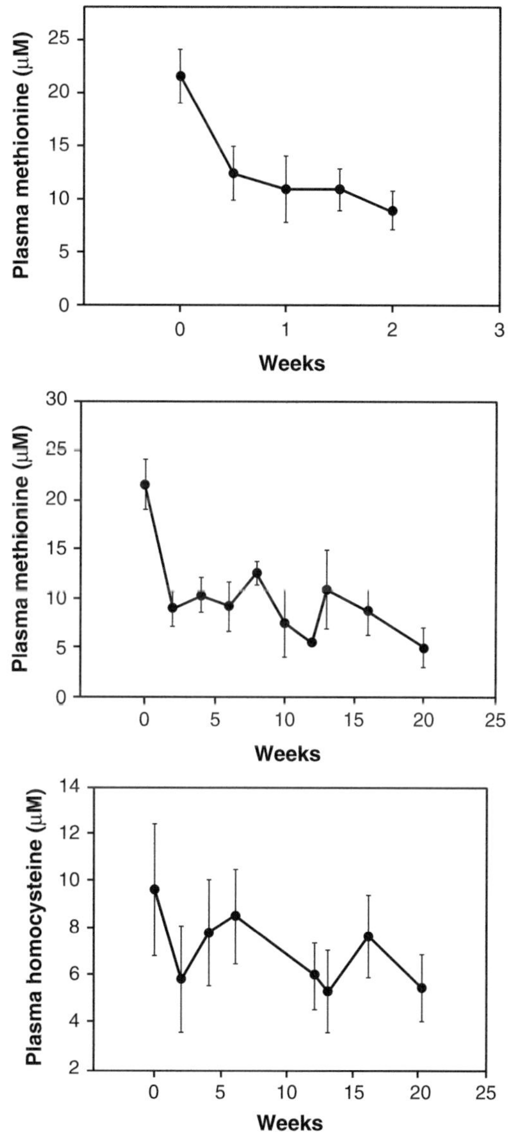

Fig. 1 Plasma amino acid levels for patients with metastatic cancer on a Phase I clinical trial of dietary MR. Top: Plasma MET levels during weeks 1 and 2. Level at week 2 was significantly different ($P = 0.005$) from baseline; levels at other time points were not. Middle panel, effect of MR diet on plasma MET over 20 weeks; lower panel, effect of MR chief on plasma HCY over 20 weeks [36]

4.3.2 MET-Free Diet Combined with FOLFOX

Eleven patients were enrolled in this study. These patients received a median number of three cycles of treatment (range 1–9 cycles). Patients consumed 92.5% of the MR diet administered at 2346 kcal/day. Plasma MET concentrations declined rapidly after the start of the MR diet. A plasma MET depletion of 58% on day 1 of the MR diet was observed (27 μm/L at 8 a.m. on day 1 vs. 11 μm/L at 12 p.m. on day 1). On D3, a plasma MET decrease of 43.3 ± 13.9% was observed (26.8 ± 8.8 μmol/L at 8 a.m. D3 vs. 14.3 ± 4.7 μmol/L at 12 p.m. D3) [37]. Patient body weight was stable during the 2-month treatment period. Plasma albumin remained normal [37]. Toxicity was grade 3 neutropenia occurring in one patient without fever. Non-hematological toxicity remained limited. Grade 2 sensory neuropathy occurred in four patients and required a dose reduction of oxaliplatinum. The other grade 2 toxicities which were observed were asthenia, diarrhea, nausea, anemia, constipation, mucositis, and leukopenia. The main reason for stopping treatment was that the diet was not palatable (10 of 11 enrolled patients) [37].

5 Notes

1. It was safely possible to decrease the level of MET in plasma, liver, and tumor tissue in vivo by infusing an amino acid mixture lacking MET and L-cysteine (CYS) for total parenteral nutrition (MR TPN), resulting in suppression of tumor growth in tumor-bearing animals [5, 7, 38].
2. MR TPN enhanced the effect of several anticancer agents [3, 4, 6, 8–10].
3. In clinical trials in gastrointestinal cancers including Phase I, early Phase II, and late Phase II, MET-depleting TPN combined with 5-FU had a significant antitumor effect in advanced gastric cancer [1, 2, 6, 11, 12]. A multicenter late Phase II randomized trial in 138 advanced gastric cancers demonstrated that MR for 14 days with 5-FU and mitomycin C showed a higher therapeutic response (26.3%) than was obtained in the control group given conventional MET-containing TPN with 5-FU and mitomycin C (8.1%); the difference was significant [12].
4. Preoperative MR TPN for 8 days with a small dose of 5-FU (4.0 g/body in total) significantly degenerated the cancer tissue with a high frequency in the AO-90 group, confirmed pathologically on the resected tumor tissue. It was reported that the histological response to chemotherapy or radiotherapy in gastrointestinal cancer tissues was greatest 2–3 weeks after completion of the treatment [39].

5. Some gastric cancer patients who received preoperative MR TPN treatment with 5-FU for more than 14 days showed a significant therapeutic response, such as complete regression of the cancer, grade 3 response [40].
6. MET-depleting TPN may act as a modulator for 5-FU [10].

References

1. Goseki N, Mori S, Habu H, Menjyo M, Murakami T (1980) Effect of intravenous methionine free hyperalimentation combined with anti-cancer drugs (RT-therapy) on adenocarcinoma of gastrointestinal tract. Jpn J Gastroenterol 77:112
2. Goseki N, Onodera T, Mori S, Menjyo M (1987) Clinical study of amino acid imbalance as an adjunct to cancer therapy. J Jpn Soc Cancer Ther 17:1908–1916
3. Goseki N, Onodera T, Kosaki G, Tsuruta K, Mori S, Tsukada K (1984) Methionine and cysteine free amino acid imbalance by total parenteral nutrition as an adjunct to cancer chemotherapy. In: Ogoshi S, Okada A (eds) Parenteral and enteral hyperalimentation. Elsevier, Amsterdam, pp 343–355
4. Goseki N, Onodera T, Tominaga T, Kosaki G, Koike M. (1985) Inhibitory effect of methionine deprived total parenteral nutrition combines with acinomycin-D on rat experimental tumors. Proc 14th Int Congr Chemother, 438–439
5. Goseki N, Onodera T, Koike M, Kosaki G (1987) Inhibitory effect of L-methionine deprived amino acid imbalance using total parenteral nutrition on growth of ascites hepatoma in rats. Tohoku J Exp Med 151:191–200
6. Goseki N, Yamazaki S, Toyoda T, Endo M, Tsukada K, Onodera T, Kosaki G, Koike M, Satou H (1987) Cancer therapy by methionine deprived total parenteral nutrition with mitomycin C and/or 5-fluorouracil. Oncologia 20:99–110
7. Goseki N, Endo M, Onodera T, Kosaki G (1989) Influence of L-methionine-deprived total parenteral nutrition on the tumor and plasma amino acids fraction and host metabolism. Tohoku J Exp Med 157:251–260
8. Goseki N, Endo M (1990) Thiol depletion and chemosensitization on nimustine hydrochloride by methionine-deprived total parenteral nutrition – experimental studies on Sato lung carcinoma bearing rats. Tohoku J Exp Med 161:227–239
9. Goseki N, Endo M, Onodera T, Kosaki G (1991) Antitumor effect of methionine-deprived total parenteral nutrition with 5-fluorouracil administration on Yoshida sarcoma-bearing rats. Ann Surg 213:83–88
10. Goseki N, Yamazaki S, Endo M, Onodera T, Kosaki G, Hibino Y, Kuwahata T (1982) Antitumor effect of methionine-depleting total parenteral nutrition with doxorubicin administration on Yoshida sarcoma-bearing rats. Cancer 69:1865–1872
11. Sugihara K, Goseki N, Yamazaki S, Endo M, Onodera T, Kosaki G, Mori S, Taguchi T, Kurihara M (1990) Early phase II study of the combined use of AO-90 methionine-free amino acid solution and anticancer agents (5-FU and MMC) in patients with advanced and recurrent gastrointestinal cancer. Jpn J Cancer Chemother 17:2405–2413
12. Taguchi T, Kosaki G, Onodera T, Endo M, Nakagawara Y, Kano K Kaibara N, Kakegawa T, Nakano S, Kurihara M, Akazawa S, Oota J, Kitamura M, Goseki N, Tokunaga K (1995) A controlled study of AO-90, a methionine-free amino acid solution, in advanced gastric cancer patients (surgery group evaluation). Jpn J Cancer Chemother in combination with 5-fluorouracil and mitomycin C. 22:753–764 (in Japanese with English abstract)
13. Goseki N, Yamazaki S, Shimojyu K, Kando F, Maruyama M, Endo M, Koike M, Takahashi H (1995) Synergistic effect of methionine-depleting total parenteral nutrition with 5-fluorouracil on human gastric cancer: a randomized, prospective clinical trial. Jpn J Cancer Res 86:484–489
14. Yoshioka T, Wada T, Uchida N, Maki H, Yoshida H, Ide N, Kasai H, Hojo K, Shono K, Maekawa R, Yagi S, Hoffman RM, Sugita K (1998) Anticancer efficacy *in vivo* and in vitro, synergy with 5-fluorouracil, and safety of recombinant methioninase. Cancer Res 58:2583–2587
15. Tan Y, Sun X, Xu M, Tan X-Z, Sasson A, Rashidi B, Han Q, Tan X-Y, Wang X, An Z, Sun F-X, Hoffman RM (1999) Efficacy of recombinant methioninase in combination with cisplatin on human colon tumors in nude mice. Clin Cancer Res 5:2157–2163

16. Kokkinakis DM, Hoffman RM, Frenkel EP, Wick JB, Han Q, Xu M, Tan Y, Schold SC (2001) Synergy between methionine stress and chemotherapy in the treatment of brain tumor xenografts in athymic mice. Cancer Res 61:4017–4023
17. Murakami T, Li S, Han Q, Tan Y, Kiyuna T, Igarashi K, Kawaguchi K, Hwang HK, Miyaki K, Singh AS, Nelson SD, Dry SM, Li Y, Hiroshima Y, Lwin TM, DeLong JC, Chishima T, Tanaka K, Bouvet M, Endo I, Eilber FC, Hoffman RM (2017) Recombinant methioninase effectively targets a Ewing's sarcoma in a patient-derived orthotopic xenograft (PDOX) nude-mouse model. Oncotarget 8:35630–35638
18. Kawaguchi K, Igarashi K, Li S, Han Q, Tan Y, Kiyuna T, Miyake Y, Murakami T, Chmielowski B, Nelson SD, Russell TA, Dry SM, Li Y, Unno M, Eilber FC, Hoffman RM (2017) Combination treatment with recombinant methioninase enables temozolomide to arrest a BRAF V600E melanoma growth in a patient-derived orthotopic xenograft. Oncotarget 8:85516–85525
19. Kawaguchi K, Igarashi K, Li S, Han Q, Tan Y, Miyake K, Kiyuna T, Miyake M, Murakami T, Chmielowski S, Nelson SD, Russell TA, Dry SM, Li Y, Unno M, Eilber FC, Hoffman RM (2018) Recombinant methioninase (rMETase) is an effective therapeutic for BRAF-V600E-negative as well as -positive melanoma in patient-derived orthotopic xenograft (PDOX) mouse models. Oncotarget 9:915–923
20. Igarashi K, Kawaguchi K, Li S, Han Q, Tan Y, Murakami T, Kiyuna T, Miyake K, Miyake M, Singh AS, Eckhadt MA, Nelson SD, Russell TA, Dry SM, Li Y, Yamamoto N, Hayashi K, Kimura H, Miwa S, Tsuchiya H, Singh RS, Eilber FC, Hoffman RM (2018) Recombinant methioninase in combination with DOX overcomes first-line DOX resistance in a patient-derived orthotopic xenograft nude-mouse model of undifferentiated spindle-cell sarcoma. Cancer Lett 417:168–173
21. Igarashi K, Li S, Han Q, Tan Y, Kawaguchi K, Murakami T, Kiyuna T, Miyake K, Li Y, Nelson SD, Dry SM, Singh AS, Elliott I, Russell TA, Eckhadt MA, Yamamoto N, Hayashi K, Kimura H, Miwa S, Tsuchiya H, Eilber FC, Hoffman RM (2018) Growth of a doxorubicin-resistant undifferentiated spindle-cell sarcoma PDOX is arrested by metabolic targeting with recombinant methioninase. J Cell Biochem 119:3537–3544
22. Kawaguchi K, Han Q, Li S, Tan Y, Igarashi K, Miyake K, Kiyuna T, Miyake M, Chmielowski B, Nelson SD, Russell TA, Dry SM, Li Y, Singh AS, Eckardt MA, Unno M, Eilber FC, Hoffman RM (2018) Intra-tumor L-methionine level highly correlates with tumor size in both pancreatic cancer and melanoma patient-derived orthotopic xenograft (PDOX) nude-mouse models. Oncotarget 9:11119–11125
23. Kawaguchi K, Han Q, Li S, Tan Y, Igarashi K, Kiyuna T, Miyake K, Miyake M, Chmielowski B, Nelson SD, Russell TA, Dry SM, Li Y, Eckhardt MA, Unno M, Eilber FC, Hoffman RM (2018) Targeting methionine with oral recombinant methioninase (o-rMETase) arrests a patient-derived orthotopic xenograft (PDOX) model of BRAF-V600E mutant melanoma: implications for clinical cancer therapy and prevention. Cell Cycle 17:356–361
24. Hoffman RM (2015) Development of recombinant methioninase to target the general cancer-specific metabolic defect of methionine dependence: a 40-year odyssey. Expert Opin Biol Ther 15:21–31
25. Yano S, Li S, Han Q, Tan Y, Bouvet M, Fujiwara T, Hoffman RM (2014) Selective methioninase-induced trap of cancer cells in S/G_2 phase visualized by FUCCI imaging confers chemosensitivity. Oncotarget 5:8729–8736
26. Yano S, Takehara K, Zhao M, Tan Y, Han Q, Li S, Bouvet M, Fujiwara T, Hoffman RM (2016) Tumor-specific cell-cycle decoy by *Salmonella typhimurium* A1-R combined with tumor-selective cell-cycle trap by methioninase overcome tumor intrinsic chemoresistance as visualized by FUCCI imaging. Cell Cycle 15:1715–1723
27. Stern PH, Hoffman RM (1986) Enhanced in vitro selective toxicity of chemotherapeutic agents for human cancer cells based on a metabolic defect. J Natl Cancer Inst 76:629–639
28. Thivat E, Farges MC, Bacin F, D'Incan M, Mouret-Reynier MA, Cellarier E, Madelmont JC, Vasson MP, Chollet P, Durando X (2009) Phase II trial of the association of a methionine-free diet with cystemustine therapy in melanoma and glioma. Anticancer Res 29:5235–5240
29. Jacquillat C, Khayat D, Banzet P, Weil M, Fumoleau P, Avril MF, Namer M, Bonneterre J, Kerbrat P, Bonerandi JJ et al (1990) Final report of the French multicenter phase II study of the nitrosourea fotemustine in 153 evaluable patients with disseminated malignant melanoma including patients with cerebral metastases. Cancer 66:1873–1878
30. Bajetta E, Del Vecchio M, Bernard-Marty C, Vitali M, Buzzoni R, Rixe O, Nova P,

Aglione S, Taillibert S, Khayat D (2002) Metastatic melanoma: chemotherapy. Semin Oncol 29:427–445
31. Galanis E, Buckner JC (2000) Chemotherapy of brain tumors. Curr Opin Neurol 13:619–625
32. Thivat E, Durando X, D'Incan M, Cure H, Mouret-Reynier MA, Madelmont JC, Souteyrand P, Chollet P (2005) Second-line chemotherapy of disseminated malignant melanoma with cystemustine at 60 mg/m^2: a phase II trial. Anticancer Drugs 16:1003–1007
33. Poirson-Bichat F, Goncalves RA, Miccoli L, Dutrillaux B, Poupon MF (2000) Methionine depletion enhances the antitumoral efficacy of cytotoxic agents in drug-resistant human tumor xenografts. Clin Cancer Res 6:643–653
34. Morvan D, Papon J, Madelmont JC, Demidem A (2002) Methionine deprivation potentiates the effect of cystemustine treatment on B16 melanoma tumor in syngenic recipients. AACR Proc 2002:3822
35. Durando X, Thivat E, Farges MC, Cellarier E, D'Incan M, Demidem A, Vasson MP, Barthomeuf C, Chollet P (2008) Optimal methionine-free diet duration for nitrosourea treatment: a phase I clinical trial. Nutr Cancer 60:23–30
36. Epner DE, Morrow S, Wilcox M, Houghton JL (2002) Nutrient intake and nutritional indexes in adults with metastatic cancer on a phase I clinical trial of dietary methionine restriction. Nutr Cancer 42:158–166
37. Durando X, Farges MC, Buc E, Abrial C, Petorin-Lesens C, Gillet B, Vasson MP, Pezet D, Chollet P, Thivat E (2010) Dietary methionine restriction with FOLFOX regimen as first line therapy of metastatic colorectal cancer: a feasibility study. Oncology 78:205–209
38. Kreis W (1979) Tumor therapy by depriving of l-methionine: rationale and results. Cancer Treat Rep 63:1069–1072
39. Shimozato Y, Oboshi S, Baba E (1971) Histopathological evaluation of effects of radiotherapy and chemotherapy for carcinomas. Jpn J Clin Oncol 1:19–35
40. Wada Y, Kando F, Shimojyu K, Aoi C, Goseki N, Okabe S, Sunagawa M, Endo M (1993) Effects of pre-operative methionine-depleting total parenteral nutrition (RT-therapy) on gastric carcinoma — pathological study in two gastrectomized cases. J Jpn Soc Cancer Ther 28:429

Chapter 10

Development of Recombinant Methioninase for Cancer Treatment

Robert M. Hoffman, Yuying Tan, Shukuan Li, Qinghong Han, Shigeo Yagi, Tomoaki Takakura, Akio Takimoto, Kenji Inagaki, and Daizou Kudou

Abstract

The elevated requirement for methionine (MET) of cancer cells is termed MET dependence. To selectively target the MET dependence of tumors for treatment on a large-scale preclinical and clinical basis, the L-methionine α-deamino-γ-mercaptomethane-lyase (EC 4.4.1.11) (methioninase, [METase]) gene from *Pseudomonas putida* has been cloned in *Escherichia coli* using the polymerase chain reaction (PCR). Purification using two DEAE Sepharose FF ion-exchange column and one ActiClean Etox endotoxin-affinity chromatography column has been established. Plasmid pMGLTrc03, which has a *trc* promoter and a spacing of 12 nucleotides between the Shine-Dalgarno sequence and the ATG translation initiation codon, was selected as the most suitable plasmid. The recombinant bacteria produced rMETase at 43% of the total proteins in soluble fraction by simple batch fermentation using a 500 L fermentor. Crystals were directly obtained from crude enzyme with 87% yield by a crystallization in the presence of 9.0% polyethylene glycol 6000, 3.6% ammonium sulfate, and 0.18 M sodium chloride using a 100 L crystallizer. After recrystallization, the enzyme was purified by anion exchange column chromatography to remove endotoxins and by gel filtration for polishing. Purified rMETase is stable to lyophilization. In order to prevent immunological reactions which might be produced by multiple dosing of rMETase and to prolong the serum half-life of rMETase, the *N*-hydroxysuccinimidyl ester of methoxypolyethylene glycol propionic acid (M-SPA-PEG 5000) has been coupled to rMETase. The PEGylated molecules (PEG-rMETase) were purified from unreacted PEG with Amicon 30 K centriprep concentrators or by Sephacryl S-300 HR gel-filtration chromatography. Unreacted rMETase was removed by DEAE Sepharose FF anion-exchange chromatography. The resulting PEG-rMETase subunit, produced from a PEG/rMETase ratio of 30/1 in the synthetic reaction, had a molecular mass of approximately 53 kda determined by matrix-assisted laser desorption/ionization mass spectrometry, indicating the conjugation of two PEG molecules per subunit of rMETase and eight per tetramer. PEG-rMETase molecules obtained from reacting ratios of PEG/rMETase of 30/1 had an enzyme activity of 70% of unmodified rMETase. PEGylation of rMETase increased the serum half-life of the enzyme in rats to approximately 160 min compared to 80 min for unmodified rMETase. PEG-rMETase could deplete serum MET levels to less than 0.1 μM for approximately 8 h compared to 2 h for rMETase in rats. A significant prolongation of in vivo activity and effective MET depletion by the PEG-rMETase were achieved by the simultaneous administration of pyridoxal 5′-phosphate. rMETase was also conjugated with methoxypolyethylene glycol succinimidyl glutarate 5000 (MEGC-PEG). Miniosmotic pumps containing various concentrations of PLP were implanted in BALB-C mice. PLP-infused mice were then injected with a single dose of 4000 or 8000 units/kg PEG-rMETase. Mice infused with 5, 50, 100, 200, and 500 mg/mL PLP-containing miniosmotic pumps increased plasma PLP to 7, 24, 34, 60,

Robert M. Hoffman (ed.), *Methionine Dependence of Cancer and Aging: Methods and Protocols*, Methods in Molecular Biology, vol. 1866, https://doi.org/10.1007/978-1-4939-8796-2_10,

and 95 μM, respectively, from the PLP baseline of 0.3 μM. PLP increased the half-life of MEGC-PEG-rMETase holoenzyme in a dose-dependent manner. The extended time of MET depletion by MEGC-PEG-rMETase was due to the maintenance of active MEGC-PEG-rMETase holoenzyme by infused PLP.

Key words Cancer, Methionine dependence, L-Methionine α-deamino, α-mercaptomethane lyase [EC4.4.1.11], Methioninase, Recombinant methioninase, rMETase, Polyethylene glycol, PEG, Methoxypolyethylene glycol, Succinimide glutarate, MEGC-PEG, Pyridoxal-L-phosphate, Methionine restriction, Anticancer efficacy, Industrial purification, Crystallization, 3-Dimensional structure

1 Introduction

Methionine (MET) is a promising metabolic target for cancer therapy, since cancer cells have an elevated requirement for MET, termed MET dependence. A MET-cleaving enzyme would lower methionine levels more than MET starvation and thereby could have more cancer therapeutic efficacy [1, 2]. For this purpose, Kreis and Hession [1] attempted to purify a methioninase (METase) from *Clostridium sporogenes.* This enzyme had a molecular weight of approximately 150 kDa. The enzyme slowed the growth of the Walker 256 carcinoma in rats more than a MET-restricted (MR) diet did. However, the enzyme preparation was highly unstable; its yield was only 2%, and it had a high K_m of 90 mM. The *C. sporogenes* enzyme therefore did not have the properties to be developed into a clinical therapeutic [1].

Ito et al. purified a METase from *Pseudomonas putida* [3]. This enzyme had a molecular weight of approximately 170 kDa and catalyzed the α, γ-elimination of MET to α-ketobutyrate, methanethiol, and ammonia in the presence of pyridoxal 5′-phosphate. Simultaneously, Nakayama isolated a METase from *Pseudomonas ovalis* [4, 5]. This group's later results showed that METase from *P. putida* comprised four identical subunits of molecular weight 43 kDa, and this enzyme had a K_m of approximately 1 mM MET [6]. Endotoxin was not removed from these rMETase preparations, precluding the METase from being a useful therapeutic.

The gene encoding METase in *P. putida* was cloned and was expressed at relatively low levels in *Escherichia coli* by Inoue et al. [7]. Hori et al. also reported the cloning of a gene from *P. putida* that they termed L-methionine-γ-deamino-α-mercaptomethane-lyase [8].

Toward the goal of developing METase into an effective antitumor therapeutic, we cloned and overexpressed the *P. putida* METase gene in *E. coli.* A protocol for high-yield, large-scale purification of recombinant METase (rMETase) was developed. The rMETase thus produced had in vitro efficacy against all of a wide variety of human tumor cell lines, but in contrast not against normal cell strains and had in vivo efficacy against human tumors in nude mice with negligible toxicity [2].

An industrial production process for recombinant methioninase was established by using an overexpression plasmid in *Escherichia coli*, large-scale cultivation, and bulk crystallization. The plasmid was optimized with a promoter and the ribosome-binding site [9].

Polyethylene glycol (PEG) conjugation of methioninase resulted in readily-purified molecules, maintained the potency of the enzyme, extended its serum half-life, reduced antigenicity, and maintained its tumor-specific efficacy [10].

rMETase has only 9 lysine residues of 398 amino acids per monomer, far lower than the normal frequency of this amino acid occurring in most proteins. In contrast, there are 37 carboxyl groups in each subunit of rMETase that can be used to couple DAB to add PEGylation sites. We designed a new strategy that can overcome the cross-linking limit to increase the extent of PEGylation of rMETase [11].

We demonstrated the dose-dependent efficacy of infused pyridoxal-L-phosphate (PLP) to significantly increase the serum half-life of the active holozyme form of PEG-rMETase and the period of maintenance of serum MET depletion in mice, suggesting the clinical potential of the combination of MEGC-PEG-rMETase and PLP treatment [12].

2 Materials

1. Restriction endonucleases.
2. T4 DNA ligase.
3. BL21(DE3) competent cells (Stratagene, San Diego, CA).
4. *GeneAmp* PCR reagent kit (Riche, Branchburg, NJ).
5. DNA purification kit (Promega, Madison, WI).
6. pT7 Blue T vector (Novagen, Madison, WI).
7. Oligonucleotide probes for PCR amplification were synthesized by IDT Inc. (Coralville, IA).
8. *Pseudomonas putida* (ATCC, Rockville, MD) [2].
9. DEAE sepharose FF (Pharmacia, Uppsala, Sweden).
10. ActiClean ETOX (Sterogen, Arcadia, CA).
11. Amicon Centriprep (Amicon, Lexington, MA).
12. Mylon Filter (Nalgene).
13. Lyophilizer (Vertis).
14. L-6200A intelligent pump (Hitachi Ltd., Tokyo, Japan).
15. Progel TSK Column (Supelco, Bellefonte, PA).
16. U2000 spectrophotometer (Hitachi).
17. Bovine serum albumin (Sigma, St. Louis, MO).

18. Sweet potato β amylase (Sigma).
19. Kaleidoscope molecular weight standards (Bio-Rad, Hercules, CA).
20. Centrifuge (Eppendorf).
21. Lowry protein reagent (Sigma).
22. LAL endotoxin test CRio Whittaker (Walkersville, MA).
23. M-SPA-PEG 5000 (NOF Corp., Tokyo, Japan).
24. Sephacryl S-300 and S-200 column (Pharmacia).
25. Cosmosil SC18-AR-II column (Niculai Tesque, Japan).
26. Osmotic pump (Durect Corp, Cupertino, CA).
27. pMOSblue T-vector (American Biosciences, Piscataway, NJ).
28. Isopropyl-β-D-thiogalactopyranoside (IPTG) (Sigma).
29. Glass-bead homogenizer (MiniBeadbeater; Biospec Products, Bartlesville, OK).
30. 30 liter and 500 liter fermenters (Marubishi, Tokyo, Japan).
31. Tangential flow filtration system (Millipore, Billerica, MA).
32. High-pressure mechanical homogenizer (Invensys Systems APV, Albertslund, Denmark).
33. Flow filtration system (Millistak, Millipore).
34. Continuous-tube centrifuge (Tomoe Engineering, Tokyo, Japan).
35. Crystallizer (100 L) (Kido, Kyogo, Japan).
36. Microfiltration membranes (Sartorius, Goettingen, Germany).
37. Ultrafiltration Membrane (Millipore).

3 Methods

3.1 Cloning of the *Pseudomonas putida* Methioninase Gene

The segment coding for the METase gene:

1. Amplify the METase gene using the PCR technique and *P. putida* DNA [2].
2. Use genomic DNA of *P. putida*, isolated by standard procedures as a template for the PCR reaction.
3. Synthesize oligonucleotide primers on the basis of the nucleic sequence of the L-METase gene determined by Inoue et al. [7].
4. Use the primers t1, 5′GCCGGTCTGTGGAATAAGCT-3′ (sense), and t2, 5′CCAGGGTCGACTCCAGCGCC-3′ (antisense) [2].
5. Use PCR reaction conditions as follows: first denaturation at 95 °C for 10 min; then five cycles of denaturation at 94 °C for 30 s; annealing at 60 °C for 30 s; and extension at 72 °C for 2 min. Follow by 25 cycles of denaturation at 94 °C for 30 s;

60 °C for 30 s; then extension at 72 °C for 1.5 min; then a final extension at 72 °C for 10 min [2].

6. Collect products consisting of two bands identified by λDNA/*Eco*RI + HindIII markers.
7. Purify and separate the PCR1365 bp band product, sequence, and confirm that it is the METase gene by sequencing.
8. Ligate the sequenced METase gene into the pT7Blue T-vector (Novagen) at the *Eco*RV T-cloning site [9].
9. Transfect this plasmid into *E. coli* DH5-α using standard procedures [2].
10. To construct an overexpression vector, use [10] the following primers for the PCR reaction: t14, 5′-GGAATTCCATATGC ACGGCTCCAACAAGC-3′ (sense), and t18, 5′-AGTCATGG ATCCTCAGGCACTCGCCTTGAGTGC-3′ (antisense).
11. Use the following PCR reaction conditions: first denaturation at 95 °C for 10 min; then five cycles of denaturation at 94 °C for 1 min; annealing at 56 °C for 1.5 min; and extension at 72 °C for 2 min. Follow by 20 cycles of denaturation at 94 °C for 30 s; 56 °C for 30 s; then extension at 72 °C for 1.5 min; then final extension at 72 °C for 10 min. Collect and purify the PCR amplified product (1220 bp), which contains the METase gene with sites modified for the *Nde* I and *Bam*H I restriction enzymes [2].
12. Digest the plasmid with the *Nde* I and *Bam*H I restriction enzymes and ligate into the PT7-7 vector at the *Nde* I and BamH I cloning sites using standard protocols.
13. Transform the resulting plasmid into *E. coli* BL21 (DE3) competent cells according to the instruction manual (Stratagene) [13].
14. Select positive clones from ampicillin-containing plates by their distinct yellow-orange color due to high enrichment of the pyridoxal phosphate-containing rMETase.
15. Select one overexpression clone and term it the pAC-1 clone [2].
16. Grow the cells from the selected colony in 5 mL LB medium at 37 °C overnight. Transfer 2×10^5 ml to a flask with 100 mL LB medium. Grow this culture at 37 °C for 8 h. Aliquot the bacteria into twenty 2 mL vials with 15% glycerol, and store at −80 °C as the Cell Bank [2].

3.2 Fermentation

1. Start every production fermentation with one vial from the Cell Bank.
2. Seed 10 mL of bacteria from the Cell Bank into 5 mL LB medium with 100 μg ampicillin and grow at 37 °C at 400 rpm overnight.

3. Transfer this culture to 800 ml terrific broth (TB) in 6 L flasks and grow overnight at 37 °C at 400 rpm at which time the OD_{600} is approximately 10.
4. Transfer the 800 ml cultures into 10,800 ml TB medium cultures in 6 L flasks and grow at 37 °C at 400 rpm for 16 h at which time the OD_{600} is approximately 10.
5. Change the medium with fresh TB and the incubate for another 6 h.
6. When the OD_{600} reaches 20, harvest the bacteria by centrifugation at 400 × *g* at 4 °C for 10 min [2].

3.3 Purification of rMETase

3.3.1 Precolumn Treatment of the Sample

1. Suspend the bacterial pellet in extraction solution (20 mM potassium phosphate, pH 9.0, 10 μM pyridoxal phosphate, and 0.01% β-mercaptoethanol).
2. Disrupt with a cavitator-type homogenizer (Microfluidics Corp., Newton, MA).
3. Treat the homogenate up to 50 °C for 1 min.
4. Centrifuge the suspension with an automatic refrigerated centrifuge (SORVALL, superspeed RC 2-B) at 4 °C at 8000 × *g* for 30 min. Collect the supernatant.
5. Ultrafiltrate with a Millipore (Bedford, MA) Prep/Scale-TFF PLHK 100 k, 2.5 ft^2 cartridge with buffer (10 mM potassium phosphate, pH 8.3) and adjust the pH to 7.2 by ultrafiltration [2].

3.3.2 Chromatographic Conditions

First Column:

6. Use DEAE Sepharose FF (pH 7.2).
7. Use the first column with 100 mm diameter and 30 cm height, with a volume of 2400 mL of DEAE Sepharose FF and elution flow rate of 15–50 mL/min.
8. Apply 40–80 g of total protein (10–20 mg/mL) on the column.
9. After loading, prewash the column with 40 mM potassium chloride in PPM buffer (10 mM potassium phosphate, pH 7.2, containing 10 μm pyridoxal phosphate and 0.01% β-mercaptoethanol) for approximately 10 vol. until the OD_{280} drops below 0.1.
10. Elute the protein with a linear gradient of 40–300 mM potassium chloride in PPM buffer and collect elution fractions of 500 ml. Identify the fractions containing rMETase by yellow color and activity assay [2].

Second Column:

11. Use DEAE Sepharose FF (pH 8.3).
12. Use the second column (XK50/30) with a height of 25 cm and a volume of 500 ml with an elution flow rate of 6–8 ml/min.
13. After 24-h dialysis in 80 mM potassium chloride and 10 mM potassium phosphate (pH 8.3), apply 5–10 g of total protein (2–5 mg/mL) on the second column.
14. After loading, prewash the column with 80 mM potassium chloride and 10 mM potassium phosphate (pH 8.3) for approximately 4 vol. until the OD_{280} drops below 0.1.
15. Elute rMETase with a linear gradient of 80–300 mM potassium chloride in 10 mM potassium phosphate buffer (pH 8.3).
16. Collect elution factions of 300 ml.
17. Identify the fractions containing rMETase by yellow color and activity assay [2].

Third Column:

18. Use ActiClean Etox as the third column to eliminate endotoxin.
19. Apply purified rMETase (10–20 mg protein/mL) in a volume of 200–300 ml on an 800 ml ActiClean Etox column (25 × 60) with a bed height of 40 cm.
20. Elute the protein with elution buffer (0.12 M sodium chloride in 10 mM sodium phosphate, pH 7.2), at a flow rate of 1 mL/min.
21. Identify the collected enzyme fractions by yellow color and activity assay [2].
22. Concentrate the final eluant with 30 K Amicon Centriprep concentrators by centrifugation at 4000 × *g* for 30 min at 4 °C. Sterilize with a 0.2 μm nylon filter (Nalgene) [2].

Formulation of rMETase:

23. Formulate rMETase in a solution consisting of 0.12 M sodium chloride and 10 mM sodium phosphate buffer (pH 7.2), at a concentration of 10–20 mg/ml. Lyophilize rMETase by first freezing on dry ice and acetone and then lyophilize (Freeze mobil 24, Vertis) at −80 °C, under a vacuum of 100 millibar for 72 h [2].

3.3.3 Analysis of rMETase

HPLC:

24. Use an Hitachi L-6200A Intelligent pump with a Supelco Progel-TSK column (G3000 SW_{XL}, 30 cm × 7.8 mm) for all HPLC experiments.

25. Load a sample of 20 μl (0.1–0.5 mg/mL) rMETase and elute (0.12 M sodium chloride in 10 mM sodium phosphate buffer, pH 7.2) at a flow rate of 1.0 ml/min.
26. Identify the protein-containing fractions with a spectrophotometer (Hitachi U2000) at a wavelength of 280 nm. Use bovine serum albumin (MW 66,000) and sweet potato β-amylase (MW 200,000) as MW standards [2].

Electrophoresis:

27. Carry out electrophoresis in 7.5% polyacrylamide-precast plates in 0.2 M Tris–glycine buffer, pH 8.3, both with and without 0.1% SDS. Use Kaleidoscope prestained molecular weight standards (Bio-Rad, Hercules, CA) [2].

Activity Assay:

28. Carry out the rMETase activity assay in a 1 ml vol of 50 mM phosphate buffer, pH 8.0, containing 10 μM pyridoxal phosphate and 10 mM MET for 10 min at 37 °C, with varying amounts of rMETase.
29. Stop the reaction by adding 0.5 ml 4.5% trichloroacetic acid (TCA). Centrifuge the suspension in an Eppendorf centrifuge at 13k rpm for 2 min.
30. Add 0.5 mg supernatant to 0.5 ml 0.05% 3-methyl-2-benzothiazolinone hydrazine in 1 ml 1 M sodium acetate, pH 5.2, and incubate at 50 °C for 30 min.
31. Determine the amount of reaction product by spectrophotometry at OD_{335}. Determine the amount of protein with the Lowry Reagent kit (Sigma) with bovine serum albumin as a standard.
32. Calculate the specific activity as units/mg protein, with one unit of enzyme defined as the amount that catalyzes the formation of 1 μmol of α-ketobutyrate [2].

Endotoxin Assay:

33. Measure the endotoxin level by the limulus amebocyte lysate (LAL) test (BioWhittaker, Walkersville, MD) [2].
34. Mix a sample of rMETase with the LAL and incubate at 37 °C for 10 min. Mix a substrate solution supplied with the kit with the sample and incubate at 37 °C for an additional 6 min [2].
35. Stop the reaction with stop reagent supplied with the kit.
36. Determine the absorbance of the sample with a spectrophotometer (Hitachi, U 2000) at 410 nm.
37. Calculate the concentration of endotoxin from a standard curve constructed from the endotoxin supplied in the kit at concentrations from 0.1 EU/mL to 1 EU/mL [2].

3.4 PEGylation of rMETase

PEG Linkers.

1. Use the M-SPA-PEG 5000 for rMETase PEGylation.

PEGylation Reaction.

2. Dissolve PEG reagents in 20 mM sodium phosphate buffer (pH 8.3) at concentrations between 2 and 20 mM.
3. Vary the molar ratios of PEG to rMETase from 10:1 to 60:1.
4. For each condition, use 0.3–0.5 g rMETase (15 mg/mL).
5. Carry out PEGylation reactions in reaction buffer (20 mM sodium phosphate buffer, pH 8.3), at 20 °C for 30 to 60 min.
6. Stop the reactions with one-tenth volume stop buffer (1 M sodium phosphate buffer, pH 6.5) at 0 °C [14]. Concentrate PEG-rMETase with a Centriprep-30.

Purification of PEG-rMETase

Sephacryl S-300.

7. Remove unreacted PEG by size-exclusion chromatography with a Sephacryl S-300 HR column (HiPrep 26/60, Pharmacia), with a diameter of 26 mm and length of 60 cm [14].
8. Load 10 ml PEGylation products (15 mg/mL) on the column, which is equilibrated, and elute with 0.15 M sodium chloride in 10 mM sodium phosphate (pH 7.4) at a flow rate of 1 mL/min.
9. Elute the fractions containing PEG-rMETase and rMETase at approximately 150–250 mL and identify by activity assay [10].

DEAE Sepharose FF.

10. Separate PEGylated rMETase from un PEGylated rMETase by anion-exchange chromatography using a DEAE Sepharose FF column (XK 16/15, Pharmacia) with a diameter of 16 mm and length of 15 cm [10, 15].
11. Equilibrate the column with equilibration buffer [50 mM sodium chloride in 10 mM sodium phosphate (pH 7.4)].
12. Elute with a 0–60% linear gradient of 300 mM sodium chloride in 10 mM sodium phosphate (pH 7.4) at a 3 mL/min flow rate.
13. Elute the fractions containing PEG-rMETase with approximately 50–80 ml equilibration buffer and identify by activity assay and electrophoresis on SDS-PAGE [10].

Sterilization and Stability of PEG-rMETase.

14. Sterilize the PEG-rMETas by filtration with a 0.2 μM micrometer membrane filter. Store PEG-rMETase at −80 °C for 6 months without loss of activity [10].

Analysis of PEG-rMETase

Electrophoresis.

15. Carry out polyacrylamide gel electrophoresis (PAGE) in 7.5% polyacrylamide-precast plates in 0.2 M Tris–glycine buffer, pH 8.3, both with 0.1% sodium dodecyl sulfate (SDS) (SDS-PAGE) and without SDS (native-PAGE) using Kaleidoscope prestained standards as molecular weight markers which contain myosin (MW 192 k), β-galactosidase (MW 127 k), bovine serum albumin (MW 73 k), carbonic anhydrase (MW 43 k), soybean trypsin inhibitor (MW 32.3 k), lysozyme (MW 17 k), and aprotinin (MW 6.6 k) [2, 10].

Matrix-Assisted Laser Desorption/Ionization Mass Spectrometry

16. Perform matrix-assisted laser desorption/ionization (MALDI) mass spectrometry with a PerSeptive Biosystems Voyager-Elite mass spectrometer with delayed extraction.
17. Irradiate samples with a nitrogen laser (Laser Science, Inc.) operated at 337 nM.
18. Attenuate the laser beam by a variable attenuator and focus on the sample target.
19. Accelerate ions produced in the ion source with a deflection voltage of 30,000 V.
20. Differentiate the ions according to the *m/z* using a time-of-flight mass analyzer [10, 14, 15].

3.5 Determination of Plasma PLP

1. Determine PLP content in plasma by HPLC using derivatization with sodium bisulfite in the mobile phase.
2. Mix the plasma sample and PLP standard solutions with an equal volume of 0.8 M $HClO_4$ as deproteinizing agent, and vortex vigorously.
3. After centrifuging at 15000 rpm for 5 min at 4 °C, transfer the supernatants to new vials. Load 50 μl of the supernatant on a reversed-phase Cosmosil 5C18-AR-II column (4.6 × 150 cm).
4. Elute the column with a gradient elution of 20–80% mobile phase B (30% acetonitrile/water v/v) in mobile phase A (0.1 M potassium dihydrogen phosphate buffer containing 0.1 M sodium perchlorate and 0.5 g/l sodium bisulfite, pH 3.0) at a flow rate of 1.0 mL/min.
5. Use a fluorescence spectrophotometer for detection: excitation at 300 nm and emission at 400 nm.
6. Identify the PLP peak by the retention time of a PLP standard. Calculate the concentration of plasma PLP using a calibration curve [19].

3.6 PLP Infusion

1. Use osmotic pumps with a 200 μl reservoir volume, pumping rate of 1.0 μl/h, and duration of 7 days (Model 2001, Durect Corporation).
2. Dissolve 500 mg of PLP and 150 mg of sodium hydroxide in 1 ml distilled water (pH 7.4).
3. Prepare other concentrations of PLP by dilution.
4. Draw the PLP solution into a 3 ml syringe attached to a blunt-tipped, 27-gauge filling tube of the minipump.
5. For s.c. placement of the pump, make a small incision in the skin between the scapulae.
6. Using a hemostat, form a small pocket by spreading the subcutaneous connective tissues apart. Insert the pump into the pocket with the flow moderator pointing away from the incision. Close the skin incision with sutures [12].

3.7 Determination of MEGC-PEG-rMETase Apoenzyme

1. Determine MEGC-PEG-rMETase apoenzyme, in the presence of PLP, as described above.

3.8 Determination of MEGC-PEG-rMETase Holoenzyme Activity

1. Determine plasma MEGC-PEG-rMETase holoenzyme activity, with no PLP added in the substrate solution and assay as described above.

3.9 Industrial Production of rMETase

3.9.1 Bacterial Strain and Plasmid Construction

1. Use *E. coli* JM109 as the host strain for expression of recombinant METase. Construct plasmid pATG3131 as an ATG vector carrying the *trc* promoter by replacing the *Eco*RI-*Xba*I fragment of pCAH4312, with the *Sma*I-*Xba*I fragment including the *trc* promoter.
2. Amplify the METase gene from *P. putida* ICR3460 with PCR using pMGL1204 [9] as a template.
3. Subclone into the pMOS*blue* T-vector to produce the MGL (-ATG)/T-vector.
4. Construct an expression plasmid designated as pMGLTrc03 by replacing the *Eco*RI-*Xba*I fragment of pATG3131 with the *Kpn*I-*Xba*I fragment of the MGL(-ATG)/T-vector [9].

3.9.2 Screening of High-Level Expression Plasmid

1. Cultivate the transformants in 10 mL production culture medium (4.0% glycerol, 2.4% yeast extract, 1.2% peptone, 1.25% K_2HPO_4, 0.23% KH_2PO_4, and 10 μg/mL tetracycline hydrochloride, pH 7.2) containing 0.02% polypropylene glycol #2000 as an antifoam in a test tube, with vigorous shaking at 28 °C [9].
2. Add isopropyl-β-D-thiogalactopyranoside (IPTG) at a final concentration of 0.3 mM after 6-h cultivation [9].

3. After cultivation for 30 h, harvest the bacteria cells by centrifugation (10,000 × *g*, 5 min, 25 °C) [9].
4. To estimate the expression levels of recombinant METase by the transformants, suspend the cells with 100 mM potassium phosphate buffer (pH 8.0) containing 1 mM EDTA, 0.5 mM PLP, 0.5 mg/mL dithiothreitol (DTT), and 0.5 mg/mL Tween 80 [9].
5. Disrupt with an homogenizer with glass beads (Mini-Beadbeater; Biospec Products, Bartlesville, OK, USA) [9] and assay rMETase as described above.

3.10 Large-Scale Cultivation of rMETase-Producing E. coli

3.10.1 First Preculture

1. Cultivate *E. coli* JM109 harboring pMGLTrc03 in 56 mL of a preculture medium (0.5% glycerol, 0.5% yeast extract, 1.0% peptone, 1.0% sodium chloride, and 10 μg/ml tetracycline hydrochloride, pH 7.4) for 7 h at 37 °C in a 500 mL Erlenmeyer flask with vigorous shaking [9].

3.10.2 Second Preculture

1. Transfer the first preculture broth to 21 L of the preculture medium containing 0.01% polypropylene glycol #2000 in a 30 l fermentor (B. E. Marubishi, Tokyo, Japan) [9].
2. Cultivate at 28 °C under agitation at 300 rpm with aeration at a rate of 21 L/min for 16 h [9].

3.10.3 Production Culture

1. Transfer the second preculture broth to 330 L of the production culture medium containing 0.05% polypropylene glycol #2000 in a 500 L fermentor (B. E. Marubishi) [9].
2. Cultivate at 28 °C under agitation at 330 rpm with aeration at a rate of 350 l/min for 24 h [9].
3. Maintain the pH of the culture broth at 7.2 with 28% aqueous ammonia [9].
4. For expression of the recombinant METase, add IPTG at a final concentration of 0.3 mM after 4-h fermentation [9].

3.11 Preparation of Crude Enzyme

1. After fermentation in production culture, harvest the bacteria cells with a tangential flow filtration system with a microfiltration membrane (0.45 μm, Millipore) [9].
5. Concentrate to 50 L as a cell suspension [9].
6. Dilute the cell suspension with 100 mM sodium phosphate buffer (pH 7.6) containing 4.4 mM EDTA, 3.3 mM PLP, and 0.16 mg/mL DTT to a turbidity of 90 at 650 nm (OD_{650}) [9].
7. Disrupt the cells by three passages through a high-pressure mechanical homogenizer (Invensys Systems APV) at 8000 psi [9].

8. Add DTT to the disrupted cells at a final concentration of 0.20 mg/ml [9].
9. Remove the cell debris by normal flow filtration system with a cellulose depth filter including an inorganic filter aid (Millistak, Millipore) [9].
10. Wash with 100 mM sodium phosphate buffer (pH 7.6) containing 4.4 mM EDTA, 3.3 mM PLP, and 0.16 mg/ml DTT [9].
11. Concentrate the clarified crude enzyme to 40 L with a tangential flow filtration system with an ultrafiltration membrane (50 kDa; Millipore) [9].
12. Adjust the pH of the concentrated crude enzyme to 7.6 with 8 M NaOH [9].

3.12 Large-Scale Purification of Recombinant L-Methionine γ-Lyase

3.12.1 Bulk Crystallization

1. To facilitate crystallization of the enzyme, add 40% PEG6000 dissolved in 100 mM sodium phosphate buffer (pH 7.6) containing 4.4 mM EDTA, 3.3 mM PLP, and 0.16 mg/mL DTT at a final PEG6000 concentration of 9.0% to 40 L of the concentrated crude enzyme with mild agitation [9].
2. Stir the solution for 30 min below 15 °C [9].
3. Remove the turbid materials by a continuous tube-type centrifuge (Tomoe Engineering, Tokyo, Japan) at 20,000 × *g* below 15 °C. To carry out the first crystallization, add ammonium sulfate to the supernatant at a final concentration of 3.6%, and then add 3.7 M sodium chloride stepwise to the solution for 15 min at a final concentration of 0.18 M with mild agitation at 130 rpm in a 100 L crystallizer (Kido, Hyogo, Japan) [9].
4. After incubation for 1 h at 33 °C, cool the solution and maintain below 15 °C overnight with mild agitation. Collect the crystals by centrifugation at 20,000 × *g* below 15 °C. Solubilize with 35 L of 20 mM sodium phosphate buffer (pH 7.2) containing 0.5 mM PLP and 0.5 mg/mL 2-mercaptoethanol (2ME) at 33 °C [9].
5. Remove the insoluble impurities by centrifugation at 20,000 × *g* below 15 °C. To carry out the second crystallization, dissolve 28% PEG6000 in 20 mM sodium phosphate buffer (pH 7.2) containing 0.5 mM PLP and 0.5 mg/mL [9].
6. Add 2-mercaptoethanol at a final PEG6000 concentration of 8.0% with mild agitation, and then add 3.7 M sodium chloride stepwise to the solution for 15 min at a final concentration of 0.18 M with mild agitation in the 100 L crystallizer [9].
7. After incubation for 1 h at 33 °C, cool the solution and maintain below 15 °C overnight with mild agitation [9].
8. Collect the crystals by centrifugation at 20,000 × *g* below 15 °C [9].

9. Solubilize with 35 L of 20 mM sodium phosphate buffer (pH 7.2) containing 0.5 mM PLP and 0.5 mg/mL β-mercaptoethanol at 33 °C [9].
10. Obtain the third batch of crystals in the same manner as the second. Crystals are stable for at least a few months with no significant loss of activity at 5 °C [9].

3.12.2 Anion-Exchange Column Chromatography

1. Solubilize the third batch of crystals with 50 mM sodium phosphate buffer (pH 7.2) containing 0.5 mM PLP and 0.5 mg/mL β-mercaptoethanol at 33 °C [9].
2. Remove the turbid materials by centrifugation at 20,000 × *g* below 15 °C [9].
3. Perform the following procedures at 15 °C unless otherwise stated. Filter the supernatant with a series of microfiltration membranes (1.2–0.45 μm; Sartorius) [9].
4. Apply a total of 1100 g of protein, corresponding to 72.1 L of the solution, to a 35 L anion-exchange column (DEAE-Sepharose FF, 30 × 50 cm), which is equilibrated with 50 mM sodium phosphate buffer (pH 7.2) [9].
5. Wash the column with 50 mM sodium phosphate buffer (pH 7.2) containing 10 μM PLP, and then elute the enzyme with 50 mM sodium phosphate buffer (pH 7.2) containing 80 mM sodium chloride and 10 μM PLP at a flow rate of 28 L/h [9].
6. Pool active fractions, concentrate by a tangential flow filtration system with an ultrafiltration membrane (10 kDa; Millipore) to 24 l, and then filter with a series of microfiltration membranes (0.45–0.20 μm; Sartorius) [9].
7. Obtain a total of 720 g of protein per batch [9].

3.12.3 Gel Filtration

1. Apply 240 g of protein from 8.0 L of solution to a gel-filtration column (Sephacryl S-200 HR), which is equilibrated with 10 mM sodium phosphate buffer (pH 8.0) [9].
2. Elute the enzyme with the same buffer at a flow rate of 30 L/h [9].
3. Pool active fractions and concentrate using a tangential flow filtration system with an ultrafiltration membrane (10 kDa; Millipore) to 6.1 l [9].
4. Add 1 mM PLP to the solution at a final concentration of 0.1 mM, and then filter the solution with a microfiltration membrane (0.22 μm; Millipore) [9].
5. Prepare 200 g purified recombinant METase per batch and store the purified enzyme at −80 °C for several months with no significant loss of activity [9].

4 Results

4.1 Small-Scale Purification of rMETase

High-Expression Clone of rMETase. The highest expression clone was selected by activity assay and termed pAC-1. pAC-1 expressed rMETase at approximately 10% of the total cell protein based on the specific activity of 20 units/mg for a 99% pure enzyme. Shaker flask cultures yielded up to 1 g rMETase per liter of medium. SDS-PAGE demonstrated a very prominent rMETase band in cell lysates, indicating rMETase overexpression [2].

Purification of rMETase from Clone pAC-1. The yield of rMETase was more than 63%, and the specific activity was 20–30 units/mg. As seen in Table 1, the simple procedure gave a yield of 85–94% for each step. There was an approximate doubling of specific activity for each step until endotoxin removal. The ActiClean endotoxin affinity step reduced endotoxin levels from more than 1000 EU/mg to less than 2 EU/mg as measured by LAL. The protocol and equipment described can readily yield 10 g rMETase [2].

Analysis of Purified rMETase. SDS-PAGE analysis of rMETase demonstrated a single band of 43 kDa identical to native METase (Fig. 1). HPLC analysis demonstrated a major peak with a retention time (RT) of 8.5 min and a purity calculated at greater than 99%. The RT of the standard of bovine serum albumin was 8.88 min and the RT of the standard sweet potato β amylase was 7.82 min [2].

Lyophilization of rMETase. Purified rMETase was lyophilized. The specific activity of rMETase in lyophilized powder and solution

Table 1
Purification of rMETase

Procedure (batch 11)	Volume (ml)	Activity (units)	Protein (g)	Specific activity (units/mg)	Yield (%)
Cell lysis	5000	82,000	29.3	2.8	100
Heat & UF[a]	4500	77,000	19.3	4.0	94
DEAE-FF (1)[b]	2200	65,400	60	10.9	80
DEAE-FF (2)[c]	800	57,500	2.9	20.0	70
ActiClean[d]	182	52,000	2.6	20.1	63

rMETase overexpression *E.coli* clone pAC-1 was grown in 10,800 ml TB medium cultures in 6 l flasks at 37°C at 400 rpm for 16 h at which time the OD600 was approximately 10. The medium was changed with fresh TB and the incubation was continued for another 6 h. When the OD600 reached 20, the bacteria were harvested by centrifugation and then lysed by cavitation. rMETase was then purified by heating to 50°C for 1 min and ultrafiltration followed by chromatography on two DEAE Sepharose Fast Flow columns and one ActiClean endotoxin-affinity column as described in the Methods (2)

[a] *UF* ultrafiltration

[b] DEAE-FF (1), DEAE Sepharose FF First column, pH 7.2

[c] DEAE-FF (2), DEAE Sepharose FF Second column, pH 8.3

[d] Endotoxin level was less than 2 EU/mg after the ActiClean step

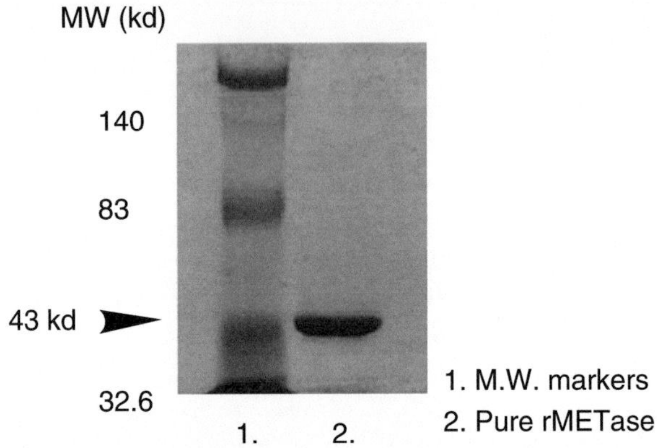

Fig. 1 SDS–PAGE of purified rMETase. rMETase was purified from the AC-1 clone with the protocol described in the Methods. 20 mg of rMETase was loaded on a 7.5% polyacrylamide SDS gel. The gel was run at 180 V for 30 min. Lane 1 contained protein molecular weight standards. Lane 2 contained native rMETase [2]

was comparable. rMETase could be stably stored as a lyophilized powder [2].

Half-Life of rMETase In Vivo. When rMETase was administered by i.v. injection in mice, the $t_{1/2}$ of rMETase was 2 h. The peak level occurred within approximately 10 min [2].

4.2 PEG-rMETase

Identity of PEG-rMETase was confirmed with electrophoresis on both SDS-PAGE and native-PAGE (Fig. 2). PEG-rMETase had a much larger molecular mass than rMETase, which is 172 kda on native-PAGE. The subunits of PEG-rMETase were also larger than the subunits of rMETase, which have a molecular mass of 43 kda [10] (*see* **Notes 1** and **2**).

Purity of PEG-rMETase. The migration rates of PEG-rMETase molecules were much slower than those of rMETase due to the conjugation of PEG molecules and subsequent hydration. SDS-PAGE demonstrated that the subunits of rMETase were all linked with PEG at P/M ratios greater than 30. There was a slight band at 43 kda on SDS-PAGE of PEG-rMETase synthesized at P/M ratios of 10–30, which might be due to PEG molecules released from some subunits during denaturation with SDS and heating to 94 °C [10].

Enzyme Activity of PEG rMETase. The enzyme activity of PEG-rMETase depended on the P/M ratio. The PEG-rMETase synthesized at P/M ratios of 20–30 had activities of approximately 60–70% that of rMETase. At higher P/M ratios of 60–120, the resulting PEG-rMETase had activities of approximately 20–40% that of rMETase (Table 2) [10].

Extent of Derivatization of rMETase with PEG. MALDI mass spectrometry results confirmed that rMETase (molecular mass

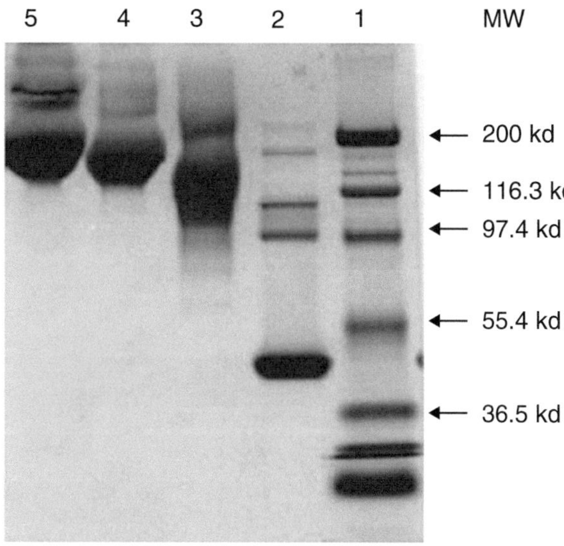

Fig. 2 SDS-PAGE of naked and PEGylated rMETase. The purified PEGylated rMETases were run on a 10% SDS-PAGE gel. The gel was stained with Coomassie Brilliant Blue. *Numbers* on the *right* indicate molecular mass. *Lane 1,* molecular mass markers. *Lane 2,* naked rMETase. *Lane 3,* PEG/rMETase synthesized at a ratio of 30/1. *Lane 4,* PEG/rMETase 60/1. *Lane 5,* PEG/rMETase 120/1 [16]

Table 2
Activity of PEG-rMETase

Enzyme	PEGylation molar ratio of PEG/rMETase	Specific activity (units/mg) ± SD	Relative activity compared to rMETase (% ± SD)
rMETase	–	20	100
PEG-rMETase	20	14.5 ± 1	75 ± 5
PEG-rMETase	30	12 ± 1	60 ± 5
PEG-rMETase	40	10 ± 1	50 ± 5
PEG-rMETase	60	8 ± 1	40 ± 5

rMETase was PEGylated with M-SPA-PEG 5000 at different molar ratios of PEG and rMETase under conditions described in the Methods. The specific activity was measured and the relative activity to rMETase was calculated as described in the Methods. The experiments were repeated twice and the standard deviations are given [10]

172 kda) comprises four identical subunits of MW 43 kda. MALDI results for PEG-rMETase indicated that PEG-rMETase contained mainly four broad peaks, corresponding to molecular weights 52,661 ± 5000 and 106,631 ± 8000 for the monomer and dimer, respectively. These molecular weights are consistent with each subunit linked to two M-SPA-PEG 5000 molecules. The broadness of the signals is due to molecular heterogeneity of M-SPA-PEG 5000 [10].

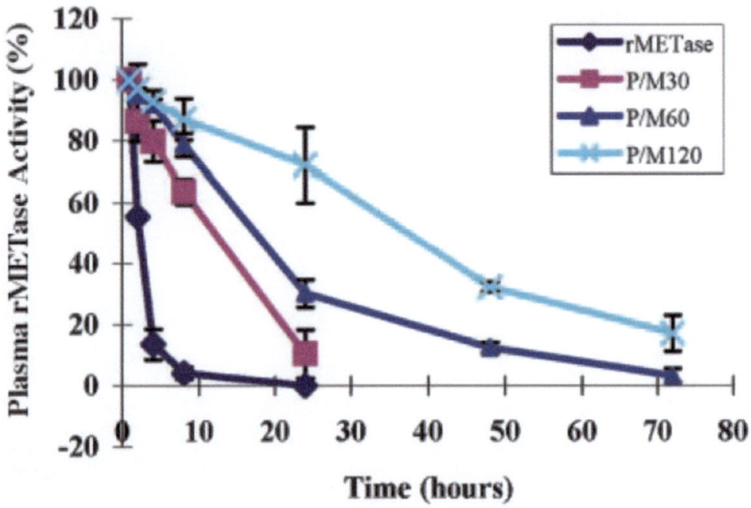

Fig. 3 Plasma rMETase enzyme activity after i.v. injection of naked and PEGylated rMETase in mice. The mice received i.v. injection of 80 units naked rMETase or the indicated PEGylated rMETase. Blood samples were collected at different time points and measured for plasma enzyme activity as described in the Methods [16]

Half-Life of PEG-rMETase In Vivo. The $t_{1/2}$ in the mouse circulation of PEG-rMETase was dependent on the extent of PEGylation (Fig. 3) [10].

Effect of PLP on PEG-rMETase Function In Vivo. rMETase is a PLP-dependent enzyme, with one molecule of PLP conjugated to each of the four subunits of rMETase. PLP delivery in vivo by mini-osmotic pump implantation significantly increased plasma PLP concentration. 80 U of naked or PEGylated rMETase was injected i.v. in animals with or without PLP supplementation from implanted mini-osmotic pumps. Blood samples were taken at different time points and measured for plasma MET concentration. Plasma MET depletion with PLP supplementation was prolonged significantly compared to MET depletion without PLP supplementation (Fig. 4), indicating PLP dependence for the in vivo MET depletion efficacy of PEG-rMETase. Plasma MET levels depleted by the three PEGylated rMETase conjugates were maintained below 5 μM for 48 h. Plasma MET levels were depleted below 5 μM for 72 h in case of PEG/rMETase 120 with PLP supplementation [16].

High-Level PEGylation of rMETase Decreases PLP Dependence In Vivo. To quantitate the effect of PEGylation on PLP dependence of rMETase, we calculated the ratios of plasma MET concentration remaining after treatment by PEGrMETase without PLP supplementation (Fig. 5) versus that remaining after treatment with PEG-rMETase with PLP supplementation. These ratios showed that

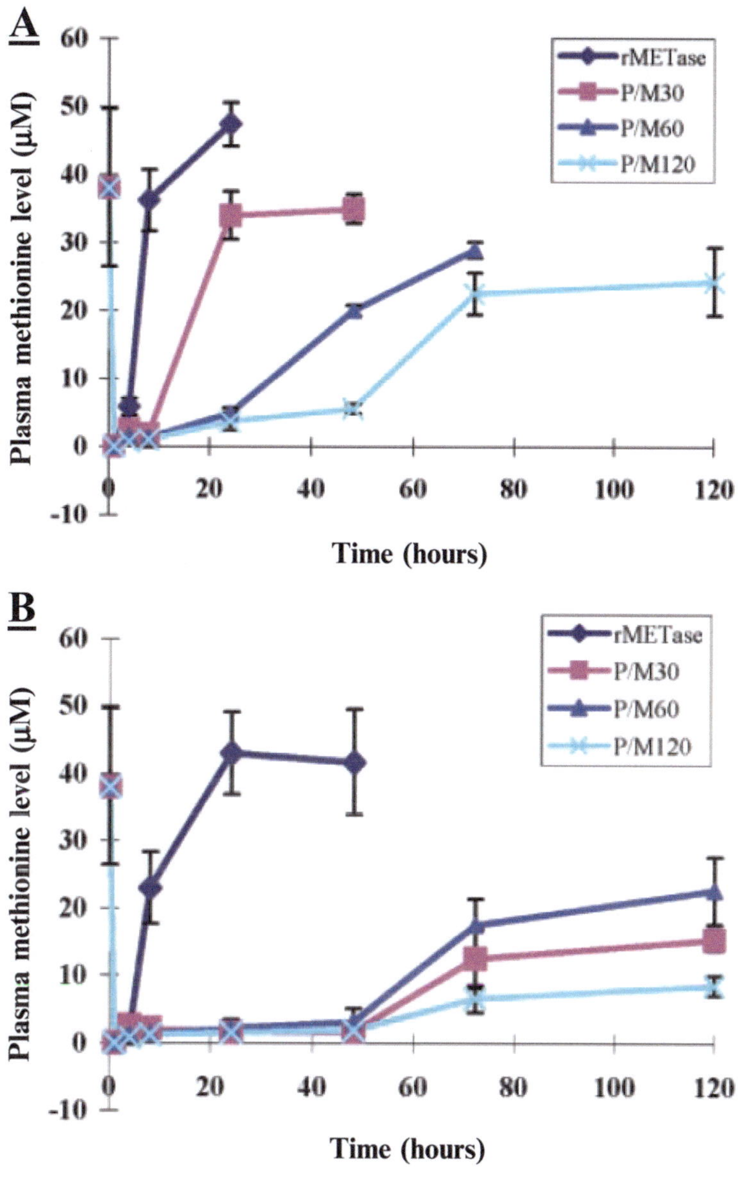

Fig. 4 (**a**) Plasma MET depletion after i.v. injection of naked and PEGylated rMETase in mice. The mice received i.v. injection with 80 units of naked rMETase or the indicated PEGylated rMETase. Blood samples were collected at different time points and measured for plasma MET concentration as described in Methods [19]. (**b**) Plasma MET depletion after PLP pump implantation and i.v. injection of naked and PEGylated rMETase. Eighty units of naked or indicated PEGylated rMETase were injected i.v. into each mouse after PLP pump implantation. Blood samples were collected at different time points and measured for plasma MET concentration as described in Methods [16]

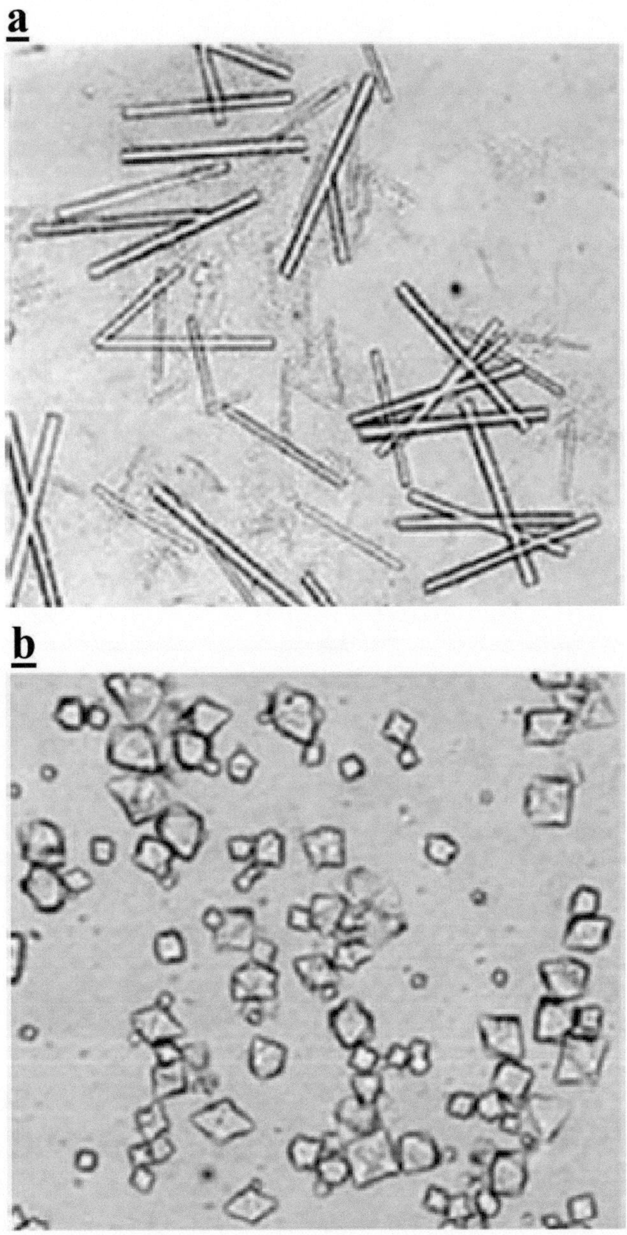

Fig. 5 Morphology of rod-shaped crystals (a) and octahedral-shaped crystals (b) of recombinant METase. (**a**) Rod-shaped crystals were obtained from the first crystallization in the presence of PEG6000, ammonium sulfate, and sodium chloride as precipitants. (**b**) Octahedral-shaped crystals were obtained from the second and third crystallizations in the presence of PEG6000 and sodium chloride as precipitants. Please see Methods for details [9]

PEG/rMETase 60 and PEG/rMETase 120 had lesser PLP dependence than PEG/rMETase-30, suggesting a protective effect of high-level PEGylation on retention of PLP by rMETase [16].

Efficacy of PLP and PEG-rMETase to maintain MET levels below 5 μm in vivo. We used 5 μM plasma MET concentration as an end point for MET depletion since it was reported that plasma MET depletion below 5 μM was an effective therapeutic level of rMETase for antitumor efficacy using mouse models of human cancer [19]. Without PLP supplementation this level of MET depletion could be achieved for 8 h by PEG/rMETase-30; 24 h by PEG/rMETase-60; and 48 h by PEG/rMETase-120. With PLP supplementation, depletion to less than 5 μM MET could be achieved for 48 h by PEG/rMETase-30 and PEG/rMETase-60, and 72 h by PEG/rMETase-120 [16] (*see* **Note 3**).

4.3 Industrial-Level Production of rMETase

Large-scale cultivation of transformant in production culture. Recombinant METase accumulated to 2.1 mg/mL as a soluble form and accounted for 43% of the total proteins in the soluble fraction after fermentation of recombination E.coli containing the rMETase gene for 24 h. Therefore, 730 g of recombinant METase was produced per batch [9].

4.4 Purification Including Bulk Crystallization

rMETase was directly crystallized from the crude enzyme overnight in a 100 L crystallizer. Yellow-colored and rod-shaped crystals were obtained by the first crystallization. The specific activity of the crystals was 54 U/mg, and the step yield of the activity by the crystallization was 87%. The second crystallization was then carried out to remove residual impurities. In this step, ammonium sulfate was not used as a precipitant. As a result, yellow-colored and octahedral-shaped crystals were obtained by the second crystallization. The third crystallization was carried out under the same conditions as the second one. Yellow-colored and octahedral-shaped crystals were also obtained by the third crystallization (Fig. 5). The enzyme was purified by repeated crystallizations without using column chromatography from the crude enzyme via SDS-PAGE analysis [9] (*see* **Note 4**).

After the three repeated crystallizations, the enzyme was further purified by a combination of anion-exchange column chromatography and gel filtration. The third batch of crystals prepared by combining two batches was subjected to anion-exchange column chromatography. More than 99.9% of endotoxins in the third-batch crystals were eliminated by the anion-exchange column chromatography. The elution concentration was divided into three parts and applied to a gel filtration column. Finally, we manufactured 600 g of purified recombinant METase with low endotoxin content by a series of two batches of fermentation and crystallization, one batch of anion-exchange column chromatography, and three batches of the gel filtration with 41% overall yield in the purification

Table 3
Purification of recombinant METase from *E. coli* JM109 harboring pMGLTrc03 [9]

Purification step	Number of batches	Total activity (MU)	Total protein (g)	Specific activity (U/mg)	Yield (%)	Endotoxin (EU/mg)
Cultivation	2	83.3	3440	24	100	ND
Debris removal	2	81.2	2680	30	97	2×10^6
First crystallization	2	70.8	1320	54	85	6×10^4
Second crystallization	2	64.2	1170	55	77	1×10^4
Third crystallization	2	61.4	1100	56	74	8×10^3
DEAE-Sepharose FF	1	40.8	720	57	49	2
Sephacryl S-200 HR	3	34.1	600	57	41	8×10^{-1}

ND not determined

process. Table 3 summarizes the purification of recombinant METase. The purified enzyme gave a single band corresponding to 42 kDa on SDS-PAGE [9] (*see* **Note 5**).

The 3-dimensional structure of rMETase determined by X-ray crystallography is shown in Fig. 6 [17].

5 Notes

1. The protective effect of PEGylation on the apparent in vivo retention of PLP by rMETase was an unexpected result as was the rapid loss in vivo of PLP by naked rMETase and low-degree PEGylated rMETase [16].
2. Reduced antigenicity of rMETase was also achieved by PEGylated rMETase [16].
3. PLP supplementation in vivo greatly extended the half-life of PEG-rMETase holoenzyme, which in turn greatly extended the time of MET depletion by PEG-rMETase in a dose-dependent manner. PLP extended the half-life of PEG-rMETase holoenzyme ~4–5-fold in a dose-dependent manner, which resulted in a ~10-fold increase in time of plasma MET depletion to $\leq$5 μm. Although PLP remains tightly bound to the enzyme in vitro, it readily dissociates from the enzyme in vivo [12].
4. Much more recombinant METase was produced in this study than those reported by Inoue et al. [7] and Tan et al. [2], with the content reaching 43% of total proteins in the soluble fraction due to high expression of rMETase in the recombinant *E. coli* clone. We were able to obtain 2.1 mg/mL of

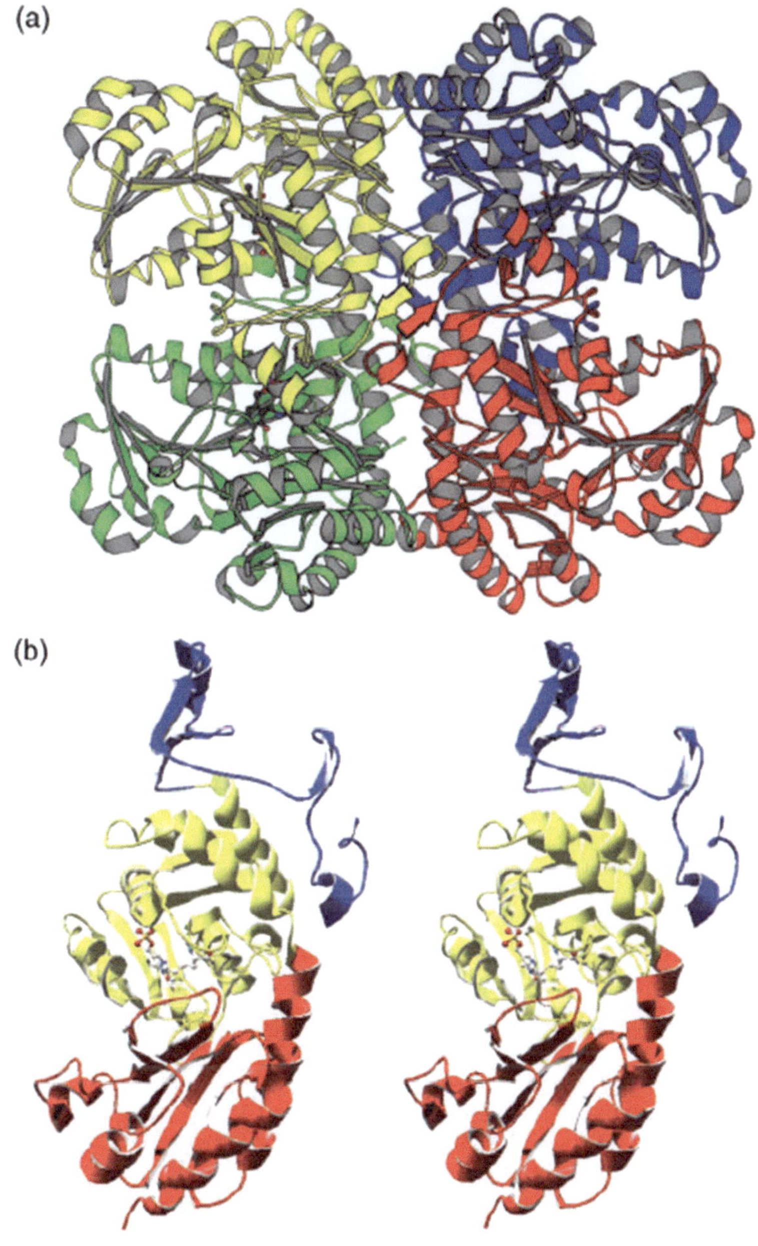

Fig. 6 Crystal structure of recombinant methioninase. (**a**) The homotetramer is built up as a dimer of active dimers, resulting in an overall 222 symmetry. The individual monomers are color coded. The PLP cofactor is mainly linked by the central domain, held in a ball-and-stick presentation. (**b**) Stereo ribbon presentation of the MGL monomer. The N-terminal domain is held in blue, the PLP-binding domain in yellow, and the C-terminal domain in red. PLP and PLP-binding Lys211 are shown in a ball-and-stick representation [17]

recombinant METase as a soluble form by simple batch fermentation using a 500 L fermentor. High-level rMETase expression enabled bulk crystallization which simplified downstream processing and the purification process, and is cost-effective, for large-scale manufacturing [9].

5. Endotoxins cause fever in humans and must be eliminated from biopharmaceuticals intended for parenteral administration. Endotoxins are produced by recombinant *E. coli*. Crystallization effectively reduced the endotoxins as well as the host cell and the culture-derived proteins from the crude enzyme. Hou and Zaniewski [20] report that anion-exchange column chromatography is useful for removal of residual endotoxins. We observed that the endotoxins could be greatly removed from a level of 8×10^3 to 2 EU/mg by anion-exchange column chromatography. Thus, the combination of crystallization and anion-exchange column chromatography is suitable for purification of the enzyme. Considering the amount of recombinant METase administration for injection, this endotoxin content is within the upper limit for the endotoxin level given in the Food and Drug Administration guidelines [9].

References

1. Kreis W, Hession C (1973) Isolation and purification of L-methionine-a-deamino-g mercaptomethane-lyase (L-methioninase) from Clostridium. Cancer Res 33:1862–1865
2. Tan Y, Xu M, Tan X-Z, Tan X-Y, Wang X, Saikawa Y, Nagahama T, Sun X, Lenz M, Hoffman RM (1997) Overexpression and large-scale production of recombinant L-methionine-α-deamino-γ-mercaptomethane-lyase for novel anticancer therapy Protein Expr Purif 9:233–245
3. Ito S, Nakamura T, Eguchi Y (1976) Purification and characterization of methoninase from P. putida. J Biochem 79:1263–1272
4. Nakamura T, Esaki N, Tanaka H, Soda K (1988) Specific labeling of the essential cysteine residue of L-methionine γ-lyase with a cofactor analogue, N-(bromo-acetyl) pyridoxamine phosphate. Biochemistry 27:1587–1591
5. Tanaka H, Esaki N, Soda K (1977) Properties of L-methionine γ-lyase from Pseudomonas ovalis. Biochemistry 16:100–106
6. Nakamura T, Esaki N, Sugiem K, Beresov T, Tanaka H, Soda K (1984) Purification of bacterial L-methionine-lyase. Anal Biochem 138:421–424
7. Inoue H, Inagaki K, Sugimoto M, Esaki N, Soda K, Tanaka H (1995) Structural analysis of the L-methionine γ lyase gene from Pseudomonas putida. J Biochem 117:1120–1125
8. Hori H, Takabayashi K, Orvis L, Carson DA, Nobori T (1996) Gene cloning and characterization of Pseudomonas put ida L-methionine-a-deamino-g-mercaptomethane-lyase. Cancer Res 56:2116–2122
9. Takakura T, Ito T, Yagi S, Notsu Y, Itakura T, Nakamura T, Inagaki K, Esaki N, Hoffman RM, Takimoto A (2006) High-level expression and bulk crystallization of recombinant L-methionine γ-lyase, an anticancer agent. Appl Microbiol Biotechnol 70:183–192
10. Tan Y, Sun X, Xu M, An Z, Tan XZ, Tan XY, Han Q, Miljkovic DA, Yang M, Hoffman RM (1998) Polyethylene glycol conjugation of recombinant methioninase for cancer therapy. Protein Expr Purif 12:45–52
11. Li S-K, Yang Z, Sun X, Tan Y, Yagi S, Hoffman RM (2004) Protein carboxyl amidation increases the potential extent of protein polyethylene glycol conjugation. Anal Biochem 330:264–272
12. Yang Z, Sun X, Li S, Tan Y, Wang X, Zhang N, Yagi S, Takakura T, Kobayashi Y, Takimoto A, Yoshioka T, Suginaka A, Frenkel EP, Hoffman RM (2004) Circulating half-life of PEGylated recombinant methioninase holoenzyme is

highly dose dependent on cofactor pyridoxal-5′-phosphate. Cancer Res 64:5775–5778

13. Weiner MP, Anderson C, Jerpseth B, Wells S, Johnson Browne B, Vaillancourt P (1994) Studier pET system vectors and hosts. Strateg Mol Biol 7:41–43
14. Bovara R, Carrea G, Gioacchini AM, Riva S, Secundo F (1997) Activity, stability and conformation of methoxypoly (ethylene glycol)-subtilisin at different concentrations of water in dioxane. Biotechnol Bioeng 54:50–57
15. Brumeanu T-D, Zaghouani H, Bona C (1995) Purification of antigenized immunoglobulins derivatized with mono methoxypolyethylene glycol. J Chromatogr A 696:219–225
16. Sun X, Yang Z, Li S, Tan Y, Zhang N, Wang X, Yagi S, Yoshioka T, Takimoto A, Mitsushima K, Suginaka A, Frenkel EP, Hoffman RM (2003) In vivo efficacy of recombinant methioninase is enhanced by the combination of polyethylene glycol conjugation and pyridoxal 5′ phosphate supplementation. Cancer Res 63:8377–8383
17. Kudou D, Misaki S, Yamashita M, Tamura T, Takakura T, Yoshioka T, Yagi S, Hoffman RM, Takimoto A, Esaki N, Inagaki K (2007) Structure of the antitumour enzyme L-methionine γ-lyase from Pseudomonas putida at 1.8Å resolution. J Biochem 141: 535–544
18. Watanabe N, Kamei S, Ohkubo A, Yamanaka M, Ohsawa S, Makino K, Tokuda K (1986) Urinary protein as measured with a pyrogallol red-molybdate complex, manually and in a Hitachi 726 automated analyzer. Clin Chem 32:1551–1554
19. Hoffman RM (2015) Development of recombinant methioninase to target the general cancer-specific metabolic defect of methioninase dependence: a 40-year odyssey. Expert Opin Biol Ther 15:21–31
20. Hou KC, Zaniewski (1991) Endotoxin removal for anion exchange polymeric matrix. Biotechnol Appl Biochem 12:315–324

Chapter 11

Methioninase Cell-Cycle Trap Cancer Chemotherapy

Robert M. Hoffman, Shuya Yano, and Kentaro Igarashi

Abstract

Cancer cells are methionine (MET) dependent compared to normal cells as they have an elevated requirement for MET in order to proliferate. MET restriction selectively traps cancer cells in the S/G_2 phase of the cell cycle. The cell cycle phase can be visualized by color coding with the fluorescence ubiquitination-based cell cycle indicator (FUCCI). Recombinant methioninase (rMETase) is an enzyme that effectively degrades MET. rMETase induces S/G_2-phase blockage of cancer cells which is identified by the cancer cells' green fluorescence with FUCCI imaging. Cancer cells in G_1/G_0 are the majority of the cells in solid tumors and are resistant to the chemotherapy. Treatment of cancer cells with standard chemotherapy drugs only led to the majority of the cancer cell population being arrested in G_0/G_1 phase, identified by the cancer cells' red fluorescence in the FUCCI system. The G_0/G_1-phase cancer cells are chemo-resistant. Tumor targeting *Salmonella typhimurium* A1-R (*S. typhimurium* A1-R) was used to decoy quiescent G_0/G_1 stomach cancer cells growing in nude mice to cycle, with subsequent rMETase treatment to selectively trap the decoyed cancer cells in S/G_2 phase, which made them highly sensitive to chemotherapy. Subsequent cisplatinum (CDDP) or paclitaxel (PTX) chemotherapy was then administered to kill the decoyed and trapped cancer cells, which completely prevented or regressed tumor growth. In a subsequent experiment, a patient-derived orthotopic xenograft (PDOX) model of recurrent CDDP-resistant metastatic osteosarcoma was eradicated by the combination of *Salmonella typhimurium* A1-R decoy, rMETase S/G_2-phase cell cycle trap, and CDDP cell kill. *Salmonella typhimurium* A1-R and rMETase pre-treatment thereby overcame CDDP resistance. These results demonstrate the effectiveness of the new chemotherapy paradigm of "decoy, trap, and kill" chemotherapy.

Key words Methionine dependence, Recombinant methioninase, rMETase, Cell cycle, S/G_2, Trap, FUCCI, Imaging, *Salmonella typhimurium* A1-R, Tumor-targeting, Decoy, Decoy-trap-kill chemotherapy, Cisplatinum, Paclitaxel

1 Introduction

Cancer cells have an excess requirement for methionine (MET) termed MET dependence, and become trapped in late S/G_2 of the cell cycle when they are selectively arrested by MET restriction (MR) [1–3].

MR of co-cultures of cancer and normal cells enabled the selective elimination of the cancer cells by chemotherapy drugs based on the S/G_2-phase cell cycle trap of the cancer cells [4].

Robert M. Hoffman (ed.), *Methionine Dependence of Cancer and Aging: Methods and Protocols*, Methods in Molecular Biology, vol. 1866, https://doi.org/10.1007/978-1-4939-8796-2_11, © Springer Science+Business Media, LLC, part of Springer Nature 2019

The fluorescence ubiquitination-based cell-cycle indicator (FUCCI) labels cycling S/G_2 cells with green fluorescent protein (GFP) and cells in G_0/G_1 with red fluorescent protein (RFP).

Tumor-targeting *S. typhimurium* A1-R decoyed quiescent G_0/G_1-phase MKN45 FUCCI-expressing cancer cells growing in nude mice, where they are the large majority in tumors, to cycle from G_0/G_1 to S/G_2 as visualized by FUCCI imaging [5]. Cancer cells treated with rMETase were selectively trapped in S/G_2 as visualized with FUCCI imaging. The S/G_2-phase trap sensitized the cancer cells to doxorubicin (DOX), cisplatinum (CDDP), or 5-fluorouracil (5-FU) [2]. This treatment strategy was termed decoy, trap, and kill chemotherapy.

In a subsequent experiment, sequential treatment of a chemotherapy-resistant osteosarcoma lung metastasis in a patient-derived orthotopic xenograft (PDOX) mouse model with *S. typhimurium* A1-R, rMETase, and CDDP eradicated the patient tumor, suggesting the clinical potential of decoy, trap, and kill cancer chemotherapy [6]. Decoy trap and kill cancer chemotherapy, is reviewed in the present chapter.

2 Materials

1. Recombinant L-methionine α-deamino-γ-mercaptomethane lyase (recombinant methioninase [rMETase] [EC 4.4.1.11]) (AntiCancer Inc., San Diego, CA).
2. pAC-1 rMETase high-expression gene clone (AntiCancer Inc.).
3. *E. coli* for expression of pAC-1 (AntiCancer Inc.).
4. *Plasmids* expressing mKO2-hCdtl (orange/red fluorescent protein) or mAG-hGem (green fluorescent protein) were obtained from the Medical and Biological Laboratory (Nagoya, Japan).
5. Athymic nu/nu nude mice (AntiCancer Inc., CA).
6. *Salmonella typhimurium* A1-R (AntiCancer Inc.).
7. Cisplatinum (CDDP).
8. Paclitaxel (PTX).
9. Doxorubicin (DOX).
10. 5-Fluorouracil (5-FU).
11. DEAE Sepharose FF (Pharmacia, Uppsala, Sweden).
12. Sephacryl S-200HR (Pharmacia).
13. ActiClean Etox (Sterogene, Arcadia, CA).
14. 10% Formalin.
15. Paraffin.
16. Hematoxylin and eosin (H&E).

17. FV1000 confocal microscope (Olympus, Tokyo, Japan).
18. INFINITY ANALYZE software (Lumenera Corporation, Ottawa, Canada).
19. 10 μL ketamine HCl, 7.6 μl xylazine, 2.4 μL acepromazine maleate, and 10 μl PBS (Henry Schein).
20. Xylene.
21. Ethanol.
22. Lipofectamine™ LTX (Invitrogen).
23. Autoclaved laboratory rodent diet (Teklad LM-485; Harlan).
24. BHS system microscope (Olympus)

3 Methods

3.1 FUCCI (Fluorescence Ubiquitination Cell Cycle Indicator)

1. Transfect plasmids expressing mKO_2-hCdtl into MKN45 human stomach cancer cells or other cancer cells using Lipofectamine™ LTX.
2. Incubate cells for 48 h after transfection and then trypsinize and seed in 96-well plates at a density of ten cells/well.
3. Sort cells into red-orange (G_0/G_1 phase) cells using a cell sorter.
4. Retransfect the sorted orange/red fluorescent cells with mAG-hGem (green) and then sort by green fluorescence [7, 8].

3.2 Mice

1. Maintain athymic *nu/nu* nude mice in a barrier facility under HEPA filtration and feed with autoclaved laboratory rodent diet.
2. Perform all mouse surgical procedures under anesthesia using s.c. administration of a ketamine mixture (10 μL ketamine HCl, 7.6 μL xylazine, 2.4 μL acepromazine maleate, and 10 μL PBS).
3. Conduct all mouse studies in accordance with the principles and procedures outlined in the National Institute of Health Guide for the Care and Use of Animals under Assurance Number A3873–1 [5].

3.3 Patient-Derived Tumors

1. Submit study protocol to an Institutional Review Board before the study begins.
2. Obtain written informed consent from the patient [9].

3.4 Surgical Orthotopic Implantation (SOI) for Establishment of a PDOX Model of a Lung-Metastatic Osteosarcoma

1. Implant an osteosarcoma patient lung metastasis in the lung of nude mice patient as follows [9]:
2. After ketamine anesthesia, put mice in a position of right lateral decubitus, with four limbs restrained.
3. Make a 1.5 cm transverse incision of skin in the left chest wall.
4. Separate chest muscles by sharp dissection and expose intercostal muscles.
5. Make a 0.8–1.0 cm intercostal incision between the sixth and seventh ribs on the chest wall and open the chest wall.
6. Take up the left lung up with a forceps and attach tumor fragments promptly into the lower lung with one suture.
7. Return the lung into the chest cavity.
8. Close the incision in the chest wall with a 6-0 surgical suture (Ethilon, Ethicon, Inc., NJ, USA). Observe the closed condition of the chest wall immediately and if a leak exists close it with additional sutures.
9. After closing the chest wall, make an intrathoracic puncture by using a 3 ml syringe and 25G 1/2 needle to withdraw the remaining air in the chest cavity.
10. After the withdrawal of air, be sure that the lung is completely inflated through the thin chest wall of the mouse. Then close the skin and chest muscle with a 6-0 surgical suture in one layer [10].

3.5 Preparation and Administration of S. typhimurium A1-R

1. Grow GFP-expressing *S. typhimurium* A1-R (AntiCancer Inc.) overnight on LB medium (Fisher Sci., Hanover Park, IL, USA) and then dilute 1:10 in LB medium.
2. Harvest bacteria at late-log phase, wash with PBS, and dilute in PBS.

3.6 rMETase Production

1. Use the pAC-1 rMETase high-expression clone for rMETase production in *E. coli*.
2. Use a fermentation procedure for host *E. coli* cells and the purification protocol for rMETase as previously described: Purify rMETase by three different steps using columns of DEAE Sepharose FF and Sephacryl S-200HR, and ActiClean Etox, which is designed for eliminating endotoxin [14].

3.7 Decoy, Trap, and Kill Chemotherapy

1. Randomize the osteosarcoma PDOX lung metastasis or other mouse models into the following groups 14 days after implantation: G1, control without treatment; G2, CDDP (6 mg/kg, intraperitoneally (i.p.) injection, weekly, for 2 weeks); G3, rMETase (100 units/mouse, i.p., daily, for 2 weeks); G4, *S. typhimurium* A1-R (5×10^7 CFU/100 μL, i.v., weekly, for 2 weeks); G5, *S. typhimurium* A1-R (5×10^7 CFU/100 μL, i. v., weekly, for 2 weeks) combined with rMETase (100 units/

mouse, i.p., daily, for 2 weeks); G6, *S. typhimurium* A1-R (5×10^7 CFU/100 μL, i.v., weekly, for 2 weeks) combined with rMETase (100 units/mouse, i.p., daily, for 2 weeks) and CDDP (6 mg/kg, i.p., weekly, for 2 weeks).

2. Measure body weight with a digital balance twice a week.
3. 14 days after initiation of treatment, sacrifice all mice and measure tumor size of the lung. Calculate tumor volume by the following formula: Tumor volume (mm^3) = length (mm) × width (mm) × width (mm) × 1/2. Present data was presented as mean ± SD [6].

3.8 Histological Examination

1. Fix fresh tumor samples in 10% formalin and embed in paraffin before sectioning and staining.
2. Deparaffin tissue sections (3 μm) in xylene and rehydrate in an ethanol series.
3. Perform hematoxylin and eosin (H&E) staining according to standard protocol.
4. Perform histological examination with a BHS system microscope.
5. Acquire images with INFINITY ANALYZE software (Lumenera Corporation, Ottawa, Canada) [9].

4 Results

4.1 Decoy, Trap, and Kill Chemotherapy of FUCCI-Expressing Stomach Cancer in Nude Mice

Decoy, trap, and kill chemotherapy on MKN45 tumor-bearing mice was tested. The mice were treated with CDDP; or *S. typhimurium* A1-R; or *S. typhimurium* A1-R and CDDP or *S. typhimurium* A1-R, rMETase, and CDDP. CDDP inhibited tumor growth ($p < 0.01$). *S. typhimurium*A1-R inhibited tumor growth more than CDDP ($p < 0.01$). *S. typhimurium* A1-R and CDDP combined had a greater inhibition of tumor growth ($p < 0.01$). The sequential combination of *S. typhimurium* A1-R, rMETase, and CDDP prevented or regressed tumor growth more than *S. typhimurium* A1-R or CDDP alone or the combination of these two agents ($p < 0.01$) (Fig. 1) [3] (*see* **Notes 1–3**).

Decoy, trap, and kill chemotherapy on MKN45 tumor-bearing mice was also tested. Paclitaxel (PTX) alone and *S. typhimurium* A1-R alone significantly inhibited tumor growth ($p < 0.05$). *S. typhimurium* A1-R combined with PTX had a similar inhibition of tumor growth compared with PTX alone or *S. typhimurium* A1-R alone. The sequential combination of *S. typhimurium* A1-R, rMETase, and PTX prevented or regressed tumor growth more than *S. typhimurium* A1-R or PTX alone or the combination of these two agents ($p < 0.05$) (Fig. 2) [3].

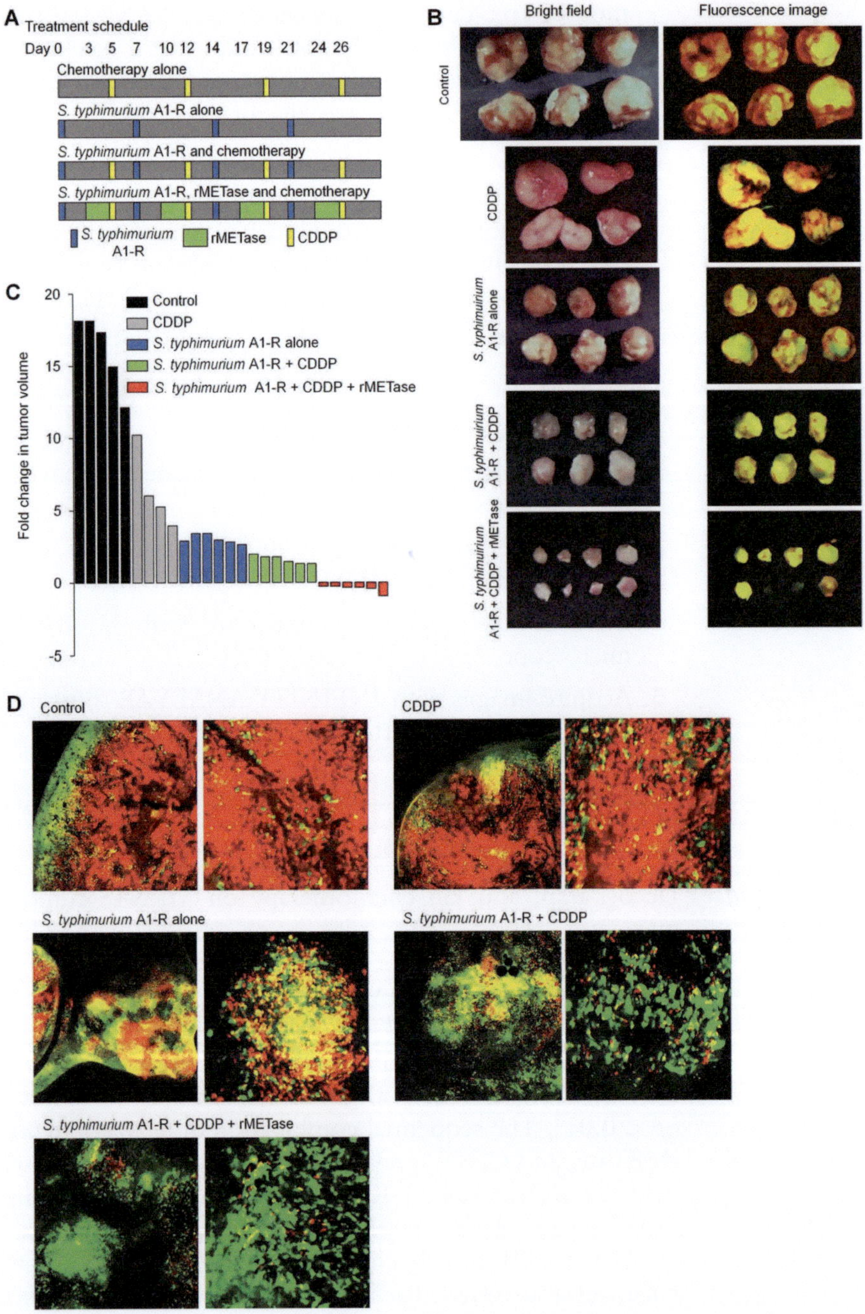

Fig. 1 Decoy, trap, and shoot chemotherapy with CDDP. (**a**) Treatment schedule. FUCCI-expressing MKN45 cells (5×10^6 cells/mouse) were injected subcutaneously into the left flank of nude mice. When the tumors reached approximately 8 mm in diameter (tumor volume, 300 mm^3), mice were administered i.v. *S. typhimurium* A1-R alone (5×10^7 CFU/mouse, i.v., qw $\times$ 4); or cisplatinum (CDDP) alone (5 mg/kg, i.p., q3d); or *S. typhimurium* A1-R followed by CDDP; or *S. typhimurium* A1-R, rMETase (200 units/mouse, i.p., qd for 3 d $\times$ 4), and CDDP in that order. (**b**) Macroscopic photographs of FUCCI-expressing tumors: untreated control; *S. typhimurium* A1-R treated; CDDP treated; *S. typhimurium* A1-R and CDDP treated; or treated with

4.2 Establishment of an Osteosarcoma Lung-Metastasis Patient-Derived Orthotopic Xenograft (PDOX) in Nude Mice

A metastatic osteosarcoma resected from the patient's lung was implanted orthotopically in the nude mouse lung [6] (*see* **Note 4**).

4.3 Decoy, Trap, and Kill Chemotherapy of Lung-Metastatic Osteosarcoma PDOX

PDOX tumor size at treatment day 14 was as follows: (G1) control: 201 ± 91 mm^3; (G2) CDDP: 174 ± 108 mm^3; (G3) rMETase: 79 ± 41 mm^3; (G4) *S. typhimurium* A1-R: 74 ± 18 mm^3; (G5) *S. typhimurium* A1-R+ rMETase 44 ± 15 mm^3; and (G6) *S. typhimurium* A1-R + rMETase + CDDP 15 ± 8 mm^3 demonstrating that decoy, trap, and kill chemotherapy with *S. typhimurium* A1-R, rMETase, and CDDP could eradicate the metastatic osteosarcoma PDOX. *P*-values were as follows: Control versus CDDP ($p = 0.586$); control versus rMETase ($p = 0.002$); control versus *S. typhimurium* A1-R ($p = 0.002$); control versus *S. typhimurium* A1-R + rMETase ($p = 0.0004$); control versus *S. typhimurium* A1-R + rMETase + CDDP ($p = 0.0001$); CDDP versus rMETase ($p = 0.045$); CDDP versus *S. typhimurium* A1-R ($p = 0.033$); CDDP versus *S. typhimurium* A1-R + rMETase ($p = 0.011$); CDDP versus *S. typhimurium* A1-R + rMETase + CDDP (decoy, trap and kill) ($p = 0.004$); rMETase versus *S. typhimurium* A1-R ($p = 0.719$); rMETase versus *S. typhimurium* A1-R + rMETase ($p = 0.048$); rMETase versus *S. typhimurium* A1-R + rMETase + CDDP ($p = 0.003$); *S. typhimurium* A1-R versus *S. typhimurium* A1-R + rMETase ($p = 0.003$); *S. typhimurium* A1-R versus *S. typhimurium* A1-R + rMETase + CDDP ($p < 0.0001$); and *S. typhimurium* A1-R + rMETase versus *S. typhimurium* A1-R + rMETase + CDDP ($p = 0.0004$) (Figs. 3 and 4) (*see* **Note 3**). There were no mouse deaths in any group. The body weight of treated mice was not significantly different in any group [6].

4.4 Histology of Osteosarcoma Lung Metastasis PDOX before and after treatment

High-power microscopy of the original patient tumor showed a neoplastic chondroid matrix occupied by anaplastic cells. The tumor had hypercellular areas populated by anaplastic cells displaying nuclear pleomorphism, coarse and hyperchromatic chromatin, and abundant mitotic figures (Fig. 5a). High-power microscopy of the untreated PDOX tumor had a solid and chondroblastic

Fig. 1 (continued) the sequential combination of *S. typhimurium* A1-R, rMETase, and CDDP. (**c**) Waterfall plot indicating fold change in tumor volume: untreated control; CDDP treated; *S. typhimurium* A1-R treated; *S. typhimurium* A1-R and CDDP treated; or treated with the sequential combination of *S. typhimurium* A1-R, rMETase, and CDDP. (**d**) Representative images of cross sections of FUCCI-expressing MKN45 subcutaneous tumors: untreated control; *S. typhimurium* A1-R treated; CDDP treated; *S. typhimurium* A1-R and CDDP treated; or treated with the sequential combination of *S. typhimurium* A1-R, rMETase, and CDDP [3]

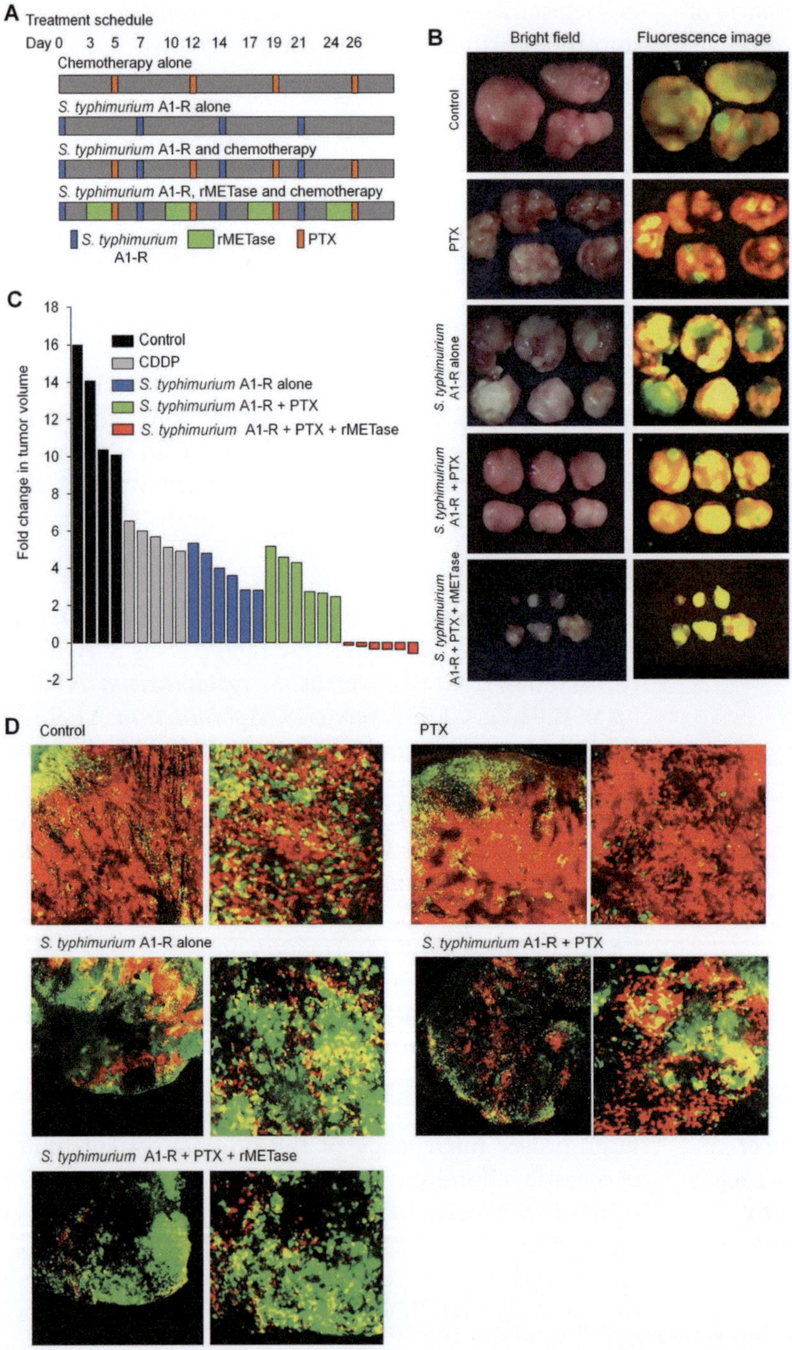

Fig. 2 Decoy, trap, and shoot chemotherapy with PTX. (**a**). Treatment schedule. FUCCI-expressing MKN45 cells (5×10^6 cells/mouse) were injected subcutaneously into the left flank of nude mice. When the tumors reached approximately 8 mm in diameter (tumor volume, 300 mm^3), mice were administered *S. typhimurium* A1-R alone (5×10^7 CFU/mouse, i.v., qw $\times$ 4); or PTX alone (6 mg/kg, i.p., q3d $\times$ 4); or *S. typhimurium* A1-R followed by PTX; or *S. typhimurium* A1-R, rMETase (200 units/mouse, i.p., qd for 3d $\times$ 4), and PTX sequentially. (**b**) Macroscopic photographs of FUCCI-expressing tumors: untreated control; *S. typhimurium*

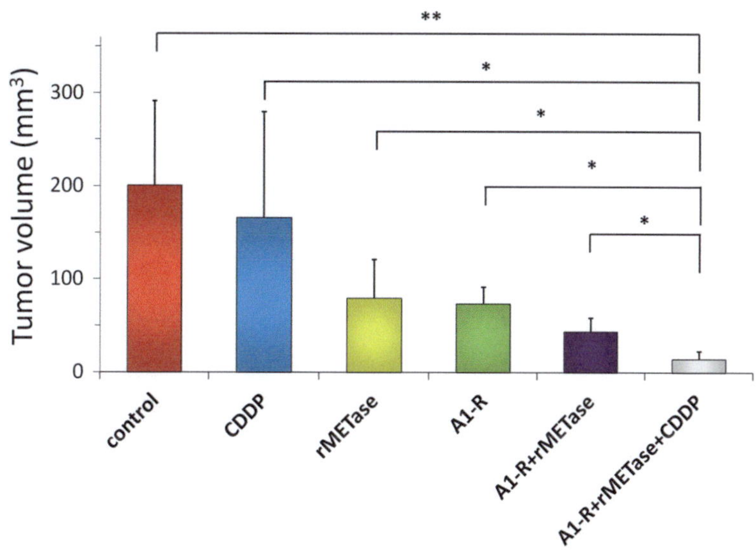

Fig. 3 Quantitative in vivo antitumor efficacy of monotherapy of CDDP, rMETase, *S. typhimurium* A1-R, and their combinations on the lung-metastatic osteosarcoma PDOX. Tumor volume was measured at day 14 at necropsy. $N = 8$ mice/group. *$p < 0.005$, **$p < 0.001$ [6]

appearance similar to the patient's original tumor with hypercellular areas filled with cancer cells displaying nuclear pleomorphism and mitotic figures (Fig. 5b). The PDOX tumor treated with CDDP comprised viable cells without apparent necrosis or inflammatory changes and almost the same features compared to the untreated control (Fig. 5c). The rMETase-treated tumor and *S. typhimurium* A1-R-treated tumor showed changes in sarcoma-cell shape (Fig. 5d, e). The *S. typhimurium* A1-R-combined-with-rMETase-treated tumor showed reduced cellularity (Fig. 5f). The *S. typhimurium* A1-R-combined-with both rMETase- and CDDP-treated tumor showed reduced cellularity and tumor necrosis (Fig. 5g) [6].

Fig. 2 (continued) A1-R treated; PTX treated; *S. typhimurium* A1-R in combination with PTX treated; or treated with the sequential combination of *S. typhimurium* A1-R, rMETase, and PTX. Scale bars, 10 mm. (**c**) Waterfall plot indicating fold change in tumor volume: untreated control; PTX treated; *S. typhimurium* A1-R treated; *S. typhimurium* A1-R in combination with PTX treated; or treated with the sequential combination of *S. typhimurium* A1-R, rMETase, and PTX. (**d**) Representative images of cross sections of FUCCI-expressing MKN45 subcutaneous tumors: untreated control; *S. typhimurium* A1-R treated; PTX treated; *S. typhimurium* A1-R in combination with PTX treated; or treated with the sequential combination of *S. typhimurium* A1-R, rMETase, and PTX [3]

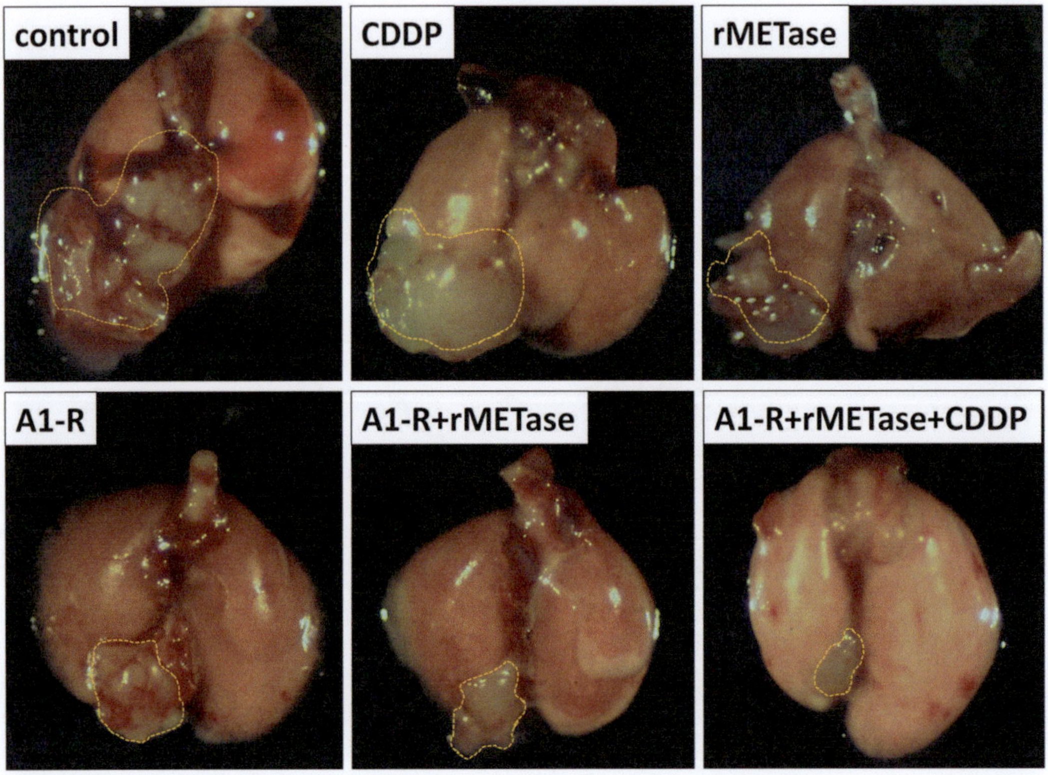

Fig. 4 Representative photos of treated and untreated osteosarcoma lung metastatic PDOX models [6]

5 Notes

1. Previously, different methods of cancer cell synchronization have been used in order to sensitize the cells to chemotherapy. Such methods include chronotherapy which attempts to target the time of day when most cancer cells in tumors are thought to be dividing [15]. Excess thymidine or its analogs have also been used to arrest cancer cells in S phase, where they are sensitized to S-phase drugs such as 5-FU or methotrexate, and after release of the block the cancer cells enter M phase synchronously where they are sensitive to M-phase drugs such as paclitaxel [16–18].
2. The critical advantage of rMETase cell synchronization (trapping) is that, unlike other methods of cancer cell synchronization, it is cancer specific [1, 4, 19–28].
3. A major problem for successful chemotherapy is the very high percentage of quiescent G_0/G_1 cancer cells in a tumor. A solution to the problem is selectively decoying G_1/G_0 cancer cells to cycle with *S. typhimurium* A1-R and then trapping

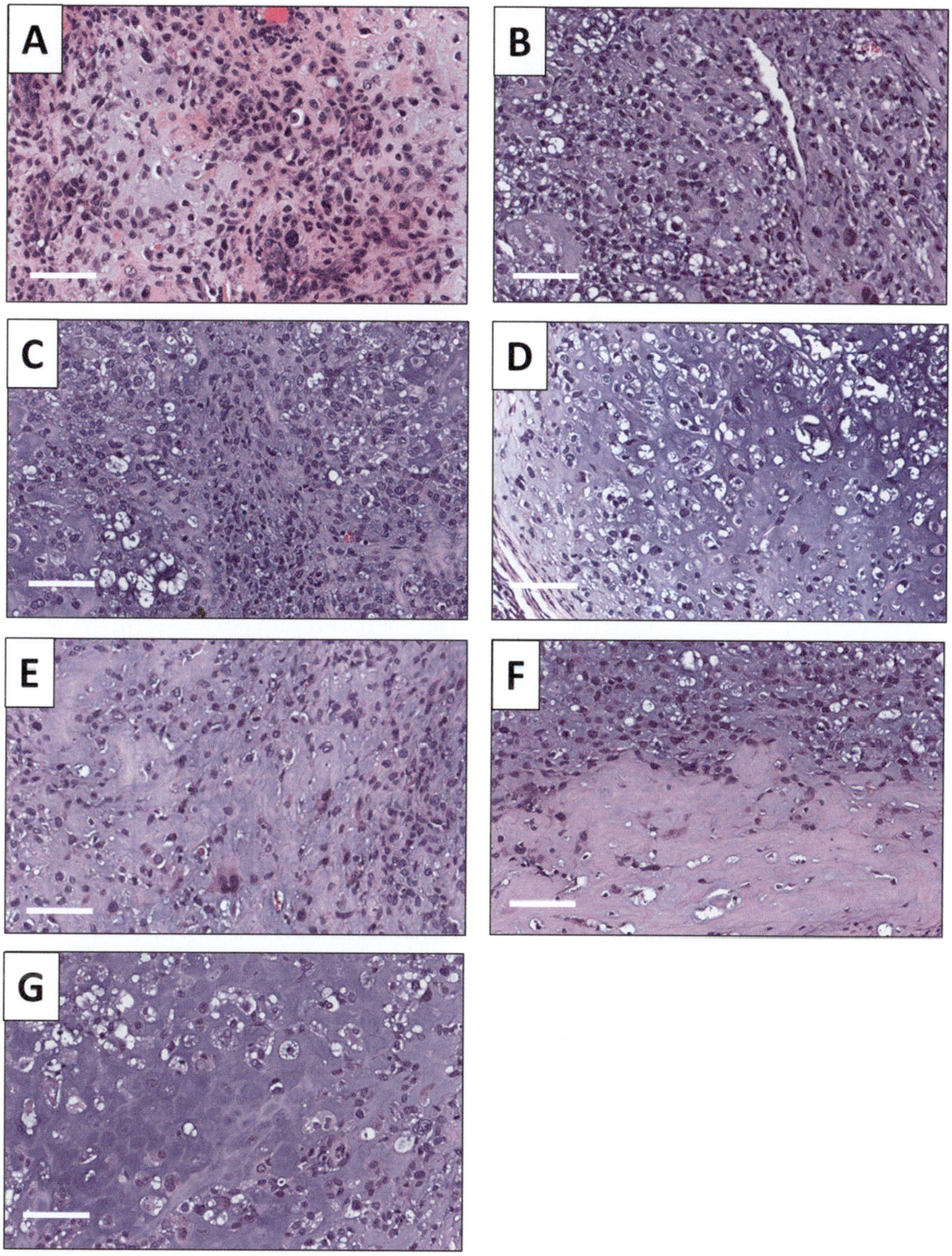

Fig. 5 Effect of treatment on osteosarcoma lung metastasis PDOX tumor histology. (**a**) Hematoxylin and eosin (H&E)-stained section of the original patient lung metastasis. (**b**) Untreated PDOX tumor. (**c**) PDOX tumor treated with CDDP. (**d**) PDOX tumor treated with rMETase. (**e**) PDOX tumor treated with *S. typhimurium* A1-R. (**f**) PDOX tumor treated with *S. typhimurium* A1-R combined with rMETase. (**g**) PDOX tumor treated with *S. typhimurium* A1-R combined with rMETase and CDDP [6]

cancer cells in S/G_2, with rMETase. The S/G_2-trapped cancer cells became sensitive to chemotherapy which targets cells in this phase of the cell cycle. Alternatively, the rMETase-induced S/G_2 block can be lifted and the cells can become sensitive to M-phase drugs, because after the lift of the S/G_2 trap the cancer cells synchronously enter mitosis. This approach has significant clinical potential since almost all cancer cell types tested are MET dependent and arrest in S/G_2 when MET restricted with an agent such as rMETase [2].

4. The PDOX model closely mimics the patient. Toward this goal, our laboratory pioneered the patient-derived orthotopic xenograft (PDOX) nude mouse model with the technique of surgical orthotopic implantation (SOI), including breast [29], ovarian [30], lung [10], cervical [31], colon [32–34], stomach [35], pancreatic [36–41], melanoma [36, 42–47], and sarcoma [6, 9, 48–63]. The PDOX model, developed by our laboratory over the past 30 years, has many advantages over subcutaneous-transplant models which are growing ectopically under the skin. Most importantly the PDOX models can metastasize [64]. The PDOX model enables precise, individualized therapy, especially for recalcitrant diseases [44], by matching the patient tumor to an effective drug identified with the PDOX models.

References

1. Hoffman RM, Jacobsen SJ (1980) Reversible growth arrest in simian virus 40-transformed human fibroblasts. Proc Natl Acad Sci U S A 77:7306–7310
2. Yano S, Li S, Han Q, Tan Y, Bouvet M, Fujiwara T, Hoffman RM (2014) Selective methioninase-induced trap of cancer cells in S/G_2 phase visualized by FUCCI imaging confers chemosensitivity. Oncotarget 5:8729–8736
3. Yano S, Takehara K, Zhao M, Tan Y, Han Q, Li S, Bouvet M, Fujiwara T, Hoffman RM (2016) Tumor-specific cell-cycle decoy by *Salmonella typhimurium* A1-R combined with tumor-selective cell-cycle trap by methioninase overcome tumor intrinsic chemoresistance as visualized by FUCCI imaging. Cell Cycle 15:1715–1723
4. Stern PH, Hoffman RM (1986) Enhanced in vitro selective toxicity of chemotherapeutic agents for human cancer cells based on a metabolic defect. J Natl Cancer Inst 76:629–639
5. Yano S, Zhang Y, Zhao M, Hiroshima Y, Miwa S, Uehara F, Kishimoto H, Tazawa H, Bouvet M, Fujiwara T, Hoffman RM (2014) Tumor-targeting *Salmonella typhimurium* A1-R decoys quiescent cancer cells to cycle as visualized by FUCCI imaging and become sensitive to chemotherapy. Cell Cycle 13:3958–3963
6. Igarashi K, Kawaguchi K, Kiyuna T, Miyake K, Miyake M, Li S, Han Q, Tan Y, Zhao M, Li Y, Nelson SD, Dry SM, Singh AS, Elliott I, Russell TA, Eckhardt MA, Yamamoto N, Hayashi K, Kimura H, Miwa S, Tsuchiya H, Eilber FC, Hoffman RM (2018) Tumor-targeting *S. typhimurium* A1-R combined with recombinant methioninase and cisplatinum eradicates an osteosarcoma cisplatinum-resistant lung metastasis in a patient-derived orthotopic xenograft (PDOX) mouse model: Decoy, trap and kill chemotherapy moves toward the clinic. Cell Cycle 17(6):801–809
7. Yano S, Zhang Y, Miwa S, Tome Y, Hiroshima Y, Uehara F, Yamamoto M, Suetsugu A, Kishimoto H, Tazawa H, Zhao M, Bouvet M, Fujiwara T, Hoffman RM (2014) Spatial-temporal FUCCI imaging of each cell in a tumor demonstrates locational dependence of cell cycle dynamics and chemoresponsiveness. Cell Cycle 13:2110–2119
8. Sakaue-Sawano A, Kurokawa H, Morimura T, Hanyu A, Hama H, Osawa H, Kashiwagi S,

Fukami K, Miyata T, Miyoshi H, Imamura T, Ogawa M, Masai H, Miyawaki A (2008) Visualizing spatiotemporal dynamics of multicellular cell cycle progression. Cell 132:487–498
9. Igarashi K, Murakami T, Kawaguchi K, Kiyuna T, Miyake K, Zhang Y, Nelson SD, Dry SM, Li Y, Yanagawa J, Russell TA, Singh AS, Tsuchiya H, Elliott I, Eilber FC, Hoffman RM (2017) A patient-derived orthotopic xenograft (PDOX) mouse model of an cisplatinum-resistant osteosarcoma lung metastasis that was sensitive to temozolomide and trabectedin: implications for precision oncology. Oncotarget 8:62111–62119
10. Wang X, Fu X, Hoffman RM (1992) A new patient-like metastatic model of human lung cancer constructed orthotopically with intact tissue via thoracotomy in immunodeficient mice. Int J Cancer 51:992–995
11. Zhao M, Yang M, Li XM, Jiang P, Baranov E, Li S, Xu M, Penman S, Hoffman RM (2005) Tumor-targeting bacterial therapy with amino acid auxotrophs of GFP-expressing Salmonella typhimurium. Proc Natl Acad Sci U S A 102:755–760
12. Zhao M, Geller J, Ma H, Yang M, Penman S, Hoffman RM (2007) Monotherapy with a tumor-targeting mutant of Salmonella typhimurium cures orthotopic metastatic mouse models of human prostate cancer. Proc Natl Acad Sci U S A 104:10170–10174
13. Zhao M, Yang M, Ma H, Li X, Tan X, Li S, Yang Z, Hoffman RM (2006) Targeted therapy with a Salmonella typhimurium leucine-arginine auxotroph cures orthotopic human breast tumors in nude mice. Cancer Res 66:7647–7652
14. Tan Y, Xu M, Tan XZ, Tan XY, Wang X, Saikawa Y, Nagahama T, Sun X, Lenz M, Hoffman RM (1997) Overexpression and large-scale production of recombinant L-methionine-α-deamino-γ-mercaptomethane-lyase for novel anticancer therapy. Protein Expr Purif 9:233–245
15. Innominato PF, Roche VP, Palesh OG, Ulusakarya A, Spiegel D, Lévi FA (2014) The circadian timing system in clinical oncology. Ann Med 46:191–207
16. Wang X, Pan L, Mao N, Sun L, Qin X, Yin J (2013) Cell-cycle synchronization reverses Taxol resistance of human ovarian cancer cell lines. Cancer Cell Int 13:77
17. Chandrasekaran B, Kute TE, Duch DS (1995) Synchronization of cells in the S phase of the cell cycle by 3′-azido-3′-deoxythymidine: implications for cell cytotoxicity. Cancer Chemother Pharmacol 35:489–495
18. Kufe DW, Egan EM, Rosowsky A, Ensminger W, Frei E 3rd (1980) Thymidine arrest and synchrony of cellular growth *in vivo*. Cancer Treat Rep 64:1307–1317
19. Hoffman RM (1984) Altered methionine metabolism, DNA methylation and oncogene expression in carcinogenesis: a review and synthesis. Biochim Biophys Acta Reviews Cancer 738:49–87
20. Hoffman RM, Erbe RW (1976) High *in vivo* rates of methionine biosynthesis in transformed human and malignant rat cells auxotrophic for methionine. Proc Natl Acad Sci U S A 73:1523–1527
21. Hoffman RM, Jacobsen SJ, Erbe RW (1978) Reversion to methionine independence by malignant rat and SV40-transformed human fibroblasts. Biochem Biophys Res Commun 82:228–234
22. Hoffman RM, Jacobsen SJ, Erbe RW (1979) Reversion to methionine independence in simian virus 40-transformed human and malignant rat fibroblasts is associated with altered ploidy and altered properties of transformation. Proc Natl Acad Sci U S A 76:I313–I317
23. Coalson DW, Mecham JO, Stem PH, Hoffman RM (1982) Reduced availability of endogenously synthesized methionine for S-adenosylmethionine formation in methionine-dependent cancer cells. Proc Natl Acad Sci U S A 79:4248–4251
24. Stem PH, Mecham JO, Wallace CD, Hoffman RM (1983) Reduced free-methionine in methionine-dependent SV40-transformed human fibroblasts synthesizing apparently normal amounts of methionine. J Cell Physiol 117:9–14
25. Mecham JO, Rowitch D, Wallace CD, Stem PH, Hoffman RM (1983) The metabolic defect of methionine dependence occurs frequently in human tumor cell lines. Biochem Biophys Res Commun 117:429–434
26. Stem PH, Wallace CD, Hoffman RM (1984) Altered methionine metabolism occurs in all members of a set of diverse human tumor cell lines. J Cell Physiol II(9):29–34
27. Stem PH, Hoffman RM (1984) Elevated overall rates of transmethylation in cell lines from diverse human tumors. In Vitro 20:663–670
28. Tan Y, Xu M, Hoffman RM (2010) Broad selective efficacy of recombinant methioninase and polyethylene glycol-modified recombinant methioninase on cancer cells *in vitro*. Anticancer Res 30:1041–1046
29. Fu X, Le P, Hoffman RM (1993) A metastatic-orthotopic transplant nude-mouse model of

human patient breast cancer. Anticancer Res 13:901–904

30. Fu X, Hoffman RM (1993) Human ovarian carcinoma metastatic models constructed in nude mice by orthotopic transplantation of histologically-intact patient specimens. Anticancer Res 13:283–286
31. Hiroshima Y, Zhang Y, Zhang N, Maawy A, Mii S, Yamamoto M, Uehara F, Miwa S, Yano S, Murakami T, Momiyama M, Chishima T, Tanaka K, Ichikawa Y, Bouvet M, Murata T, Endo I, Hoffman RM (2015) Establishment of a patient-derived orthotopic xenograph (PDOX) model of HER-2-positive cervical cancer expressing the clinical metastatic pattern. PLoS One 10:e0117417
32. Fu X, Besterman JM, Monosov A, Hoffman RM (1991) Models of human metastatic colon cancer in nude mice orthotopically constructed by using histologically intact patient specimens. Proc Natl Acad Sci U S A 88:9345–9349
33. Metildi CA, Kaushal S, Luiken GA, Talamini MA, Hoffman RM, Bouvet M (2014) Fluorescently-labeled chimeric anti-CEA antibody improves detection and resection of human colon cancer in a patient-derived orthotopic xenograft (PDOX) nude mouse model. J Surg Oncol 109:451–458
34. Hiroshima Y, Maawy A, Metildi CA, Zhang Y, Uehara F, Miwa S, Yano S, Sato S, Murakami T, Momiyama M, Chishima T, Tanaka K, Bouvet M, Endo I, Hoffman RM (2014) Successful fluorescence-guided surgery on human colon cancer patient-derived orthotopic xenograft mouse models using a fluorophore-conjugated anti-CEA antibody and a portable imaging system. J Laparoendosc Adv Surg Tech A 24:241–247
35. Furukawa T, Kubota T, Watanabe M, Kitajima M, Hoffman RM (1993) Orthotopic transplantation of histologically intact clinical specimens of stomach cancer to nude mice: correlation of metastatic sites in mouse and individual patient donors. Int J Cancer 53:608–612
36. Kawaguchi K, Han Q, Li S, Tan Y, Igarashi K, Miyake K, Kiyuna T, Miyake M, Chmielowski B, Nelson SD, Russell TA, Dry SM, Li Y, Singh AS, Eckardt MA, Unno M, Eilber FC, Hoffman RM (2018) Intra-tumor L-methionine level highly correlates with tumor size in both pancreatic cancer and melanoma patient-derived orthotopic xenograft (PDOX) nude-mouse models. Oncotarget 9:11119–11125
37. Kawaguchi K, Miyake K, Han Q, Li S, Tan Y, Igarashi K, Lwin TM, Higuchi T, Kiyuna T, Miyake M, Oshiro H, Bouvet M, Unno M, Hoffman RM (2018) Targeting altered cancer methionine metabolism with recombinant methioninase (rMETase) overcomes partial gemcitabine-resistance and regresses a patient-derived orthotopic xenograft (PDOX) nude mouse model of pancreatic cancer. Cell Cycle 21:1–6
38. Hiroshima Y, Zhang Y, Murakami T, Maawy A, Miwa S, Yamamoto M, Yano S, Sato S, Momiyama M, Mori R, Matsuyama R, Chishima T, Tanaka K, chikawa Y, Bouvet M, Endo I, Zhao M, Hoffman RM (2014) Efficacy of tumor-targeting *Salmonella typhimurium* A1-R in combination with anti-angiogenesis therapy on a pancreatic cancer patient-derived orthotopic xenograph (PDOX) and cell line mouse models. Oncotarget 5:12346–12357
39. Fu X, Guadagni F, Hoffman RM (1992) A metastatic nude-mouse model of human pancreatic cancer constructed orthotopically with histologically intact patient specimens. Proc Natl Acad Sci U S A 89:5645–5649
40. Hiroshima Y, Maawy A, Zhang Y, Murakami T, Momiyama M, Mori R, Matsuyama R, Katz MH, Fleming JB, Chishima T, Tanaka K, Ichikawa Y, Endo I, Hoffman RM, Bouvet M (2014) Metastatic recurrence in a pancreatic cancer patient derived orthotopic xenograft (PDOX) nude mouse model is inhibited by neoadjuvant chemotherapy in combination with fluorescence-guided surgery with an anti-CA 19–9-conjugated fluorophore. PLoS One 9:e114310
41. Hiroshima Y, Maawy AA, Katz MH, Fleming JB, Bouvet M, Endo I, Hoffman RM (2015) Selective efficacy of zoledronic acid on metastasis in a patient-derived orthotopic xenograph (PDOX) nude-mouse model of human pancreatic cancer. J Surg Oncol 111:311–315
42. Kawaguchi K, Igarashi K, Li S, Han Q, Tan Y, Kiyuna T, Miyake Y, Murakami T, Chmielowski B, Nelson SD, Russell TA, Dry SM, Li Y, Unno M, Eilber FC, Hoffman RM (2017) Combination treatment with recombinant methioninase enables temozolomide to arrest a BRAF V600E melanoma growth in a patient-derived orthotopic xenograft. Oncotarget 8:85516–85525
43. Kawaguchi K, Han Q, Li S, Tan Y, Igarashi K, Kiyuna T, Miyake K, Miyake M, Chmielowski B, Nelson SD, Russell TA, Dry SM, Li Y, Eckhardt MA, Unno M, Eilber FC, Hoffman RM (2018) Targeting methionine with oral recombinant methioninase (o-rMETase) arrests a patient-derived orthotopic xenograft (PDOX) model of BRAF-V600E mutant melanoma: implications for clinical

cancer therapy and prevention. Cell Cycle 17 (3):356–361

44. Kawaguchi K, Murakami T, Chmielowski B, Igarashi K, Kiyuna T, Unno M, Nelson SD, Russell TA, Dry SM, Li Y, Eilber FC, Hoffman RM (2016) Vemurafenib-resistant BRAF-V600E mutated melanoma is regressed by MEK targeting drug trametinib, but not cobimetinib in a patient-derived orthotopic xenograft (PDOX) mouse model. Oncotarget 7:71737–71743
45. Kawaguchi K, Igarashi K, Murakami T, Chmiewloski B, Kiyuna T, Zhao M, Zhang Y, Singh A, Unno M, Nelson SD, Russell T, Dry SM, Li Y, Eilber FC, Hoffman RM (2016) Tumor-targeting *Salmonella typhimurium* A1-R combined with temozolomide regresses malignant melanoma with a BRAF-V600 mutation in a patient-derived orthotopic xenograft (PDOX) model. Oncotarget 7:85929–85936
46. Kawaguchi K, Igarashi K, Murakami T, Zhao M, Zhang Y, Chmielowski B, Kiyuna T, Nelson SD, Russell TA, Dry SM, Li Y, Unno M, Eilber FC, Hoffman RM (2017) Tumor-targeting *Salmonella typhimurium* A1-R sensitizes melanoma with a BRAF-V600E mutation to vemurafenib in a patient-derived orthotopic xenograft (PDOX) nude mouse model. J Cell Biochem 118:2314–2319
47. Yamamoto M, Zhao M, Hiroshima Y, Zhang Y, Shurell E, Eilber FC, Bouvet M, Noda M, Hoffman RM (2016) Efficacy of tumor-targeting *Salmonella typhimurium* A1-R on a melanoma patient-derived orthotopic xenograft (PDOX) nude-mouse model. PLoS One 11:e0160882
48. Murakami T, Li S, Han Q, Tan Y, Kiyuna T, Igarashi K, Kawaguchi K, Hwang HK, Miyaki K, Singh AS, Hiroshima Y, Lwin TM, DeLong JC, Chishima T, Tanaka K, Bouvet M, Endo I, Eilber FC, Hoffman RM (2017) Recombinant methioninase effectively targets a Ewing's sarcoma in a patient-derived orthotopic xenograft (PDOX) nude-mouse model. Oncotarget 8:35630–35638
49. Igarashi K, Kawaguchi K, Li S, Han Q, Tan Y, Murakami T, Kiyuna T, Miyake K, Miyake M, Singh AS, Eckhadt MA, Nelson SD, Russell TA, Dry SM, Li Y, Yamamoto N, Hayashi K, Kimura H, Miwa S, Tsuchiya H, Singh RS, Eilber FC, Hoffman RM (2018) Recombinant methioninase in combination with DOX overcomes first-line DOX resistance in a patient-derived orthotopic xenograft nude-mouse model of undifferentiated spindle-cell sarcoma. Cancer Lett 417:168–173
50. Igarashi K, Li S, Han Q, Tan Y, Kawaguchi K, Murakami T, Kiyuna T, Miyake K, Li Y, Nelson SD, Dry SM, Singh AS, Elliott I, Russell TA, Eckhadt MA, Yamamoto N, Hayashi K, Kimura H, Miwa S, Tsuchiya H, Eilber FC, Hoffman RM (2018) Growth of a doxorubicin-resistant undifferentiated spindle-cell sarcoma PDOX is arrested by metabolic targeting with recombinant methioninase. J Cell Biochem 119:3537–3544
51. Kawaguchi K, Igarashi K, Kiyuna T, Miyake K, Miyake M, Murakami T, Chmielowski B, Nelson SD, Russell TA, Dry SM, Li Y, Singh AS, Unno M, Eilber FC, Hoffman RM (2018) Individualized doxorubicin sensitivity testing of undifferentiated soft tissue sarcoma (USTS) in a patient-derived orthotopic xenograft (PDOX) model demonstrates large differences between patients. Cell Cycle 17(5):627–633
52. Murakami T, DeLong J, Eilber FC, Zhao M, Zhang Y, Zhang N, Singh A, Russell T, Deng S, Reynoso J, Quan C, Hiroshima Y, Matsuyama R, Chishima T, Tanaka K, Bouvet M, Chawla S, Endo I, Hoffman RM (2016) Tumor-targeting *Salmonella typhimurium* A1-R in combination with doxorubicin eradicate soft tissue sarcoma in a patient-derived orthotopic xenograft PDOX model. Oncotarget 7:12783–12790
53. Hiroshima Y, Zhao M, Zhang Y, Zhang N, Maawy A, Murakami T, Mii S, Uehara F, Yamamoto M, Miwa S, Yano S, Momiyama M, Mori R, Matsuyama R, Chishima T, Tanaka K, Ichikawa Y, Bouvet M, Endo I, Hoffman RM (2015) Tumor-targeting *Salmonella typhimurium* A1-R arrests a chemo-resistant patient soft-tissue sarcoma in nude mice. PLoS One 10:e0134324
54. Kiyuna T, Murakami T, Tome Y, Kawaguchi K, Igarashi K, Zhang Y, Zhao M, Li Y, Bouvet M, Kanaya F, Singh A, Dry S, Eilber FC, Hoffman RM (2016) High efficacy of tumor-targeting *Salmonella typhimurium* A1-R on a doxorubicin- and dactolisib-resistant follicular dendritic-cell sarcoma in a patient-derived orthotopic xenograft PDOX nude mouse model. Oncotarget 7:33046–33054
55. Murakami T, Singh AS, Kiyuna T, Dry SM, Li Y, James AW, Igarashi K, Kawaguchi K, DeLong JC, Zhang Y, Hiroshima Y, Russell T, Eckardt MA, Yanagawa J, Federman N, Matsuyama R, Chishima T, Tanaka K, Bouvet M, Endo I, Eilber FC, Hoffman RM (2016) Effective molecular targeting of CDK4/6 and IGF-1R in a rare FUS-ERG fusion CDKN2A-deletion doxorubicin-resistant Ewing's sarcoma in a patient-derived

orthotopic xenograft (PDOX) nude-mouse model. Oncotarget 7:47556–47564

56. Hiroshima Y, Zhang Y, Zhang N, Uehara F, Maawy A, Murakami T, Mii S, Yamamoto M, Miwa S, Yano S, Momiyama M, Mori R, Matsuyama R, Chishima T, Tanaka K, Ichikawa Y, Bouvet M, Endo I, Hoffman RM (2015) Patient-derived orthotopic xenograft (PDOX) nude mouse model of soft-tissue sarcoma more closely mimics the patient behavior in contrast to the subcutaneous ectopic model. Anticancer Res 35:697–701
57. Igarashi K, Kawaguchi K, Kiyuna T, Murakami T, Miwa S, Nelson SD, Dry SM, Li Y, Singh A, Kimura H, Hayashi K, Yamamoto N, Tsuchiya H, Eilber FC, Hoffman RM (2017) Temozolomide combined with irinotecan caused regression in an adult pleomorphic rhabdomyosarcoma patient-derived orthotopic xenograft (PDOX) nude-mouse model. Oncotarget 8:75874–75880
58. Igarashi K, Kawaguchi K, Murakami T, Kiyuna T, Miyake K, Nelson SD, Dry SM, Li Y, Yanagawa J, Russell TA, Singh AS, Yamamoto N, Hayashi K, Kimura H, Miwa S, Tsuchiya H, Eilber FC, Hoffman RM (2017) Intra-arterial administration of tumor-targeting *Salmonella typhimurium* A1-R regresses a cisplatin-resistant relapsed osteosarcoma in a patient-derived orthotopic xenograft (PDOX) mouse model. Cell Cycle 16:1164–1170
59. Murakami T, Kiyuna T, Kawaguchi K, Igarashi K, Singh AS, Hiroshima Y, Zhang Y, Zhao M, Miyake K, Nelson SD, Dry SM, Li Y, DeLong JC, Lwin TM, Chishima T, Tanaka K, Bouvet M, Endo I, Eilber FC, Hoffman RM (2017) The irony of highly-effective bacterial therapy of a patient-derived orthotopic xenograft (PDOX) model of Ewing's sarcoma, which was blocked by Ewing himself 80 years ago. Cell Cycle 16:1046–1052
60. Igarashi K, Kawaguchi K, Murakami T, Kiyuna T, Miyake K, Singh A, Nelson SD, Dry SM, Li Y, Yamamoto N, Hayashi K, Kimura H, Miwa S, Tsuchiya H, Eilber FC, Hoffman RM (2017) High efficacy of pazopanib on an undifferentiated spindle-cell sarcoma resistant to first-line therapy is identified with a patient-derived orthotopic xenograft (PDOX) nude mouse model. J Cell Biochem 118:2739–3743
61. Kiyuna T, Murakami T, Tome Y, Kawaguchi K, Igarashi K, Miyake K, Kanaya F, Singh A, Eilber FC, Hoffman RM (2017) Analysis of stroma labeling during multiple passage of a sarcoma imageable patient-derived orthotopic xenograft (iPDOX) in red fluorescent protein transgenic nude mice. J Cell Biochem 118:3367–3371
62. Igarashi K, Kawaguchi K, Murakami T, Kiyuna T, Miyake K, Yamamoto N, Hayashi K, Kimura H, Nelson SD, Dry SM, Li Y, Singh AS, Miwa S, Odani A, Eilber FC, Tsuchiya H, Hoffman RM (2017) A novel anionic-phosphate-platinum complex effectively targets an undifferentiated pleomorphic sarcoma better than cisplatinum and doxorubicin in a patient-derived orthotopic xenograft (PDOX). Oncotarget 8:63353–63359
63. Miyake K, Murakami T, Kiyuna T, Igarashi K, Kawaguchi K, Miyake M, Li Y, Nelson SD, Dry SM, Bouvet M, Elliott IA, Russell TA, Singh AS, Eckardt MA, Hiroshima Y, Momiyama M, Matsuyama R, Chishima T, Endo I, Eilber FC, Hoffman RM (2017) The combination of temozolomide-irinotecan regresses a doxorubicin-resistant patient-derived orthotopic xenograft (PDOX) nude-mouse model of recurrent Ewing's sarcoma with a *FUS-ERG* fusion and CDKN2A deletion: direction for third-line patient therapy. Oncotarget 8:103129–103136
64. Hoffman RM (2015) Patient-derived orthotopic xenografts: better mimic of metastasis than subcutaneous xenografts. Nat Rev Cancer 15:451–452

Chapter 12

High Efficacy of Recombinant Methioninase on Patient-Derived Orthotopic Xenograft (PDOX) Mouse Models of Cancer

Robert M. Hoffman, Takashi Murakami, Kei Kawaguchi, Kentaro Igarashi, Yuying Tan, Shukuan Li, and Qinghong Han

Abstract

Methionine (MET) is a general target in cancer due to the excess requirement of MET by cancer cells. MET has been effectively restricted by recombinant methioninase (rMETase) in mouse models of cell-line tumors. This chapter reviews the efficacy of rMETase on patient-derived orthotopic xenograft (PDOX) mouse models of human cancer. Ewing's sarcoma is a recalcitrant disease even though development of multimodal therapy has improved patients' outcome. A Ewing's sarcoma was implanted in the right chest wall of nude mice to establish a PDOX model. rMETase effectively reduced tumor growth compared to the untreated control. The MET level both of plasma and supernatants derived from sonicated tumors was lower in the rMETase treatment group. Body weight did not significantly differ at any time points between the two groups. A PDOX nude mouse model of a BRAF V600E-mutant melanoma was established in the chest wall of nude mice and also tested with rMETase in combination with a first-line melanoma drug, temozolomide (TEM). Combination therapy of TEM and rMETase was significantly more efficacious than either monotherapy. The results reviewed in this chapter demonstrate the clinical potential of rMETase.

Key words Methionine dependence, Patient-derived orthotopic xenograft, PDOX, Recombinant methioninase, rMETase, Chemotherapy, Combination

1 Introduction

Methionine (MET) dependence is the enhanced requirement of MET for cancer cells in order to proliferate compared to normal cells. MET dependence may be the only known general and widespread metabolic defect in cancer [1] (*see* **Note 1**).

The elevated MET requirement of cancer cells is possibly due to excessive MET use for aberrant transmethylation reactions [1–5]. The excessive use of MET by cancer cells is observed clinically in [^{11}C]MET PET imaging, where high uptake of [^{11}C]MET results in a very strong and selective tumor signal compared with normal tissue background. [^{11}C]MET is superior to [^{18}F]

Robert M. Hoffman (ed.), *Methionine Dependence of Cancer and Aging: Methods and Protocols*, Methods in Molecular Biology, vol. 1866, https://doi.org/10.1007/978-1-4939-8796-2_12,

fluorodeoxyglucose (FDG) for PET imaging, suggesting that MET dependence is more tumor specific than glucose dependence [6–9].

Ewing's sarcoma is a rare and aggressive malignancy. Previously, a Ewing's sarcoma tumor from the chest wall of a patient with a cyclin-dependent kinase inhibitor 2A/B (CDKN2A/B) loss and FUS-ERG fusion was implanted in the right chest wall of nude mice to establish a patient-derived orthotopic xenograft (PDOX) model. The Ewing's sarcoma PDOX model was sensitive to the CDK4/6 inhibitor, palbociclib, and the IGF-R inhibitor, linsitinib. The PDOX tumor was resistant to first-line therapy doxorubicin (DOX) as was the patient [10] (*see* **Note 2**).

Melanoma becomes a recalcitrant cancer when it metastasizes to regional lymph nodes, with a 5-year survival rate of 29%; and 7% when it metastasizes to organs [11]. There is still no cure for stage III and IV melanoma due to drug resistance, tumor heterogeneity, and an immune-suppressed tumor microenvironment [11–15]. Temozolomide (TEM), an alkylating agent, is first-line chemotherapy for melanoma but with limited efficacy [11–15]. Targeted chemotherapy and immunotherapy are also of limited efficacy in melanoma [11–15]. Melanin may also interfere with therapy [14, 15] (*see* **Note 3**).

L-Methionine α-deamino-γ-mercaptomethane lyase (recombinant methioninase [rMETase, EC 4.4.1.11]) was first used as a cancer therapeutic by Kreis and Hession [16]. METase has since been cloned from *Pseudomona putida* and used as a therapeutic against cell-line mouse models of human cancer [17–20].

MET restriction (MR) therapy, using rMETase, sensitized a human brain tumor cell line to TEM in xenografts in nude mice [18] (*see* **Note 4**).

This chapter reviews the use of rMETase in PDOX models of recalcitrant cancer, such as Ewing's sarcoma and metastatic melanoma.

2 Materials

1. Athymic male *nu/nu* nude mice (AntiCancer Inc., San Diego, CA), 4–6 weeks old.
2. Ketamine mixture: 20 mg/kg ketamine, 15.2 mg/kg xylazine, and 0.48 mg/kg acepromazine maleate (Henry Schein).
3. DEAE Sepharose FF (Pharmacia, Uppsala, Sweden).
4. Sephacryl S-200HR (Pharmacia).
5. ActiClean Etox chromatography columns (Sterogene, Arcadia CA).
6. HPLC (Hitachi L-6200A Intelligent pump; Hitachi, Ltd., Tokyo, Japan).
7. Phosphate-buffered saline (PBS).

8. Protein assay reagent (Bio-Rad, Hercules, CA).
9. U-2000 spectrophotometer (Hitachi, Tokyo, Japan).
10. Bovine serum albumin (BSA).
11. BHS system microscope (Olympus Corp., Tokyo, Japan).
12. INFINITY ANALYZE software (Lumenera Corporation, Ottawa, Canada).
13. SPSS statistics version 21.0 was used for all statistical analyses (IBM, New York City, NY, USA).
14. 6-0 Nylon suture (Ethilon, Ethicon, Inc., NJ, USA).
15. Formalin.
16. Paraffin.
17. Xylene.
18. Ethanol.
19. Hematoxylin and eosin (H&E).
20. Fluoraldehyde reagent.
21. Recombinant L-methionine α-deamens-γ-mercaptomethano-lyase (recombinant methioninase [rMETase, EC 4.4.1.11])
22. HPLC with an L-6200A Intelligent pump or equivalent (Hitachi Ltd., Tokyo, Japan).

2.1 Patient-Derived Ewing's Sarcoma Tumor and Establishment of PDOX

A female patient was diagnosed with metastatic Ewing's sarcoma in the right chest wall. She underwent surgery in the Department of Surgery, University of California, Los Angeles (UCLA). Written informed consent was obtained from the patient, and the Institutional Review Board (IRB) of UCLA approved this experiment [10, 21].

2.2 Patient-Derived Melanoma Tumor and Establishment of PDOX

A 75-year-old female patient was previously diagnosed with a BRAF-V600E melanoma of the right chest wall. The tumor was previously resected in the Department of Surgery, University of California, Los Angeles (UCLA). Written informed consent was provided by the patient, and the Institutional Review Board (IRB) of UCLA approved this experiment [9, 22–24].

3 Methods

3.1 Mice

1. Use athymic male *nu/nu* nude mice (AntiCancer Inc., San Diego, CA), 4–6 weeks old.
2. Conduct all animal studies in accordance with the principals and procedures outlined in the Guide for the Care and Use of Laboratory Animals, eighth edition, under Public Health Service Assurance Number A3873-1.

3. House animals with no more than five per cage and house in a barrier facility on a high-efficiency particulate arrestance (HEPA)-filtered rack under standard conditions of 12-h light/dark cycles.
4. Feed the animals an autoclaved laboratory rodent diet.
5. Perform all mouse surgical procedures and imaging with the animals anesthetized by subcutaneous injection of the ketamine mixture [21].

3.2 Establish PDOX Model of Metastatic Ewing's Sarcoma

1. Anesthetize mice with the ketamine mixture.
2. Make a 7 mm skin incision on the right chest wall.
3. Orthotopically implant a single tumor fragment (4 mm^3) into the layer between the pectoral muscle and intercostal muscle in the right chest wall of nude mice to establish the PDOX model representative of the patient's metastasis [10] and close the wound with a 6-0 suture.

3.3 Establishment of PDOX Model of BRAF V600E Mutant Melanoma

1. Harvest subcutaneously grown melanoma and cut into small fragments (3 mm^3).
2. After nude mice have been anesthetized with the ketamine solution (above), make a 5 mm skin incision on the right chest into the chest wall and split the wall to make space for the melanoma tissue fragment.
3. Orthotopically implant a single tumor fragment into the space to establish the PDOX model that matches the patient's metastasis.
4. Close the wound with a 6-0 nylon suture (Ethilon, Ethicon, Inc., NJ, USA) [9, 22–24].

3.4 rMETase Production

1. Use the pAC-1 rMETase high-expression clone for rMETase production in *E. coli* [25].
2. Ferment host *E. coli* cells as previously described [25].
3. Purify rMETase as previously described: rMETase is purified by three different steps using DEAE Sepharose FF and Sephacryl S-200HR, and ActiClean Etox columns. The latter is designed for eliminating endotoxin [25].

3.5 Treatment Study Design for the Ewing's Sarcoma PDOX

1. Randomize the PDOX mouse models into an rMETase treatment group and an untreated control group when tumor volume reaches 60 mm^3.
2. Administer rMETase (100 units) by intraperitoneal (i.p.) injection, every 24 h for 14 consecutive days.

3.6 Treatment Study Design of the Melanoma PDOX Model

1. Randomize PDOX mouse models into four groups of ten mice each: untreated control ($n = 10$); temozolomide (TEM) (25 mg/kg, oral [p.o.], 14 consecutive days, $n = 10$); rMETase (100 units, intraperitoneal [i.p.], 14 consecutive days, $n = 10$); and TEM + rMETase (TEM: 25 mg/kg, p.o., rMETase: 100 units, i.p., 14 consecutive days, $n = 10$).

3.7 Measurement of Tumor Response to rMETase

1. Measure tumor length, width, and mouse body weight twice a week [21].
2. Calculate tumor volume by the following formula: Tumor volume (mm^3) = length (mm) × width (mm) × width (mm) × 1/2 [21].
3. Define tumor volume ratio as the ratio of tumor volume on each measurement day relative to day 0 [21].

3.8 Measurement of Plasma L-MET Levels

1. Collect 50 μL blood from the retro-orbital plexus with heparinated capillary tubes before treatment and 3, 6, 12, and 24 h after treatment [21].
2. Obtain plasma from blood by centrifugation at 4000 rpm for 5 min [21].
3. Measure plasma L-MET levels with an HPLC after derivatization of serum amino acids with the fluoraldehyde reagent OPA as described previously [25, 26]. Show L-MET levels as the percentage of the initial plasma L-MET level [21].

3.9 Tumor Protein and MET-Level Measurement

1. Place each PDOX tumor in phosphate-buffered saline (PBS) (1 mL) [21].
2. Sonicate tumors on ice for 30 s and subsequently centrifuge at 12,000 rpm for 10 min [21].
3. Dilute supernatants to concentrations ranging from 200 to 1500 μl/mL [21].
4. Prepare protein assay reagent as a fourfold dilution and add to each tube with the sonicated tumor supernatants [21].
5. Measure the absorbance of 595 nm with a spectrophotometer [21].
6. Calculate protein levels from the standard curve obtained by protein standard, bovine serum albumin (BSA) [21].

3.10 Measurement of Tumor L-MET Levels

1. Determine L-MET levels as nmol/mL with the HPLC procedure described above [26].
2. Calculate standardized L-MET levels using the following formula: standardized L-MET level (nmol/mg protein) = L-MET level (nmol/mL)/protein level (mg protein/mL) [21].

3.11 Histological Analysis

1. Fix fresh tumor samples in 10% formalin and embed in paraffin before sectioning and staining.
2. Deparaffin tissue sections (5 μm) in xylene and rehydrate in an ethanol series.

3. Perform hematoxylin and eosin (H&E) staining according to a standard protocol.
4. Perform histological analysis with a BHS system microscope.
5. Acquire images with INFINITY ANALYZE software [10].

3.12 Statistical Analysis

1. Use SPSS statistics version 21.0 for all statistical analyses.
2. Determine significant differences for continuous variables using the Student's *t*-test.
3. Express both line graphs and bar graphs with mean values with an error bar to show standard deviation (SD).
4. Calculate a probability value (P) between the control and treatment groups with $P < 0.05$ considered statistically significant [21].

4 Results

4.1 Established Ewing's Sarcoma PDOX Tumor Recapitulates the Original Patient Tumor

The PDOX tumor in the right chest wall of nude mice histologically recapitulated the original patient tumor [10].

4.2 Ewing's Sarcoma PDOX Tumor Growth Is Suppressed by rMETase Treatment

The tumor volume ratio in the rMETase-treated group was significantly smaller from days 10 to 15 compared to the untreated control mice ($P < 0.05$) (Fig. 1a). Tumor weight was also significantly smaller in the rMETase-treated group (Fig. 1b)

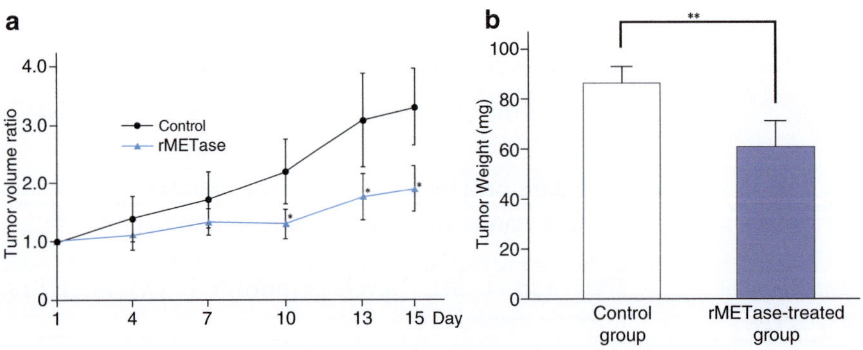

Fig. 1 Response of Ewing's sarcoma PDOX to rMETase. (**a**) Line graph shows tumor volume ratio of both groups. Tumor volume ratios at the indicated times relative to tumor volume at day 0 in the rMETase-treated group was significantly smaller from days 10 to 15 compared to control. (**b**) Bar graph shows resected tumor weight. Tumor weight was also significantly less in the rMETase-treated group than in the control group. **$P < 0.01$, *$P < 0.05$. Error bars: ±1 SD. *SD* standard deviation. $N = 4$ for each group [21]

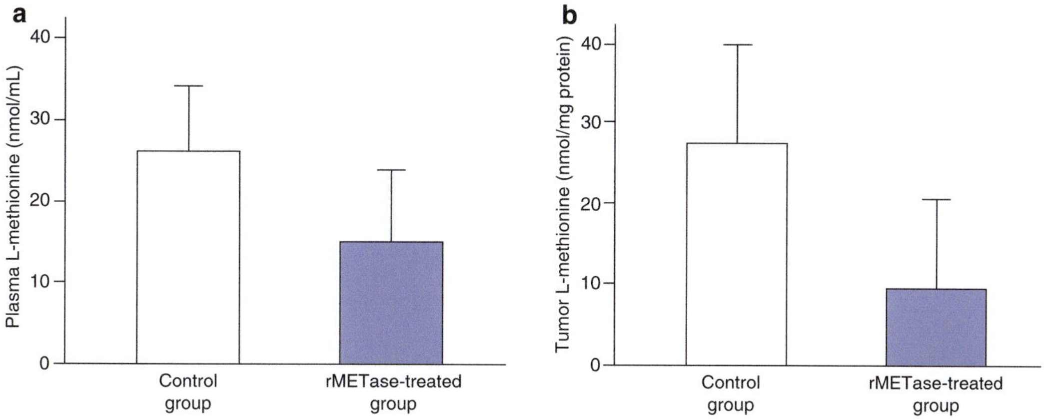

Fig. 2 Plasma and Ewing's sarcoma PDOX tumor L-methionine levels at termination of the experiment. Bar graphs show (**a**) plasma L-methionine level and (**b**) tumor L-methionine level standardized by tumor protein concentration. Both plasma and tumor L-methionine levels in the rMETase-treated animals were lower than the untreated control. Error bars: ±1 SD. $N = 4$ for each group [21]

(60.6 ± 10.6 mg) than in the untreated control group (86.1 ± 6.8 mg) ($P < 0.01$). Mouse body weight was not significantly reduced in the rMETase group [21] (*see* **Notes 1** and **2**).

4.3 Plasma and Tumor L-MET Were Reduced by rMETase in the Ewing's Sarcoma PDOX

Plasma L-MET levels in the rMETase-treated Ewing's sarcoma PDOX (15.0 ± 8.8 nmol/mL) trended to be lower than in the untreated control (26.0 ± 8.1 nmol/mL). L-MET levels were reduced in the rMETase-treated tumors (9.5 ± 11.3 nmol/mg protein) compared to the untreated control tumor (27.5 ± 12.2 nmol/mg protein) (Fig. 2). It should be noted that the MET levels were measured 24 h after the last rMETase administration during which time MET levels could have increased from both endogenous MET synthesis and mouse chow [21].

4.4 Efficacy of rMETase Alone and in Combination with Temozolomide (TEM) in the BRAF V600E-Mutant Melanoma PDOX

Both TEM and rMETase inhibited growth of the BRAF V600E-mutant melanoma PDOX. Combination therapy of TEM and rMETase had significantly better efficacy than either therapy alone (TEM: $p = 0.0051$, rMETase: $p = 0.0051$). There was no significant difference between TEM and rMETase monotherapy ($p = 0.1282$) (Figs. 3 and 4) [9] (*see* **Notes 3–5**).

4.5 Tumor MET Levels in the BRAF V600E-Mutant Melanoma PDOX

Posttreatment MET levels in tumors treated with rMETase alone or along with TEM significantly decreased compared to untreated control ($p < 0.0001$) (Fig. 5). These results showed that the BRAF V600E-mutant melanoma PDOX is MET dependent and rMETase thereby suppresses its growth [9] (*see* **Notes 1–5**).

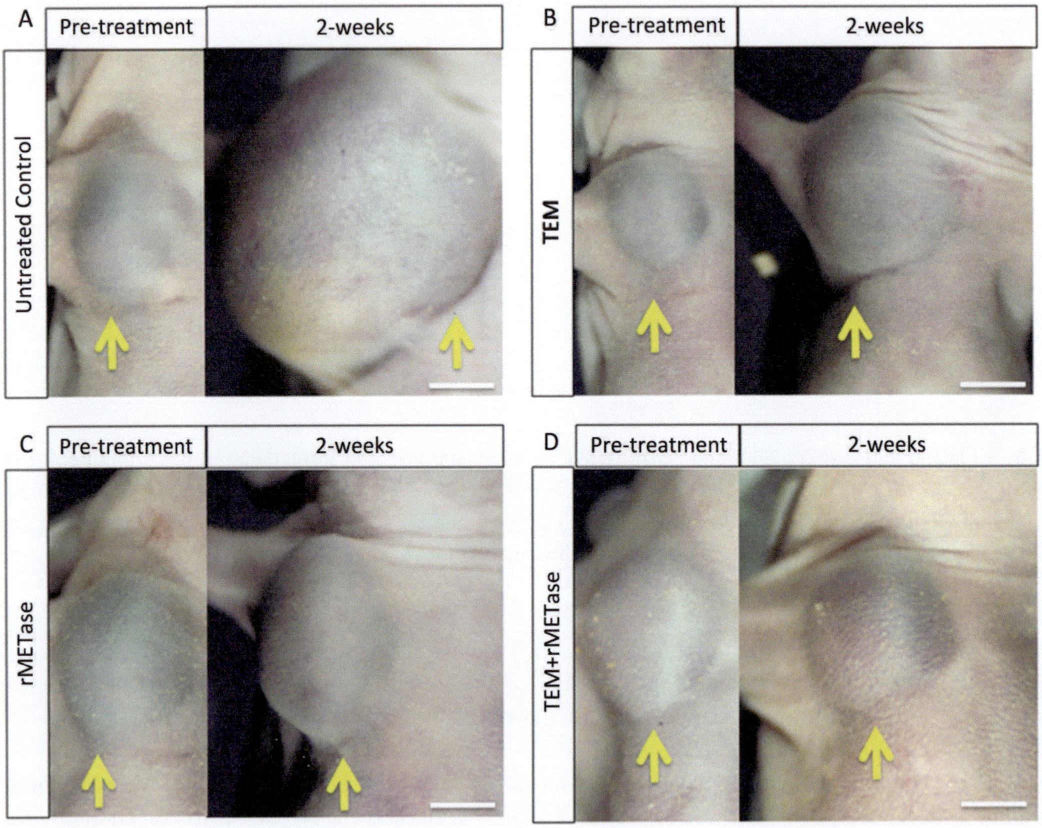

Fig. 3 Macroscopic evaluation of therapeutic efficacy of TEM, rMETase, and their combination on a BRAF V600E-mutant melanoma. (**a**) Tumor in untreated control. (**b**) TEM. (**c**) rMETase. (**d**) Combination of TEM and rMETase. Yellow arrows show PDOX tumor growing on right chest wall. Scale bar: 5 mm [9]

4.6 Effect of rMETase on Body Weight

Body weight loss was observed only in the treatment groups including TEM. rMETase alone did not cause body weight loss. There were no animal deaths in any group [9].

4.7 Effect of rMETase on Tumor Histology

Histologically, the control untreated BRAF V600E-mutant melanoma PDOX tumor mainly comprised viable cells. Epithelioid melanoma cells, devoid of melanin, with a high mitotic index, were observed [24]. In the tumors treated with rMETase only, there were still mitotic figures present indicating that rMETase did not completely arrest the tumor. The same degree of necrosis was observed in tumors treated with TEM and rMETase as monotherapy. Tumors treated with the combination of TEM and rMETase showed extensive necrosis, suggesting that tumor necrosis is a major pathway of tumor growth arrest, but apoptosis may play a role as well (Fig. 6) [9].

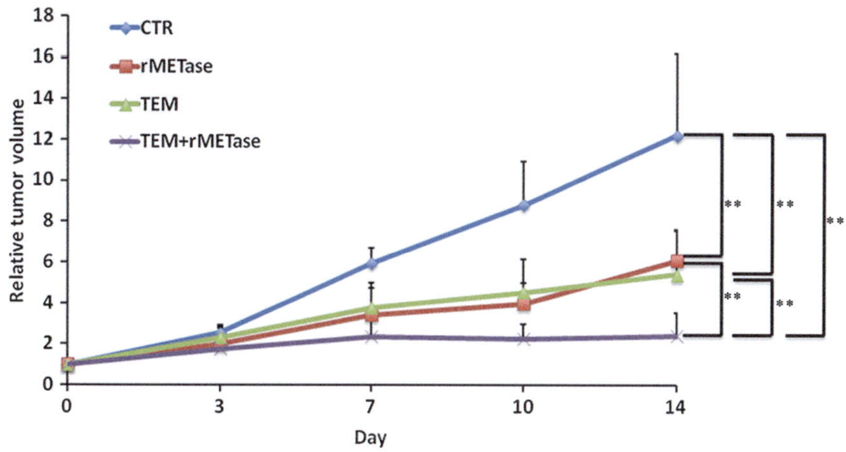

Fig. 4 Time-course treatment efficacy of TEM, rMETase, and their combination in the BRAF V600E-mutant melanoma PDOX. Line graphs show relative tumor volume at each time point relative to the initial tumor volume. All treatments significantly inhibited tumor growth compared to the untreated control (TEM: $p = 0.0081$; rMETase: $p = 0.0037$; TEM-rMETase: $p = 0.0024$). In addition, TEM and rMETase combination therapy was significantly more efficacious than either TEM ($p = 0.0051$) or rMETase ($p = 0.0051$) alone at day 14. There was no significant difference between TEM and rMETase. $^{**}p < 0.01$. Error bars: ±SD [9]

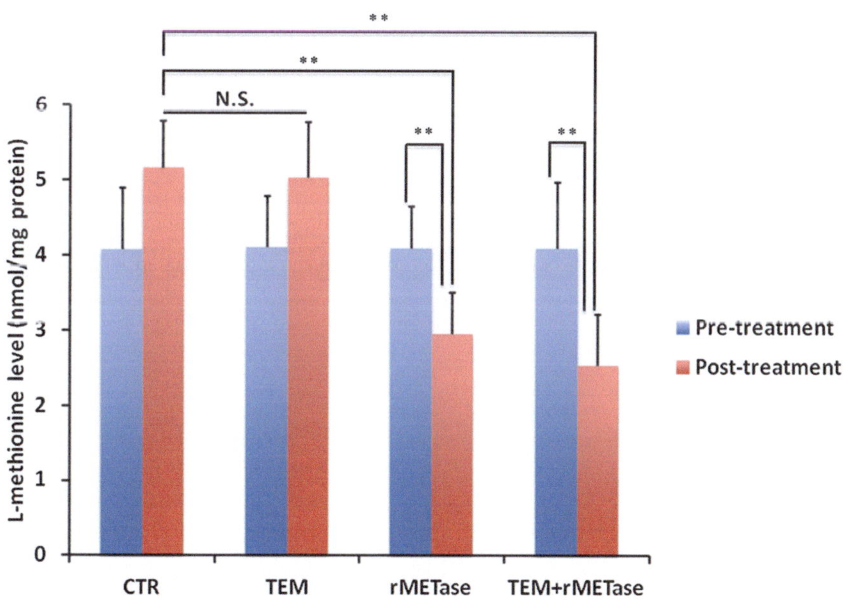

Fig. 5 Intra-tumor MET levels after rMETase or TEM or their combination treatment in the BRAF V600E mutant melanoma PDOX. Bar graphs show MET levels in each treatment group for rMETase or TEM pre- and posttreatment. rMETase or the combination of rMETase and TEM significantly decreased intra-tumor MET levels $^{**}p < 0.01$ [9]

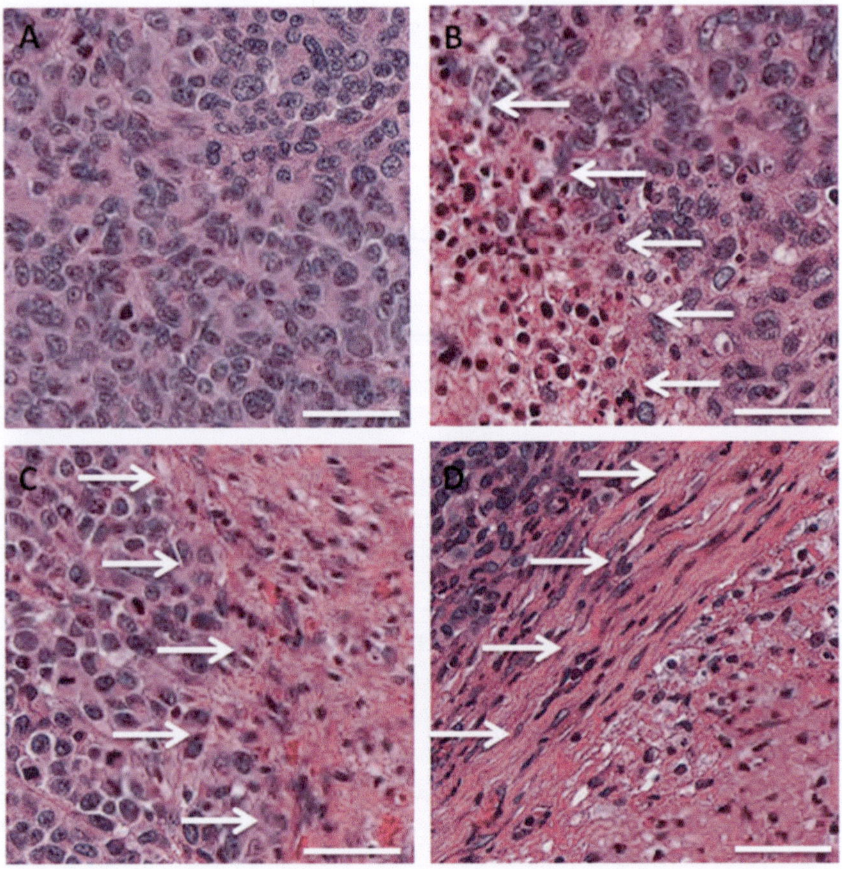

Fig. 6 Tumor histology in untreated and TEM and rMETase-treated BRAF V600E-mutant melanoma PDOX models. (**a**) Untreated control comprised viable cells without obvious necrosis. Epithelioid melanoma cells, devoid of melanin, with a high mitotic index are present. (**b**) Tumor treated with TEM showed partial necrosis. (**c**) Tumor treated with rMETase. Mitotic figures are present, indicating that rMETase did not completely arrest the cell cycle. Tumor treated with rMETase showed partial necrosis similar to TEM. (**d**) Tumor treated with the combination of TEM and rMETase showed extensive necrosis. White arrows: necrotic areas. Scale bars: 50 μm [9]

5 Notes

1. The first hint that MET metabolism is perturbed in cancer came almost 60 years ago when Sugimura et al. [27] observed that rat tumor growth was slowed by giving the rats a defined diet depleted of MET. Approximately 45 years ago, it was observed that L5178Y mouse leukemia cells in culture required very high levels of MET to proliferate [28]. Subsequently, most cancer cell lines were found to be MET dependent [19, 29]. Normal unestablished cell strains grow well under conditions of MET restriction [19].

2. Human patient tumors, including tumors of the colon, breast, ovary, prostate, and a melanoma, were also found to be MET dependent in Gelfoam® histoculture [30].
3. TEM is a first-line chemotherapy for melanoma; however, with limited response rMETase combined with TEM had increased efficacy in the PDOX model of BRAF V600E melanoma, a recalcitrant cancer. We had previously demonstrated that rMETase potentiates TEM in a mouse model of a human glioma cell line [18].
4. Cell cycle analysis demonstrated that cancer cells are arrested in the S/G_2 phases of the cell cycle upon MET restriction [30–34]. This is important for potential efficacy of drugs active against cells in S/G_2.
5. Recently, a paper appeared with the title "The new anticancer era: tumor metabolism targeting" [35]. This "new anticancer era" started in 1959 with the observation of Sugimura et al. [27] that depriving animals of MET arrested tumor growth.

References

1. Hoffman RM (2015) Development of recombinant methioninase to target the general cancer-specific metabolic defect of methionine dependence: a 40-year odyssey. Expert Opin Biol Ther 15:21–31
2. Stern PH, Mecham JO, Wallace CD, Hoffman RM (1983) Reduced free-methionine in methionine-dependent SV40-transformed human fibroblasts synthesizing apparently normal amounts of methionine. J Cell Physiol 117:9–14
3. Stern PH, Wallace CD, Hoffman RM (1984) Altered methionine metabolism occurs in all members of a set of diverse human tumor cell lines. J Cell Physiol 119:29–34
4. Stern PH, Hoffman RM (1984) Elevated overall rates of transmethylation in cell lines from diverse human tumors. In Vitro 20:663–670
5. Coalson DW, Mecham JO, Stern PH, Hoffman RM (1982) Reduced availability of endogenously synthesized methionine for S-adenosylmethionine formation in methionine dependent cancer cells. Proc Natl Acad Sci U S A 79:4248–4251
6. Hoffman RM (2017) The wayward methyl group and the cascade to cancer. Cell Cycle 16:825–829
7. Hoffman RM (2017) Is DNA methylation the new guardian of genome? Mol Cytogenetics 10:11
8. Xu W, Gao L, Shao A, Zheng J, Zhang J (2017) The performance of [^{11}C]-methionine PET in the differential diagnosis of glioma recurrence. Oncotarget 8.91030–91039
9. Kawaguchi K, Igarashi K, Li S, Han Q, Tan Y, Kiyuna T, Miyake Y, Murakami T, Chmielowski B, Nelson SD, Russell TA, Dry SM, Li Y, Unno M, Eilber FC, Hoffman RM (2017) Combination treatment with recombinant methioninase enables temozolomide to arrest a BRAF V600E melanoma growth in a patient-derived orthotopic xenograft. Oncotarget 8:85516–85525
10. Murakami T, Singh AS, Kiyuna T, Dry SM, Li Y, James AW, Igarashi K, Kawaguchi K, DeLong JC, Zhang Y, Hiroshima Y, Russell T, Eckardt MA, Yanagawa J, Federman N, Matsuyama R, Chishima T, Tanaka K, Bouvet M, Endo I, Eilber FC, Hoffman RM (2016) Effective molecular targeting of CDK4/6 and IGF-1R in a rare FUS-ERG fusion CDKN2A-deletion doxorubicin-resistant Ewing's sarcoma in a patient-derived orthotopic xenograft (PDOX) nude-mouse model. Oncotarget 7:47556–47564
11. Chapman PB, Hauschild A, Robert C, Haanen JB, Ascierto P, Larkin J, Dummer R, Garbe C, Testori A, Maio M, Hogg D, Lorigan P, Lebbe C et al (2011) Improved survival with vemurafenib in melanoma with BRAF V600E mutation. N Engl J Med 364:2507–2516
12. Flaherty LE, Othus M, Atkins MB, Tuthill RJ, Thompson JA, Vetto JT, Haluska FG, Pappo AS, Sosman JA, Redman BG, Moon J, Ribas A,

Kirkwood JM, Sondak VK (2014) Southwest Oncology Group S0008: a phase III trial of high-dose interferon Alfa-2b versus cisplatin, vinblastine, and dacarbazine, plus interleukin-2 and interferon in patients with high-risk melanoma--an intergroup study of cancer and leukemia Group B, Children's Oncology Group, Eastern Cooperative Oncology Group, and Southwest Oncology Group. J Clin Oncol 32:3771–3778

13. Tang H, Wang Y, Chlewicki LK, Zhang Y, Guo J, Liang W, Wang J, Wang X, Fu YX (2016) Facilitating T Cell infiltration in tumor microenvironment overcomes resistance to PD-L1 blockade. Cancer Cell 29:285–296
14. Brozyna AA, Jóźwicki W, Roszkowski K, Filipiak J, Slominski AT (2016) Melanin content in melanoma metastases affects the outcome of radiotherapy. Oncotarget 7:17844–17853
15. Slominski AT, Carlson JA (2014) Melanoma resistance: a bright future for academicians and a challenge for patient advocates. Mayo Clin Proc 89:429–433
16. Kreis W, Hession C (1973) Isolation and purification of L-methionine-alpha-deamino-gamma-mercaptomethane-lyase (L-methioninase) from *Clostridium sporogenes.* Cancer Res 33:1862–1865
17. Tan Y, Sun X, Xu M, Tan X-Z, Sasson A, Rashidi B, Han Q, Tan X-Y, Wang X, An Z, Sun F-X, Hoffman RM (1999) Efficacy of recombinant methioninase in combination with cisplatin on human colon tumors in nude mice. Clin Cancer Res 5:2157–2163
18. Kokkinakis DM, Hoffman RM, Frenkel EP, Wick JB, Han Q, Xu M, Tan Y, Schold SC (2001) Synergy between methionine stress and chemotherapy in the treatment of brain tumor xenografts in athymic mice. Cancer Res 61:4017–4023
19. Mecham JO, Rowitch D, Wallace CD, Stern PH, Hoffman RM (1983) The metabolic defect of methionine dependence occurs frequently in human tumor cell lines. Biochem Biophys Res Commun 117:429–434
20. Yoshioka T, Wada T, Uchida N, Maki H, Yoshida H, Ide N, Kasai H, Hojo K, Shono K, Maekawa R, Yagi S, Hoffman RM, Sugita K (1998) Anticancer efficacy *in vivo* and *in vitro*, synergy with 5-fluorouracil, and safety of recombinant methioninase. Cancer Res 58:2583–2587
21. Murakami T, Li S, Han Q, Tan Y, Kiyuna T, Igarashi K, Kawaguchi K, Hwang HK, Miyaki K, Singh AS, Nelson SD, Dry SM, Li Y, Hiroshima Y, Lwin TM, DeLong JC, Chishima T, Tanaka K, Bouvet M, Endo I, Eilber FC, Hoffman RM (2017) Recombinant methioninase effectively targets a Ewing's sarcoma in a patient-derived orthotopic xenograft (PDOX) nude-mouse model. Oncotarget 8:35630–35638
22. Kawaguchi K, Murakami T, Chmielowski B, Igarashi K, Kiyuna T, Unno M, Nelson SD, Russell TA, Dry SM, Li Y, Eilber FC, Hoffman RM (2016) Vemurafenib-resistant BRAF-V600E mutated melanoma is regressed by MEK targeting drug trametinib, but not cobimetinib in a patient-derived orthotopic xenograft (PDOX) mouse model. Oncotarget 7:71737–71743
23. Kawaguchi K, Igarashi K, Murakami T, Chmiewloski B, Kiyuna T, Zhao M, Zhang Y, Singh A, Unno M, Nelson SD, Russell T, Dry SM, Li Y et al (2016) Tumor-targeting *Salmonella typhimurium* A1-R combined with temozolomide regresses malignant melanoma with a BRAF-V600 mutation in a patient-derived orthotopic xenograft (PDOX) model. Oncotarget 7:85929–85936
24. Kawaguchi K, Igarashi K, Murakami T, Zhao M, Zhang Y, Chmielowski B, Kiyuna T, Nelson SD, Russell TA, Dry SM, Li Y, Unno M, Eilber FC, Hoffman RM (2017) Tumor-targeting *Salmonella typhimurium* A1-R sensitizes melanoma with a BRAF-V600E mutation to vemurafenib in a patient-derived orthotopic xenograft (PDOX) nude mouse model. J Cell Biochem 118:2314–2319
25. Tan Y, Xu M, Tan XZ, Tan XY, Wang X, Saikawa Y, Nagahama T, Sun X, Lenz M, Hoffman RM (1997) Overexpression and large-scale production of recombinant L-methionine-α-deamino-γ-mercaptomethane-lyase for novel anticancer therapy. Protein Expr Purif 9:233–245
26. Sun X, Tan Y, Yang Z, Li S, Hoffman RM (2005) A rapid HPLC method for the measurement of ultra-low plasma methionine concentrations applicable to methionine depletion therapy. Anticancer Res 24:59–62
27. Sugimura T, Birnbaum SM, Winitz M, Greenstein JP (1959) Quantitative nutritional studies with water-soluble, chemically defined diets. VIII. The forced feeding of diets each lacking in one essential amino acid. Arch Biochem Biophys 81:448–455
28. Chello PL, Bertino JR (1973) Dependence of 5-methyltetrahydrofolate utilization by

L5178Y murine leukemia cells *in vitro* on the presence of hydroxycobalamin and transcobalamin II. Cancer Res 33:1898–1904

29. Tan Y, Xu M, Hoffman RM (2010) Broad selective efficacy of recombinant methioninase and polyethylene glycol-modified recombinant methioninase on cancer cells *in vitro*. Anticancer Res 30:1041–1046
30. Guo HY, Herrera H, Groce A, Hoffman RM (1993) Expression of the biochemical defect of methionine dependence in fresh patient tumors in primary histoculture. Cancer Res 53:2479–2483
31. Guo H, Lishko VK, Herrera H, Groce A, Kubota T, Hoffman RM (1993) Therapeutic tumor-specific cell cycle block induced by methionine starvation *in vivo*. Cancer Res 53:5676–5679
32. Hoffman RM, Jacobsen SJ (1980) Reversible growth arrest in simian virus 40-transformed human fibroblasts. Proc Natl Acad Sci U S A 77:7306–7310
33. Yano S, Li S, Han Q, Tan Y, Bouvet M, Fujiwara T, Hoffman RM (2014) Selective methioninase-induced trap of cancer cells in S/G_2 phase visualized by FUCCI imaging confers chemosensitivity. Oncotarget 5:8729–8736
34. Yano S, Takehara K, Zhao M, Tan Y, Han Q, Li S, Bouvet M, Fujiwara T, Hoffman RM (2016) Tumor-specific cell-cycle decoy by *Salmonella typhimurium* A1-R combined with tumor-selective cell-cycle trap by methioninase overcome tumor intrinsic chemoresistance as visualized by FUCCI imaging. Cell Cycle 15:1715–1723
35. Borriello A, Della Ragione F (2017) The new anticancer era: tumor metabolism targeting. Cell Cycle 16:310–311

Chapter 13

Total Methionine Restriction Treatment of Cancer

Robert M. Hoffman, Demetrius M. Kokkinakis, and Eugene P. Frenkel

Abstract

This chapter reviews how total methionine (MET) restriction (MR) of a human brain tumor xenograft, effected by the combination of recombinant L-methionine-α-deamino-γ-lyase (rMETase) and a MET-free diet, greatly potentiates standard chemotherapy for brain tumors in mouse models. The growth of human brain tumor Daoy, SWB77, and D-54 xenografts in nude mice was arrested after the depletion of mouse plasma methionine (MET) with a combination of an MR diet and rMETase and homocysteine to rescue normal cells and tissues. MET was depleted to below 5 μm by this treatment. MR for 10–12 days inhibited tumor growth, but did not prevent tumor regrowth after treatment cessation. A single dose of N,N′-bis (2-chloroethyl)-N-nitrosourea (BCNU), which was ineffective alone, was administered at the end of the MR regimen, and caused a more than 80-day growth delay for Daoy and D-54 and a 20-day growth delay for SWB77. The total MR treatment regimens also increased the efficacy of temozolomide (TMZ) against the SWB77 xenograft when administered at the end of the MET regimen.

Key words Cancer, Methionine dependence, Methionine, Homocysteine, Choline, Restriction, Nude mice, Recombinant methioninase, BCNU, Temozolomide, Combination, Rescue

1 Introduction

The prognosis for patients with glioblastoma and anaplastic astrocytoma is very poor [1]. No treatment has been developed that can eradicate glioblastoma which remains after surgery or radiation therapy [2]. Bis-chloroethylnitrosourea (BCNU) [3] has only modest efficacy in patients with anaplastic gliomas [3]. The limited of response appears to be due to mechanisms of resistance [4–6]. Temozolomide (TMZ) has shown promise against astrocytomas and glioblastomas, but efficacy is also limited [7–9].

This chapter reviews the efficacy of MET restriction (MR) on the growth of human brain tumor xenografts in nude mice in combination chemotherapy with first line drugs BCNU and TMZ, compared to chemotherapy alone. MR was achieved by the combination of recombinant L-methionine-α-deamino-γ-lyase (methioninase [rMETase] and an MR diet) [9].

Robert M. Hoffman (ed.), *Methionine Dependence of Cancer and Aging: Methods and Protocols*, Methods in Molecular Biology, vol. 1866, https://doi.org/10.1007/978-1-4939-8796-2_13,

2 Materials

1. Recombinant methioninase (rMETase) (AntiCancer Inc., San Diego, CA).
2. *Escherichia coli.*
3. DEAE-Sepharose (fast flow) (Pharmacia, Uppsala, Sweden).
4. ActiClean Etox (Sterogene, Arcadia, CA).
5. Nude athymic mice (4 weeks old) (AntiCancer Inc., San Diego, CA).
6. Human MET-dependent human glioblastomas cancer cell lines D-54 and SWB77 and MET-dependent human medulloblastoma Daoy cancer cell line.
7. Fetal bovine serum (Life Technologies, Inc., Gaithersburg, MD).
8. Eagle's MEM (Life Technologies, Inc.) supplemented with lysine, valine, MET, and leucine (100 mM each); nonessential amino acids (1:100 dilution of stock from Life Technologies, Inc.); 1 mM sodium pyruvate; 1 μM α-hydroxycobalamin; 10 μM folic acid; and 0.2 mg/mL gentamicin.
9. Lombardi diet without homocysteine (HCY) (diet 518,786) (Dyets, Bethlehem, PA). The DL-HCY, choline-deficient diet (diet 518,763), is referred to as MET(+)HCYS(−)CHOL(−).
10. Diet 518,787 containing 1.7 g/kg HCY and is MET and choline deficient. It is referred to as MET(−)HCY(+)CHOL (−) (Dyets, PA). Diet 518,788 was devoid of MET, HCY, and choline and is referred to as MET(−)HCY(−)CHOL(−) [10].
11. Sephacmyl S-200 HR
12. Basal diet (Teklad Laboratory diet; Harlan, Indianapolis, IN).
13. *N*,*N*′-bis(2-chloroethyl)-*N*-nitrosourea (BCNU).
14. Temozolomide (TMZ).
15. Dimethyl sulfoxide (DMSO).
16. HPLC with a Coularray detector equipped with a four-channel 5010 graphite electrode (ESA, Chelmsford, MA).
17. Tris 2-carboxy-ethyl-phosphine.

3 Methods

3.1 Diets

1. Administer all experimental animals a basal MET-containing Harlan Teklad laboratory mouse diet until they weigh 16–18 g. At that time, inoculate animals s.c. with cancer cells.

2. Switch to the MET(−)HCY(+)CHOL(−) or the MET(−)HCY(−)CHOL(−) diets.
3. Supplement the HCY-free diet with 20 mg/kg daily i.p. injections of HCY to maintain normal tissue function.

3.2 Cancer Cell Lines

1. Grow the human MET-dependent human glioblastoma cancer cell lines D-54 and SWB77 and human medulloblastoma Daoy cancer cell lines in 5% fetal bovine serum in Eagle's MEM supplemented with lysine, valine, MET, and leucine (100 mM each); nonessential amino acids; 1 mM sodium pyruvate; 1 μM α-hydroxycobalamin; 10 μM folic acid; and 0.2 mg/mL gentamicin.

3.3 Drug Treatment

1. Administer rMETase i.p. at a dose of 1500 units/kg every 8 h for 10–12 days in animals receiving MR diets.
2. Administer BCNU i.p. in ethanol in water from a stock solution of 20 mg/mL in anhydrous ethanol.
3. Dissolve TMZ in DMSO and administer i.p. in a volume of 20 mL/m^2.
4. Calculate drug doses as mg/m^2 using the formula $m^2 = weight\ (g)^{2/3} \times K \times 10^{-4}$, where K is 10.5 for mice [11].

3.4 Tumor Implantation and Treatment

1. Inject 3×10^6 D-54, SWB77, or Daoy cells in 200 μL 5% serum media s.c. in the left flank of 6-week-old athymic nude mice weighing between 18 and 20 g. Visible tumors will appear in most of the animals within 3–5 weeks after implantation.
2. Measure the tumors in two perpendicular dimensions and estimate their volumes using the formula $(\alpha^2 \times \beta)/2$, where α is the shorter of the two dimensions and β is the longer of the two dimensions.
3. Administer treatment to animals with tumors ranging between 120 and 160 mm^3, approximately 4–5 weeks after implantation, depending on the tumor.
4. Measure tumor mass every other day or as otherwise indicated until tumor volume exceeds 5× the volume of the tumor at the onset of treatment.
5. Analyze the data using Wilcoxon's rank-sum test.
6. Use T − C where T is the time to reach a designated tumor size is the treated group and C is the time to reach a designated tumor size in the control groups.
7. Score tumor regression as a >10% maintained reduction of original tumor size over three consecutive daily measurements.
8. Define a complete response as the disappearance of measurable tumor mass (<1 mm) at some point within a 12-week period after initiation of treatment. Define a maintained complete

response as no tumor regrowth within 12 weeks of completing the treatment regimen.

9. Evaluate toxicity by animal weight reduction after treatment with MR or MR combined with the chemotherapy drug.
10. Compare tumor regression among groups with the two-tailed Fisher's exact test.
11. Treat experimental groups with (*a*) MR alone, (*b*) MR followed by a single injection of BCNU, or (*c*) MR followed by a single injection of TMZ.
12. Control animal groups include (*a*) animals treated with BCNU alone, (*b*) animals treated with TMZ alone, and (*c*) animals treated with the vehicle (15% ethanol or DMSO) alone. Administers control animals either a MET(+)HCY(−)CHOL(+) or a MET(+)HCY(−)CHOL(−) diet throughout.

3.5 Determination of MET and HCY

1. Determine MET and HCY content in plasma by HPLC with electrochemical detection using a Coularray detector equipped with a four-channel 5010 graphite electrode set at 520, 650, 750, and 850 mV operating potentials according to the following method:
2. Mix 150 μl of plasma with 75 μL of penicillamine (internal standard) and 25 μL 60 mg/ml Tris 2-carboxy-ethyl-phosphine.
3. Cap tubes, vortex for 60 s, and allow to stand for 10 min at room temperature.
4. Cool the samples on ice, and add 500 μL ice-cold 0.3 N perchloric acid.
5. Cap the tubes tightly, vortex for 30 s, and centrifuge for 5 min at 10,000 rpm.
6. Transfer a 100 μL aliquot of the supernatant into an ESA 542 autosampler operating at 5 °C, and inject 20 μL onto an 80 × 4.6 mm ESA HR-80 C-18 3 μm HPLC column equilibrated at 30 °C.
7. Elute the sample isocratically with a mixture of 10% acetonitrile in 0.15 M phosphate buffer (pH 2.9) containing 1.0 mM SDS, HCY, and penicillamine.
8. Elute MET at 5.1, 6.7, and 8.6 min, respectively, and identify and quantitate by the ratios of the detector's response at the operating potentials.

3.6 Histology

1. Harvest fresh tumors and livers from animals in the different dietary groups immediately after sacrifice.
2. Fix in 10% neutral-buffered formalin.

3. After overnight fixation, dehydrate the tissue in graded alcohol solutions to xylene and embed in paraffin. Cut sections (6 μm) from the paraffin blocks on a standard rotary microtome, stain with H&E, and evaluate by light microscopy by an observer blinded to the dietary and treatment status of the animal.

4 Results

4.1 Effect of Dietary MET and Choline Restriction on Mouse Body Weight

The growth rate of the mice did not change when the basal diet was replaced with complete amino-acid synthetic diets. Replacement of dietary MET with HCY in the absence of choline resulted in a slower growth rate. Restriction of MET, choline, and HCY resulted in extensive initial weight loss of 0.9 g/day and death in 10–14 days. When mice fed a MET-, choline-, and HCY-restricted diet were injected i.p. with 20 mg/kg homocysteine (HCY) on a daily basis, weight loss was minimized to 0.2–0.3 g/day for the first 10 days and the mice were alive and healthy for at least 40 days [9] (Table 1).

4.2 Effect of Dietary MET and Choline Restriction on Tumor Growth

None of the tumors, Daoy, D-54, and SWB77, grew in nude mice fed a MR- and choline-restricted diet, even when HCY was supplied either in the diet or i.p. In animals fed synthetic diets containing MET and choline, the tumors grew at rates comparable with those observed in animals fed a basal diet [9].

Table 1
Dietary and pharmacological modulation of MET and total HCY in plasma of athymic mice bearing human medulloblastoma (Daoy) xenografts [9]

Diet/treatment	MET (μM)	HCY (μM)
Basal[a]	60.3 ± 3.4	3.1 ± 0.8[b]
MET(+)HCY(−)CHOL(+)	67.2 ± 3.2	5.7 ± 0.1
MET(+)HCY(−)CHOL(−)	18.5 ± 1.1	7.3 ± 0.8
MET(−)HCY(+)CHOL(−)	24.3 ± 4.3	89.6 ± 13.3
MET(−)HCYS(−)CHOL(−)/HCY[c]	9.0 ± 0.9	5.8 ± 0.8
MET(+)HCY(−)CHOL(−)/rMETase[d]	15.2 ± 2.9	3.0 ± 0.8
MET(−)HCY(+)CHOL(−)/rMETase	15.6 ± 1.3	13.3 ± 3.8
MET(−)HCY(−)CHOL(−)/rMETase+HCYSS	4.3 ± 1.1	7.9 ± 2.1

[a]Diet fed for at least 7 days before determination
[b]Mean of six determinations (animals) ± SD
[c]HCY (20 mg/kg) once per day i.p. (measurement made 8 h after dosing)
[d]rMETase, 1500 units/kg i.p. every 8 h (measurement 4 h after fourth treatment)

4.3 Efficacy of Depletion of Plasma MET on Tumor Growth

Reduction of plasma MET below 5 μM arrested human xenograft growth in athymic mice [10]. To lower plasma MET below 5 μM, it was necessary to restrict dietary MET, HCY, and choline and administer 1500 units of rMETase i.p. every 8 h. HCY, 20 mg/kg once a day i.p., was used as a rescue agent. Supplementing HCY i.p. during administration of the MET(−)HCY(−)CHOL(−) diet did not raise the level of plasma HCY over that of mice fed the MET(+)HCY(−)CHOL(+) diet [9] (*see* **Note 1**).

4.4 Efficacy of MR and BCNU on Daoy Xenografts

Restriction of plasma MET with the combination of dietary MR and rMETase resulted in the arrest of tumor growth of Daoy medulloblastoma xenografts. The tumors continued to regress as long as the animals were treated with rMETase and HCY. However, tumor growth resumed when treatment was discontinued and mice were given a MET-sufficient diet. Treatment with a low dose of BCNU 8 h after discontinuation of MR resulted in a maintained complete response of five of six tumor xenografts. BCNU alone had no effect on the rate of growth of the Daoy xenograft. Tumors that were deprived of MET for 12 days responded to the low dose of BCNU (35 mg/m^2) by further regression and by delayed regrowth for at least a period of 90 days after the initiation of MR (Fig. 1) [9] (*see* **Note 2**).

4.5 Efficacy of MR and BCNU on D-54 Xenografts

MR of D-54 xenografts resulted in a 26-day tumor growth delay. MR combined with a single treatment of 35 mg/m^2 BCNU resulted in a sustained complete response for at least 90 days [9].

4.6 Efficacy of MR and BCNU on SWB77 Xenografts

The combination of MR + BCNU (35 mg/m^2) induced a 20-day tumor growth delay compared with untreated animals and an 18-day delay compared with animals treated with 35 mg/m^2 BCNU [9].

The combination of MR followed by TMZ resulted in a tumor delay of 39 days versus a delay of 11 days for MR alone. TMZ was significantly more effective when combined with MR [9].

4.7 Toxicity of MET Restriction

Only the liver was affected in mice subjected to MR. Hepatocellular lipid accumulation (steatosis) occured in all animals. A 12-day administration of a MET(−)HCY(−)CHOL(−) diet with concomitant treatment with i.p. HCY and rMETase was associated with mild steatosis [9] (Fig. 2) (*see* **Note 3**).

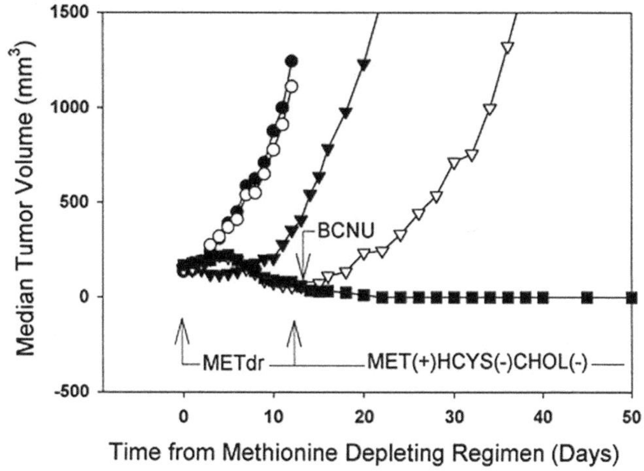

Fig. 1 Effect of a 12-day MET-restriction and subsequent BCNU treatment on the growth of human (Daoy) medulloblastoma xenografts implanted s.c. in athymic mice. The MR animals were fed a MET(−)HCY(−)CHOL(−) diet and treated with 1500 units/kg rMETase i.p. every 8 h and 20 mg/kg HCY i.p. every 24 h. Treatment was initiated when tumors reached a volume of 120–160 mm^3. Animals were given a MET(+)HCY(−)CHOL(−), diet before MR and returned to the same diet after 12 days of treatment. Open circles, untreated controls fed a MET(+)HCYS(−)CHOL(−) diet; filled circles, animals given BCNU (35 mg/m^2) with a MET(+)HCYS(−)CHOL(−) diet throughout; filled triangles, animals given BCNU (65 mg/m^2) with a MET(+)HCY(−)CHOL(−) diet throughout; open triangles, animals on a 12-day MR diet followed by a MET(+)HCY(−)CHOL(−) diet; filled squares, animals on MR followed by a MET(+)HCY(−)CHOL(−) diet + a single treatment with BCNU (35 mg/m^2) administered 8 h after termination of MET restriction [9]

5 Notes

1. Tumor regressions can be induced by reduction of the plasma MET level to a steady state of <5 μM in athymic mice bearing human tumor xenografts [10]. These levels can be achieved with the use of rMETase during restriction of dietary MET, HCY, and choline, combined with the rescue of normal tissue with i.p. HCY.
2. Even when tumor regression was achieved with prolonged MR, discontinuation of MR resulted in tumor regrowth. Therefore, combination of MR with chemotherapy is necessary for complete regression.
3. MR causes liver steatosis, but these changes are diet related and reversible. Thus the reduction of the animal weight during MR regimens is due to nutritional imbalances rather than the toxicity of the regimen.

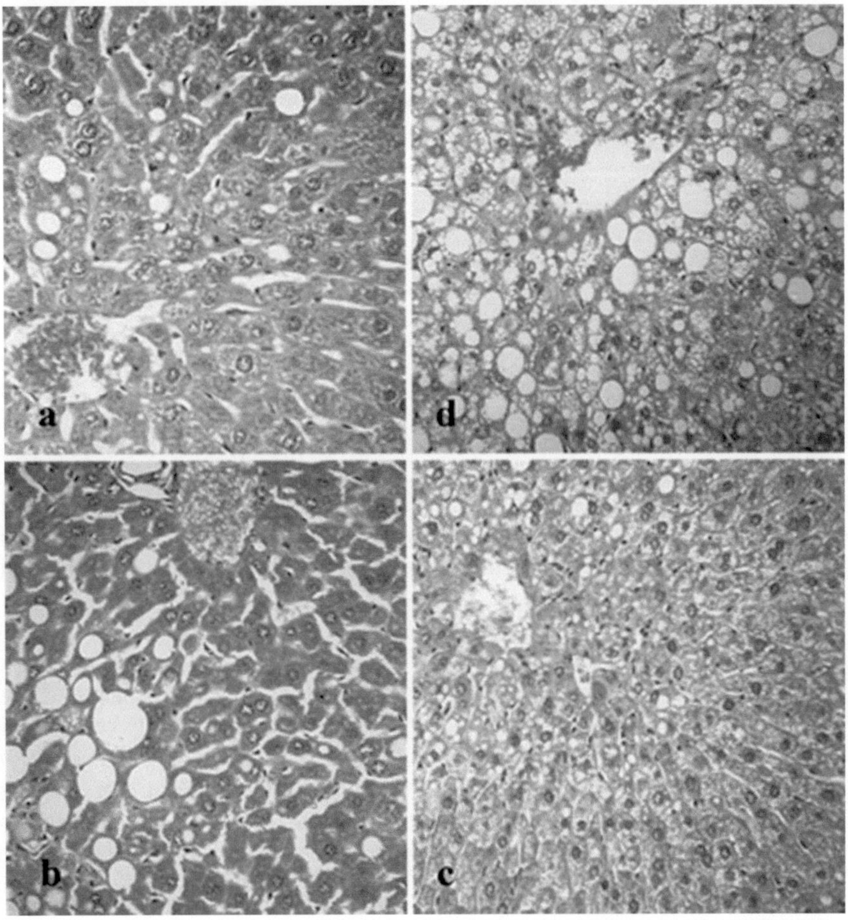

Fig. 2 Toxicity of MR on the liver of athymic mice. (**a**) Liver from an animal maintained on a MET(−)HCY(−)CHOL(−) diet and i.p. HCY (20 mg/kg) daily while on treatment with rMETase for 12 days, demonstrating very mild macrovesicular fat accumulation within hepatocytes (stained with H&E; original magnification, ×150). (**b**) Liver from an animal maintained on a MET(−)HCY(+)CHOL(−) diet while on treatment with rMETase for 12 days, demonstrating the presence of large lipid droplets within hepatocytes, most conspicuously within the mid-zonal region (stained with H&E; original magnification, ×150). (**c**) Liver from an animal initially maintained on a MET(−)HCY(−)CHOL(−) diet + i.p. HCY (20 mg/kg) while on treatment with rMETase for 12 days followed by reintroduction of dietary MET for 10 days reveals a mixed macro- and microvesicular steatosis pattern (stained with H&E; original magnification, ×100). (**d**) Liver from an animal initially maintained on MET(−)HCY(+)CHOL(−) diet while treated with rMETase for 12 days followed by reintroduction of dietary MET for 10 days. A widespread accumulation of small fat droplets (microvesicular steatosis) is present, in addition to the macrovesicular fat noted in MR animals (stained with H&E; original magnification, ×100) [9]

References

1. Wick W, Gorlia T, Bendszus M, Taphoorn M, Sahm F, Harting I, Brandes AA, Taal W, Domont J, Idbaih A, Campone M, Clement PM, Stupp R, Fabbro M, Le Rhun E, Dubois F, Weller M, von Deimling A, Golfinopoulos V, Bromberg JC, Platten M, Klein M, van den Bent MJ (2017) Lomustine and bevacizumab in progressive glioblastoma. N Engl J Med 377:1954–1963

2. Silbergeld DL, Chicoine MR (1997) Isolation and characterization of human malignant glioma cells from histologically normal brain. J Neurosurg 86:525–531
3. Levin VA, Prados MR, Wara WM, Davis RL, Gutin PH, Phillips TL, Lamborn K, Wilson C, B (1995) Radiation therapy and bromodeoxyuridine chemotherapy followed by procarbazine, lomustine, and vincristine chemotherapy for the treatment of anaplastic gliomas. Int J Radiat Oncol Biol Phys 32:75–83
4. Belanich M, Pastor M, Randall T, Guerra D, Kibitel J, Alas L, Li B, Citron M, Wasserman P, White A, Eyre H, Jaeckle K, Schulman S, Rector P, Prados M, Coons S, Shapiro W, Yarosh D (1996) Retrospective study of the correlation between DNA repair protein alkyltransferase and survival of brain tumor patients treated with carmustine. Cancer Res 56:783–788
5. Jaeckle KA, Eyre HJ, Townsend JJ, Schulman S, Knudson HM, Belanich M, Yarosh DB, Bearman SI, Giroux DJ, Schold SC (1998) Correlation of tumor O6-methylguanine-DNA methyltransferase levels with survival of malignant astrocytoma patients treated with bis-chloroethylnitrosourea: a Southwest Oncology Group study. J Clin Oncol 16:3310–3315
6. Pegg AE, Dolan ME, Moschel RC (1995) Structure, function, and inhibition of O6-alkylguanine-DNA alkyltransferase. Prog Nucleic Acid Res Mol Biol 51:167–223
7. Yung WK, Prados MD, Yaya-Tur R, Rosenfeld SS, Brada M, Friedman HS, Albright R, Olson J, Chang SM, O'Neill AM, Friedman AH, Bruner J, Yue N, Dugan M, Zaknoen S, Levin VA (1999) Multicenter Phase II trial of temozolomide in patients with anaplastic astrocytoma or anaplastic oligoastrocytoma at first relapse. J Clin Oncol 17:2762–2771
8. Bower M, Newlands ES, Bleehen NM, Brada M, Begent RJ, Calvert H, Colquhoun I, Lewis P, Brampton MH (1997) Multicentre CRC Phase II trial of temozolomide in recurrent or progressive high-grade glioma. Cancer Chemother Pharmacol 40:484–488
9. Kokkinakis DM, Hoffman RM, Frenkel EP, Wick JB, Han Q, Xu M, Tan Y, Schold SC (2001) Synergy between methionine stress and chemotherapy in the treatment of brain tumor xenografts in athymic mice. Cancer Res 61:4017–4023
10. Kokkinakis DM, Schold SC Jr, Hori H, Nobori T (1997) Effect of long-term depletion of plasma methionine on the growth and survival of human brain tumor xenografts in athymic mice. Nutr Cancer 29:195–204
11. Hawks CT, Leary SL (1995) Formulary for laboratory animals. Iowa State University Press, Ames, IA

Chapter 14

Methioninase Gene Therapy

Robert M. Hoffman, Kenji Miki, Waddah Al-Refaie, Mingxu Xu, and Yuying Tan

Abstract

Recombinant methioninase (rMETase) derived from *Pseudomonas putida* targets the elevated methionine (MET) requirement of cancer cells (methionine dependence) and has shown efficacy against a variety of cancer types in mouse models. To enhance the efficacy of rMETase, we constructed the pLGFP-METSN retrovirus encoding the *P. putida* methioninase (METase) gene fused with the green fluorescent protein (GFP) gene. pLGFP-METSN or control vector pLGFPSN was introduced into the human lung cancer cell line H460. The retrovirus-mediated METase gene transfer decreased the intracellular MET level of the cancer cells and consequently enhanced the efficacy of treatment with the rMETase protein. The rMETase gene was introduced into an adenovirus. rAd-METase transduction of human OVACAR-8 ovarian cancer cells and human fibrosarcoma HT1080 cells in vitro and in vivo resulted in high levels of METase expression up to 10% or more of the total protein of the cells, depending on the multiplicity of infection. The combination of rAd-METase and rMETase was synergistic to kill these cells. Normal fibroblasts, on the other hand, appeared relatively resistant to the METase gene in the presence of rMETase. Adenoviral METase-transduced cancer cells were used in combination with selenomethionine, releasing highly toxic methylselenol, which killed both the cancer cells containing the METase gene and bystanders. Methylselenol damaged the mitochondria via oxidative stress and caused cytochrome c release into the cytosol, thereby activating the caspase cascade and cancer-cell apoptosis. Adenoviral METase-gene/SeMET treatment also inhibited tumor growth in rodents and significantly prolonged their survival. AdMETase/SeMET therapy was effective against Bcl-2-overproducing A549 lung cancer cells, which were resistant to staurosporine-induced apoptosis, with a strong bystander effect. The combination of Ad-METase/SeMET and doxorubicin (DOX) delayed the growth of the H460 human lung cancer, growing subcutaneously in nude mice. These results demonstrate the potential of methionine restriction (MR) for cancer treatment.

Key words Cancer, Methionine dependence, Gene cloning, Methioninase, Adenovirus, GFP, Gene therapy, Selenomethionine, Prodrug, Methylselenol, By-stander effect

1 Introduction

There have been several therapeutic strategies to target the methionine (MET) dependence of cancer cells. MET starvation therapy such as with a methionine-restricted (MR) diet or MR total parenteral nutrition prolonged the survival time of tumor-bearing

Robert M. Hoffman (ed.), *Methionine Dependence of Cancer and Aging: Methods and Protocols*, Methods in Molecular Biology, vol. 1866, https://doi.org/10.1007/978-1-4939-8796-2_14, © Springer Science+Business Media, LLC, part of Springer Nature 2019

rodents [1–3]. MR total parenteral nutrition in combination with chemotherapeutic drugs showed preliminary evidence that MR enhanced the activity of chemotherapy of patients with high-stage gastric cancer [4]. Recombinant methioninase (rMETase), cloned from *Pseudomonas putida* [5, 6], which degrades methionine to α-ketobutyrate, ammonia, and methanethiol, has antitumor efficacy in vitro and in vivo [7, 8]. rMETase has synergistic efficacy in combination with 5-fluorouracil [7] and cisplatinum [8] on rodent and human tumors in mouse models.

rMETase was also highly effective on human cell-line-derived orthotopic mouse models of colon cancer and brain cancer [7–9] and in patient-derived orthotopic xenograft (PDOX) models of cancer [10–12].

We have introduced the *P. putida methioninase* (*METase*) gene into a retroviral vector [13]. To increase the *METase* gene transduction efficiency, we have constructed a recombinant adenoviral vector with the *METase* gene (rAdMETase).

We determined the synergistic efficacy of the combination of rAd-METase and exogenous administration of rMETase on human ovarian cancer cells and human fibrosarcoma cells compared with the efficacy of the combination on normal fibroblasts in vitro [13].

We have taken advantage of the production of methylselenol from selenomethionine (SeMET) by the *METase* gene product to design a gene-directed enzyme prodrug therapy system for cancer [14].

We also determined the efficacy of the combination of both DOX and Ad-METase/SeMET on cancer cells [15].

We also determined the potential of rAdMETase/SeMET therapy against Bcl-2-overproducing cancer cells which are apoptosis resistant [16].

2 Materials

1. Doxorubicin (DOX) (Sigma, St. Louis, MO).
2. Selenomethionine (SeMET) (Sigma, St. Louis, MO).
3. Phosphate-buffered saline (PBS).
4. Athymic nude mice (male) (AntiCancer Inc., San Diego, CA).
5. Recombinant adenovirus rAdMETase, in which the *METase* gene is driven by the CMV-5 promoter and enhancer.
6. Human non-small cell lung adenocarcinoma cell line H460.
7. N1S1 rat hepatoma tumor cells.
8. RPMI 1640 with 10% fetal bovine serum (FBS).
9. 100 U/mL Penicillin.

10. 100 mg/mL streptomycin.
11. NIH-3T3-based amphotropic retroviral, packaging cell line PT67.
12. Dulbecco's modified Eagle's medium (DME) with 10% FBS.
13. Balb/c nude mice.
14. Animal diets (Harlan Teklad, Madison, WI).
15. RPMI 1640 medium with 10% fetal bovine sera (FBS), 100 U/mL penicillin, and 100 mg/mL streptomycin.
16. *Nhe*I.
17. *Hpa*I.
18. DOTAP (Boehringer Mannheim, Mannheim, Germany).
19. Dimethylsulfoxide.
20. 293A cells (Quantum, Montreal, Canada)
21. AdCMV5GFPΔE1/ΔE3 (Quantum).
22. Sephadex G25 column (Amersham Pharmacia Biotech, Piscataway, NJ).
23. DEAE Sepharose FF column (Amersham Pharmacia).
24. HPLC.
25. OVCAR-8 cells (AntiCancer Inc.).
26. Bcl-2 cDNA.
27. Lipofectamine (Gibco BRL Life Technologies, Rockville, MD).
28. Bcl-2 retroviruses.
29. G-418.
30. Cell Fractionation Kit (Clontech, Palo Alto, CA).
31. Nitrocellulose membranes (Amersham Life Science).
32. 7% Powdered nonfat milk
33. Tris SDS gels (Invitrogen, Carlsbad, CA).
34. Quantikine human cytochrome *c* kit (Alexis, San Diego, CA).
35. Staurosporine (Alexis, San Diego, CA).
36. Chamber slides (Nalge Nunc International, Naperville, IL).
37. Selenomethionine (SeMET).
38. Hoechst 33258 (Sigma).
39. Model BH-2 fluorescence microscope (Olympus, Tokyo, Japan).
40. G418 (Life Technologies, Grand Island, NY).
41. Supercosil LC-18-DB (Supelco, Bellefonte, PA).
42. Fluorescence F1000 spectrophotometer (Hitachi, Tokyo, Japan).

43. Benchmark Microplate Reader (BioRad Laboratories, Hercules, CA).
44. pGFP-1 (Clontech).
45. pAC-1 rMETase plasmid (AntiCancer Inc.).
46. pGFPC-3 (Clontech) plasmid vector.
47. pLXSN (Clontech).
48. pQBI-AdCMV5GFP (Quantum).
49. *Cla*I (Quantum).
50. SeaPlaque agarose (FMC BioProducts, Rockland, ME).
51. Lowry Reagent kit (Sigma Chemical Co., St. Louis, MO).
52. SDS-PAGE (Novex, San Diego, CA).
53. Coomassie Brilliant Blue R.
54. pLXIN-Bcl-2 and pVSV-G vectors (Clontech, Palo Alto, CA),
55. GP-293 retroviral packaging cells (Clontech, Palo Alto, CA).
56. Type-B pestle (Fisher, Pittsburgh, PA).
57. (Microfuge® 18) centrifuge (Beckman).
58. U-2000 spectrophotometer (Hitachi).
59. Rabbit polyclonal primary antibody against Bcl-2 (Santa Cruz Biotechnology, Santa Cruz, CA).
60. Donkey anti-rabbit secondary antibody (Amersham).
61. Chemiluminescence reagent ECL + Plus (Amersham).
62. Cytochrome *c* (BD Biosciences Clontech, Palo Alto, CA).
63. Bcl-2 ELISA kit (R&D Systems Inc., Minneapolis, MN).
64. Microplate Manager-4.0 PC Data Analysis software (Bio-Rad Laboratories).
65. O-phthaldialdehyde (OPA).
66. 3-(4,5-dimethylthiazol-2-yl)-2,5-dimethyltetrazolium bromide (MTT) Sigma.
67. Microplate reader (Benchmark).
68. Lowry protein reagent kit.
69. Doxorubicin (DOX).
70. ELISA kit for Bcl-2 and Cytochrome C.
71. Staurosporine.
72. Hoechst 33258 DNA strain.
73. Ampicillin (Sigma).
74. Mitosensor dye (Clontech).

3 Methods

3.1 Cell Lines

1. Maintain cancer cell lines in RPMI 1640 with 10% fetal bovine sera (FBS), 100 U/mL penicillin, and 100 mg/mL streptomycin.
2. Maintain the NIH-3T3-based amphotropic retroviral packaging cell line PT67 in Dulbecco's modified Eagle's medium with 10% FBS, 100 U/mL penicillin and, 100 mg/mL streptomycin [13].

3.2 Plasmid Construction

1. Construct pLGFP-METSN and pLGFPSN, which are both based on the pLXSN plasmid.
2. Generate pLGFP-METSN by inserting the GFP-METase gene, which is a fusion of the jellyfish *Aequorea victoria* green fluorescent protein (GFP) with the METase gene derived from *P. putida* [5].
3. Amplify the METase gene with the polymerase chain reaction using the pAC-1 rMETase gene clone [5] as a template and two oligonucleotide primers:

   59-CCGCTCGAGATGCACGGCTCCAACAAGCTCCCA-39 and 59-CGCGGATCCTTAGGCACTCGCCTTGAGTG CCTG-39 [13].
4. Ligate the 1.2 kb METase DNA into the pGFPC-3 plasmid vector downstream of the GFP gene at the *Xho*I/*Bam*HI site.
5. Digest the resulting plasmid with *Nhe*I and then digest with *Bam*HI.
6. Digest the retroviral expression vector pLXSN with *Hpa*I, blunt-ended, and then digest with *Bam*HI.
7. Ligate the GFP-METase cassette into pLXSN at the blunt-ended *Hpa*I and *Bam*HI site [13].
8. Drive the GFP-METase gene with the Moloney murine leukemia virus long terminal repeat. Drive the neomycin-resistance gene with the simian virus 40 early promoter gene.
9. Construct pLGFPSN by inserting the GFP gene purified from pGFP-1 into the pLXSN retroviral vector [13].

3.3 Retrovirus Preparation

1. Culture PT67 cells in Dulbecco's modified Eagle's medium supplemented with 10% FBS, 100 U/ml penicillin and 100 mg/ml streptomycin.
2. For retroviral vector production, transfect packaging cells at 70% confluence in 6-well culture dishes and transfect using DOTAP liposomal reagent containing saturating amounts of pLGFPSN or pLGFP-METSN plasmid.

3. After 18 h of incubation, replace the culture medium with fresh medium. For the selection of stable virus-producing cells, culture the cells in the presence of 0.8 mg/mL G418 at 2 days post-transfection for an additional 2 weeks [13].

3.4 Retroviral Transduction of H460 Cells

1. Expose H460 cells to PT67/pLGFP-METSN or pLGFPSN supernatants at a 1:1 ratio of RPMI 1640 medium containing 10% FBS in the presence of 8 mg polybrene for 12 h.
2. Maintain the cells in fresh RPMI 1640 containing 400 mg/mL G418 to select for transduced cells.
3. Monitor the expression level of both vectors by GFP fluorescence.
4. Isolate the high-expression clones with each vector using cloning cylinders and amplify for further experiments [13].

3.5 Methionine Levels in Cancer Cells

1. Determine the methionine level in the cell lysates of amino acids with the fluorescent reagent *O*-phthaldialdehyde (OPA) [17, 18].
2. Precipitate the cell lysate (200 mL) with acetonitrile (800 mL).
3. Mix a total of 10 mL supernatant with 5 mL OPA.
4. After 1 min, add 50 mL 0.1 M sodium acetate (pH 7.0), and load 20 mL sample on a reversed-phase Supercosil LC-18-DB column at room temperature.
5. Resolve the amino acid derivatives with solution A (tetrahydrofuran/methanol/0.1 M sodium acetate (pH 7.2): 5/95/900) and solution B (methanol).
6. Run a gradient from 20 to 60% at a flow rate of 1.5 mL/min.
7. Read the eluate with a fluorescence spectrophotometer at 350–450 nm [13].

3.6 Production of rMETase

1. Use the pAC-1 rMETase high-expression clone, derived from *P. putida*, for the production of rMETase in host *Escherichia coli* cells [5].
2. Construct pAC-1 with the pT7-7 vector containing the T7 RNA polymerase promoter for high expression of the *rMETase* gene in *E. coli* [5].
3. Purify rMETase with a DEAE Sepharose FF column. The rMETase was 98% pure upon HPLC analysis and a single band of M_r 43,000 on SDS-PAGE. The specific activity was ~20 units/mg protein [13].

3.7 In Vitro Efficacy of rMETase

1. Use the 3-(4,5-dimethylthiazol-2-yl)-2,5-dimethyltetrazolium bromide (MTT) assay [19] to determine the in vitro growth inhibition of cancer cells treated with rMETase.

2. Plate cells (2000 cells/well) in 96-well culture plates in 100 mL culture medium.
3. After 24 h, add various concentrations of rMETase to the wells.
4. After 3 days incubation with rMETase, measure cytotoxicity with the MTT assay.
5. Use MTT at a concentration of 0.2 mg/mL.
6. Solubilize the resulting formazan product in dimethyl sulfoxide and measure absorbance at 540 nm in a microplate reader using plastic spectrophotometer cells.
7. Express growth inhibition as the percentage of absorbance of treated cultures with respect to untreated cells.
8. Measure the resulting formazan product in dimethyl sulfoxide and absorbance at 540 nm in a microplate reader using 1 cm path length plastic spectrophotometer cells.
9. Express growth inhibition as the percentage of absorbance of treated cultures with respect to untreated cells [13].

3.8 In Vivo Evaluation of the Efficacy of the METase Gene

1. Implant tumor fragments (1 mm in diameter) derived from H460-GFP or H460-GFP-MET tumors growing subcutaneously in nude mice using surgical orthotopic implantation (SOI) into the left lungs of nude mice [20, 21].
2. Administer 100 U rMETase intraperitoneally twice a day from days 2 to 13 post-operation.
3. Choose 4–5 mice in each group and sacrifice.
4. Measure the primary tumor weights and evaluate the incidence of metastasis in relevant organs under fluorescence microscopy of fresh tissue.
5. Determine the statistical significance for tumor weights with the Student's *t*-test.
6. Monitor the remaining 10–12 mice in each group for survival.
7. Compare differences in survival at 30 days.
8. Analyze the overall survival with the log-rank test [13].

3.9 Construction of METase-Expressing rAd

1. Amplify the *METase* gene cloned from *P. putida* [22] by the PCR using the pAC-1 rMETase plasmid [5] as a template and two oligonucleotide primers, 5′-GGAAGATCTATGCACGGCTCCAACAAGCTCCCA-3′ and 5′-CGCGGATCCTTAGGCACTCGCCTTGAGTGCCTG-3′.
2. Ligate the 1.2 kb *METase* gene into the transfer vector pQBI-AdCMV5GFP downstream of the CMV-5 promoter at the *Bgl*II/*Pme*I site.

3. In the resulting pQBI-AdCMV5 MET-CMVGFP shuttle vector, drive the *METase* gene and *GFP* gene with the CMV-5 promoter and CMV promoter, respectively.
4. Co-transfect shuttle vectors into 293A cells using the calcium phosphate method [23] along with the AdCMVLacZΔE1/ΔE3 viral DNA cut with *Cla*I [13].
5. Overlay transfected cells with 1.25% SeaPlaque agarose and incubate at 37 °C for 14–21 days.
6. Isolate primary plaques and use them to infect 293A cells to generate a primary crude viral lysate.
7. Confirm *METase* gene expression in the viral lysate with a METase activity assay [22].
8. After a second plaque purification, amplify a single plaque in 293A cells. Use AdCMV5GFPΔE1/ΔE3 as a control vector (control-rAd).
9. Expand rAds in 293A cells, and purify by CsCl gradient centrifugation and subsequent fractionation on a Sephadex G25 column [13].

3.10 Cells and Cell Culture

1. Maintain OVCAR-8 human ovarian cancer cells [24] and HT-1080 human fibrosarcoma cells [25] in RPMI 1640 with 10% heat-inactivated fetal bovine serum, 100 units/mL of penicillin, and 100 μg/mL of streptomycin at 37 °C, and 5% CO_2.
2. Maintain FS6 human normal foreskin fibroblasts in DMEM with 10% heat-inactivated fetal bovine serum, 100 units/mL of penicillin, and 100 μg/mL of streptomycin at 37 °C, and 5% CO_2 [13].

3.11 rAd-MET Transduction

1. Transduce OVCAR-8 and HT1080 cells (2×10^6) with rAd-METase at multiplicity of infection (MOI) of 10, 30, 100, and 300.
2. Harvest cells 48 h after infection.
3. Lyse the cells by sonication for 1 min in 0.5 mL PBS.
4. Measure rMETase activity after centrifugation at 13,000 rpm, in the supernatants, using the method of Tanaka et al. [22], which determines α-ketobutyrate production in the presence of 10 mM methionine using 3-methyl-2-benzo-thiazoline hydrazone.
5. Calculate specific rMETase activity as units/mg protein, with one unit of enzyme defined as the amount that catalyzes the formation of 1 μmol of α-ketobutyrate/min.
6. Determine the protein concentrations of cell lysates with the Lowry Reagent kit [13].

3.12 SDS Gel Electrophoreses of rAd-METase-Produced rMETase

1. Lyse rAd-METase-transduced OVCAR-8 cells with sonication for 1 min in 0.5 mL PBS.
2. After centrifugation at 13,000 rpm, analyze the supernatants containing a total of 15 μg of total protein with 12% SDS-PAGE and stain with Coomassie Brilliant Blue R [13].

3.13 Combination Therapy Using rAd-MET and rMETase

1. Seed cells at 4000 cells/well in 96-well plates.
2. Twenty-four hours later, add rAd-METase or control-Ad at different doses ranging from 5×10^5 to 8×10^6 pfu/well for cancer cell lines and from 10^6 to 10^8 pfu/well for normal fibroblasts.
3. Three hours later, add rMETase at different doses in a range of concentrations from 0.025 to 0.1 units/mL for cancer cell lines and from 0.06 to 5.4 units/mL for normal fibroblasts.
4. Evaluate a total of 12 different combinations (three concentrations of rMETase and four titers of rAd-METase or control-rAd) on OVCAR-8.
5. Evaluate 35 different combinations (7 concentrations of rMETase and 5 titers of rAds) on HT-1080.
6. Evaluate 45 different combinations (5 concentrations of rMETase and 9 titers of rAds) on the normal fibroblasts.
7. Three days after the transduction, quantify surviving cells with the MTT assay [13].

3.14 Preparation and Use of Drugs

1. Prepare doxorubicin (DOX) 250 mg/mL for use in final dosage of 2 mg/kg body weight as an i.p. injection.
2. Prepare SeMET as a 20 mM solution in PBS, and inject 50 μL intra-tumorally.
3. Use 50 μL PBS in appropriate control groups for intra-tumor injections.
4. Administer Ad-METase and control-Ad in 50 μL intra-tumor injections containing 3×10^8 PFU virus [15].

3.15 Bcl-2 Transfection

1. Ligate Bcl-2 cDNA (0.8 Kb) into the pLXIN retroviral vector at the *Eco*R-I site using T4 ligase.
2. Co-transfect pLXIN-Bcl-2 and pVSV-G vectors into GP-293 retroviral packaging cells using Lipofectamine.
3. Use supernatants, of transfected GP-293 cells, containing Bcl-2 retroviruses, to infect A549 cells to establish Bcl-2-overexpressing clones of A549.
4. Select Bcl-2-transformed cells using G-418 up to 2.2 mg/mL.
5. Select two clones, named BB for Bcl-2 moderate expression and B1S for Bcl-2 high expression [16].

3.16 Western Blotting for Detection of Bcl-2 and Cytochrome c

1. To detect Bcl-2 expression, harvest 5×10^7 cells and collect by centrifugation.
2. After washing twice with ice-cold PBS, treat the cell pellet according to the manufacturer's protocol with the Cell Fractionation Kit.
3. Disrupt the cells by douncing 100 times using a tissue grinder with a type B pestle on ice.
4. Obtain supernatants by centrifugation at 700 $\times g$ for 10 min in a Beckman (Microfuge® 18) centrifuge.
5. Determine protein concentrations at OD-280 with a Hitachi U-2000 spectrophotometer [16].
6. Load protein (25 μg) per lane on a 10–20% SDS-polyacrylamide gel at 125 V.
7. After electrophoresis, electrotransfer the proteins to nitrocellulose membranes at 200 mA for 1 h.
8. Block the membranes for 3 h in a solution of 7% powdered nonfat milk in TTBS (0.1% Tween 20, 150 mM NaCl, and 10 mM Tris–HCl pH 7.6).
9. After gently rinsing with TTBS, probe the membranes with a rabbit polyclonal primary antibody against Bcl-2 at a concentration of 3 μL/mL at 4 °C overnight.
10. After washing three times, treat the membrane with donkey anti-rabbit secondary antibody at a concentration of 1 μL/ 5 mL for 1 h.
11. For signal detection, use chemiluminescence reagent ECL + Plus according to the manufacturer's protocol [16].
12. For cytochrome *c* extraction, harvest 5×10^7 cells for each cell line and treat with the Cell Fractionation Kit.
13. Disrupt the cells by douncing 60 times using a tissue grinder with a type A pestle on ice.
14. After centrifugation at 700 $\times g$ for 10 min, centrifuge this supernatant at 10,000 $\times g$ for 25 min to obtain the cytosol fraction.
15. Load supernatant protein (30 μg) in each lane on 10–20% Tris-glycine SDS gels at 120 V.
16. After membrane transfer and blocking, probe the membrane with rabbit monoclonal primary antibody against cytochrome *c* at a concentration of 4 μL/mL.
17. For detection, use a chemiluminescence reagent ECL + Plus with donkey anti-rabbit secondary antibody [16].

1. Quantitate Bcl-2 and cytochrome *c* with ELISA.
2. Use a Bcl-2 ELISA kit for Bcl-2.

3.17 ELISA for Detection of Bcl-2 and Cytochrome c

3. Use the Quantikine human cytochrome *c* kit for cytochrome *c*.
4. Carry out each procedure according to the manufacturer's protocols.
5. Read absorbance at 450 nm on a Benchmark Microplate Reader.
6. Analyze the data with Microplate Manager-4.0 PC Data Analysis software on an IBM PC [16].

3.18 Hoechst 33258 Staining for Apoptosis

1. Use Hoechst 33258 DNA stain, as a nuclear marker of apoptosis.
2. Use staurosporine to introduce apoptosis.
3. Seed cells (5×10^4) on chamber slides in wells with culture medium (RPMI 1640 with 10% FBS).
4. Add staurosporine the next day to each well at a concentration of 3 μM and incubate for 3 h.
5. Change the medium to a medium containing Hoechst 33258 at a concentration of 2 μM with incubation for 20 min.
6. After gently washing with PBS, observe fluorescent nuclei with an Olympus model BH-2 fluorescence microscope with a 360 nm filter for excitation and 500 nm filter for emission.
7. Use morphology of the stained nuclei to determine apoptosis.
8. Seed the parental A549 clone and derived clones, BB and B1S (5×10^3 cells), in culture medium in each well of four chamber plates.
9. After 24 h, add rAdMETase (MOI 20) to the cells. At 24 h after transfection, add SeMET to each well at the final concentration of 20 μM.
10. After 12 h, stain cells with Hoechst 33258 to observe nuclear condensation [16].

3.19 IC_{50} Determination of rAdMETase/SeMET

1. Test human cancer cell lines for the in vitro efficacy of rAdMETase/SeMET.
2. Evaluate cytotoxicity using the MTT assay.
3. Seed cells (4×10^3) in 96-well plates transduced with rAdMETase or control-rAd.
4. Twenty-four hours after transduction, add SeMET.
5. After 3 days' incubation, replace the medium with 0.5 mg/mL MTT for 2 h.
6. Remove the supernatants, add 200 μL of isopropanol to each well, and measure absorbance at 540 nm in a microtiter plate reader. Determine IC_{50} values by the median-effect equation [14, 26].

3.20 In Vivo Efficacy of rAdMETase/SeMET

1. Implant N1S1 rat hepatoma tumor cells (1×10^6 cells) into the peritoneal cavities of female nude mice [27].
2. Two days after implantation, inject rAdMETase (5×10^8 pfu), control-rAd (5×10^8 pfu), or mock controls every other day for a total of five doses.
3. Treat mice i.p. with either SeMET (1 μmol/mouse) or normal saline as a control, every day from day 3 to day 13. Evaluate ascites tumor growth by body weight gain.
4. Conduct all animal studies in accordance with the principles and procedures outlined in the NIH Guide for the Care and Use of Laboratory Animals under assurance number A3873–1 [14].
5. Breed and maintain the animals in a high-efficiency particulate air-filtered environment.
6. Sterilize cages, food, and bedding by autoclaving.
7. Add a total of 5.0% (vol/vol) ampicillin to the autoclaved drinking water [13].

3.21 Bystander Effect

1. To evaluate the bystander effect of rAdMETase/SeMET gene therapy for Bcl-2-overexpressing clones, co-culture rAdMETase-transduced cells and nontransduced cells at various ratios for each clone.
2. Mix the cells at various ratios and seed onto 96-well plates adjusted to 5×10^3 cells in each well.
3. After 24 h, add SeMET to each well at a final concentration of 20 μM.
4. After 3 days of incubation, evaluate the surviving cell ratio with the MTT assay as described above [16].

4 Results

4.1 Transduction of H460 with GFP-MET or GFP Genes

H460 cells transduced with either the GFP-METase or the GFP genes were able to grow in vitro. High-expression clones containing these vectors were isolated and selected by the extent of their GFP fluorescence. The GFP fluorescence was evenly distributed in cells with the GFP gene. In contrast, in GFP-MET cells, the fluorescence was localized only in the cytoplasm and not in the nuclei. The reason for localization of GFP-MET expression only in the cytoplasm remains unclear. There were no significant differences in the cell growth rates between GFP cells and GFP-MET cells as determined by comparing their doubling time in vitro (data not shown) [13] (*see* **Note 1**).

4.2 METase Activity and Methionine Levels

The METase activity of GFP-MET cells was 33 mU/mg protein. METase activity was not detectable in the H460 parent cells or in H460-GFP cells. Pure rMETase has a specific activity of ~20 U/mg protein, which means that the GFP-MET cells expressed METase at ~0.17% of their total protein. The free methionine level of H460-GFP-MET was determined to be ~33% of that of H460-GFP cells or H460 parent cells [13] (*see* **Note 2**).

4.3 In Vitro Efficacy of rMETase

The efficacy of rMETase in vitro on H460-GFP or H460-GFP-MET was determined with the MTT assay. H460-GFP-MET cells were more sensitive to low concentrations of rMETase compared with H460-GFP cells or H460 cells. In the presence of 0.08 U/mL rMETase, the survival of H460-GFP-METase cells was 10% compared with the untreated cells. In contrast, H460 and H460-GFP cells were only slightly affected by this concentration of rMETase. These results indicated that the MET gene increased the methionine requirement of these cancer cells, making them more sensitive to rMETase [13] (*see* **Note 3**).

4.4 In Vivo Efficacy of the METase Gene and rMETase

Animals with GFP-METase-transduced tumors treated with rMETase had the longest median survival time among the four groups in two repeat experiments. There was a 50% increase in the survival of the rMETase-treated animals with H460-GFP-METase tumors over rMETase-treated animals with H460-GFP tumors (Fig. 1) [13] (*see* **Notes 1, 3–5**).

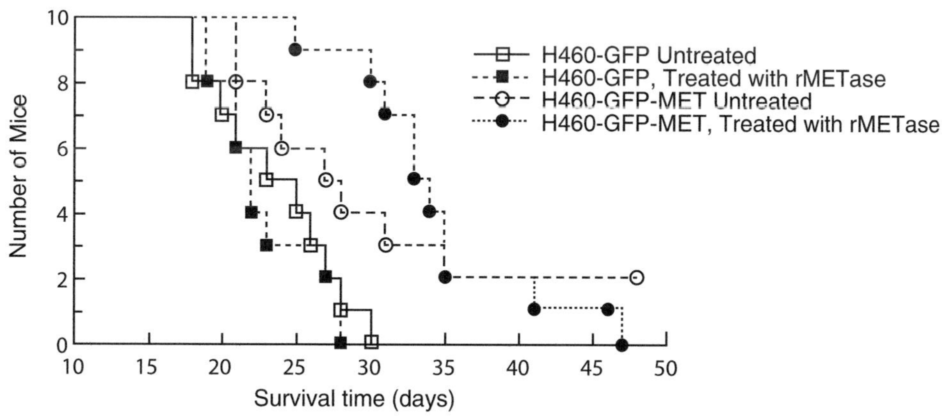

Fig. 1 Survival curves of four groups of mice orthotopically implanted with H460. Untreated animals with an H460-GFP tumor had a median survival of 23 days. rMETase-treated animals with an H460-GFP tumor had a median survival of 22 days. Untreated animals with an H460-GFP-METase tumor had a median survival of 27 days. rMETase-treated animals with an H460-GFP-METase tumor had a median survival of 33 days, a 50% increase over rMETase-treated animals with H-460-GFP tumors. Overall survival of rMETase-treated animals with H460-GFP-MET tumors was significantly longer than either rMETase-treated or -untreated animals with H460-GFP tumors ($P < 0.05$ in log-rank test) [13]

4.5 METase Expression in rAd-METase-Infected Cells

The activity of the rAd-*METase* gene was measured in cell lysates of OVCAR-8 and HT1080 cells infected with this vector. The METase activities were positively dependent on the MOI of rAd-METase. At the lowest MOI of 10, the METase activity in OVCAR-8 was 0.26 unit/mg protein, which was nine times higher than the activity using retroviral vectors [13]. At an MOI of 300, the METase activity for both OVCAR-8 and HT 1080 was ~2 units/mg protein in the crude lysate, indicating that METase was expressed at ~10% of the total protein of the cells. High-level rAd-MET expression in infected OVCAR-8 cells can also be seen by the predominant M_r 43,000 METase monomer band in SDS-PAGE [13].

4.6 Efficacy of rAd-METase

The percentage of surviving cells was determined after transduction with various MOIs of rAd-METase or control-rAd. The IC_{50} for rAd-METase on OVACAR-8 and HT-1080 was 2.0×10^6 and 4.6×10^6 pfu/well, respectively. In contrast, the IC_{50} for control-rAd in OVACAR-8 and HT-1080 was 4.0×10^7 and 2.3×10^7 pfu/well, respectively, which was 20 and 5 times higher than that of rAd-MET, respectively. The IC_{50} for rAd-METase and control-rAd on normal fibroblasts was 4.7×10^7 and over 1×10^8 pfu/well, respectively (Fig. 2) [13].

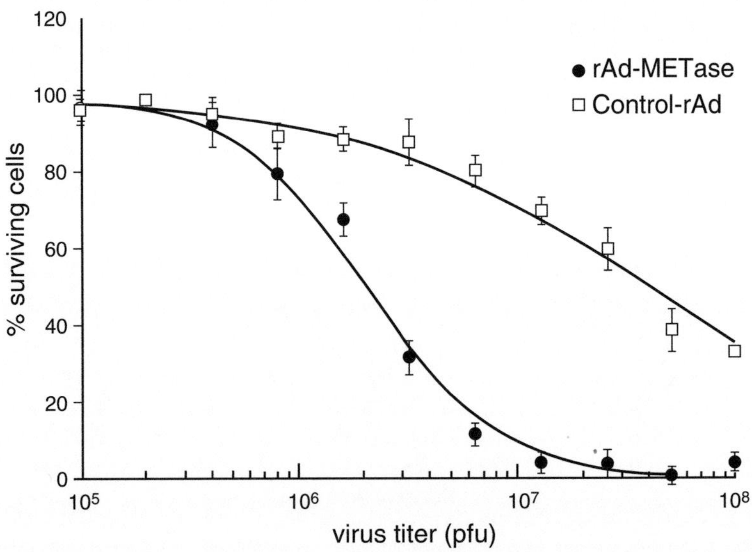

Fig. 2 Efficacy of rAd-METase and control-rAd on OVCAR-8 1080 cells. Cells (4000) were infected with rAd-METase (*A, closed circles*) or control-rAd (*A, open squares*) at various titers. Three days after infection, the percentage of surviving cells was determined with the MTT assay. Dose-response curves for rAd-METase and control-rAd were plotted. The IC_{50} of rAd-METase was 2×10^6 pfu. The IC_{50} of control-rAd was 4×10^7. *Bars,* SD [13]

4.7 Efficacy of rMETase

A dose-response relationship was observed for rMETase on both OVCAR-8 and HT1080 cells with an IC_{50} of 0.1 unit/mL and 0.15 unit/mL, respectively. In contrast, the IC_{50} on the normal fibroblasts was 1.68 units/mL, >10 times higher than tumor cells [13].

4.8 Combination Therapy of Ad-METase and rMETase

In the presence of the IC_{50} of 2×10^6 pfu of rAd-METase, the addition of 0.025 unit/mL of rMETase, which was one-fourth of the IC_{50} dose, inhibited OVCAR-8 cell growth by 90%. This level of rMETase on untransduced cells or control-Ad-transduced cells had an efficacy of only 10%. The normal fibroblasts, on the other hand, appeared relatively resistant to the *METase* gene because, in the presence of rMETase, 2.5×10^7 pfu/well of rAd-METase or control-rAd had almost an identical effect on cell survival [13].

Synergistic efficacy of rAd-METase and rMETase was determined by calculating the combination index (CI). All of the CIs of the combinations of rMETase and rAd-METase tested on OVCAR-8 were <0.7, with a mean of 0.5 ± 0.13. Therefore, this combination has strong synergy. In contrast, the CIs of rMETase and control-rAd for OVCAR-8 had a mean of $0.97 + 0.13$. This combination had only an additive effect. The mean value of CIs for the combination of rMETase and rAd-METase on HT1080 was 0.74 ± 0.13, indicating synergy. In contrast, the combination of rMETase and control-rAd on HT-1080 had a mean of 1.11 ± 0.20. Therefore, rMETase and rAd-METase had synergistic efficacy on OVCAR-8 and HT-1080, whereas rMETase and control-rAd did not. There were significant differences in the mean CI values between the test and control combinations on both cell lines using the Student's *t*-test ($P < 0.0001$). The CIs of the combination of rMETase and rAd-METase and combination of rMETase and control-rAd on normal fibroblasts were 0.89 ± 0.43 and 1.25 ± 1.30, respectively. There were no significant differences in the mean CIs between the two combinations on normal fibroblasts, again suggesting relative resistance of the normal fibroblasts to the *METase* gene [13].

rMETase protein therapy degrades extracellular methionine but cannot block the synthesis of methionine inside the cells, whereas *METase* gene delivery via rAd-METase degrades intracellular MET but cannot block the uptake of methionine. Perhaps MET depletion in both the extracellular space and within the cell accounts for the synergy in the cancer cells. Tisdale [23] has speculated that exogenous MET and intracellularly biosynthesized MET may be differentially used in cancer cells [13] (*see* **Notes 5** and **6**).

4.9 Cellular Toxicity of the Ad-METase and SeMET Combination

The addition of subtoxic levels of SeMET (20 μM) resulted in approximately a 100-fold enhancement of the toxicity of rAdMETase to human tumor cells in vitro attributable to the release of toxic methylselenol by the rAdMETase gene product, rMETase [14].

The IC_{50} values of SeMET for nontransduced or control-rAd-transduced human cancer cells (MOI, 50) were between 100 and 1000 μM. In contrast, the IC_{50} values of SeMET on rAdMETase-transduced (MOI, 50) cells were greatly reduced to 0.3–5 μM. Thus, rAdMETase increased the toxicity of SeMET up to 1000-fold in tumor cells. The combination was highly toxic on all of the human cancer cell lines tested, including A549 lung cancer cells, OVCAR-8 ovarian cancer cells, Mia-PaCa and BxPC3 pancreatic cancer cells, Hep-2 head and neck cancer cells, and EKVX lung cancer cells [14] (*see* **Note 2**).

4.10 Bystander Effect of rAdMETase/SeMET

To evaluate the bystander effect of the *METase* gene/SeMET combination, we co-cultured nontransduced A549 cells with rAdMETase-transduced A549 cells (MOI 50) at various ratios. The administration of SeMET (20 μM) to cultures containing just 3% rAdMETase-transduced cells resulted in the killing of more than 80% of the total cells in the culture. This strong bystander effect was thought to be caused by the diffusion of methylselenol from the *METase*-gene-transduced cells to the nontransduced cells [14] (*see* **Note 7**).

4.11 Apoptosis Induction by rAdMETase/SeMET

Twelve hours after exposure to SeMET, sub-G_0 populations of A549 cells appeared, indicating apoptosis. Nucleosomal DNA fragmentation also occurred in the rAdMETase/SeMET-treated A549 cells. To investigate the mechanism of rAdMETase/SeMET induction of apoptosis, we first determined the extent of reactive oxygen species (ROS) generation as measured by lucigenin-dependent chemiluminescence (CL) [28]. The level of CL in rAdMETase-treated A549 cells was dependent on the SeMET concentration. At 160 μM SeMET, CL was 100-fold higher than control and was completely inhibited by addition of SOD. In contrast, nontransduced cells did not produce ROS, even at the highest concentration of SeMET tested. Extracellular superoxide released from the treated cells was detected by lucigenin. Detection of CL started immediately after adding lucigenin, suggesting that the reaction between lucigenin and superoxide occurred in the cell culture medium. Therefore, SOD probably depleted extracellular superoxide (*see* **Note 8**).

ROS, especially the superoxide anion, may be formed during the oxidation of methylselenol by ambient dioxygen [29], followed by the oxidation of glutathione (GSH) by the oxidized diselenide, which is retransformed to methylselenol [29]. Indeed, the rAdMETase/SeMET-treated cells had marked depletion of GSH in contrast to control-rAd/SeMET-treated cells [14] (*see* **Note 9**).

4.12 rAdMETase/SeMET-Induced Mitochondrial Permeability and Release of Cytochrome c

The mitochondrial permeability transition is activated by oxidants, which causes mitochondrial swelling and loss of membrane potential [30, 31], resulting in mitochondrial cytochrome *c* release to the cytosol. The released cytochrome *c* binds to Apaf-1 and activates caspase-9 [32], which in turn activates downstream caspases and induces apoptosis [30–33]. rAdMETase/SeMET induces this apoptotic pathway in A549 human lung adenocarcinoma cells. Mitochondrial membrane potential is lowered by rAdMETase/SeMET treatment but not by rAdMETase or SeMET alone, as determined with the Mitosensor fluorescent dye (Clontech). A significant release of cytochrome *c* to the cytosolic fraction was observed beginning 6 h after rAdMETase/SeMET treatment, and it increased in a time-dependent manner. rAdMETase/SeMET activated caspase-9 and caspase-3 in the treated cells up to 15-fold and 45-fold of untreated control, respectively. Caspase-8 was activated only fivefold. Control-rAd/SeMET did not activate these caspases. Mitochondrial swelling was visualized by electron microscopy in rAdMETase/SeMET-treated cells after 12 h [14].

4.13 In Vivo efficacy of rAdMETase/SeMET

Treatment of rat hepatoma N1S1 ascites in nude mice with rAdMETase/SeMET inhibited ascites tumor growth as measured by body weight gain relative to similar nontumor-bearing animals. rAdMETase/SeMET significantly prolonged their survival with three of five rAdMETase/SeMET animals alive at day 72. In contrast, all of the rAdMETase or SeMET-only-treated mice were dead by day 24 (Fig. 3) [14] (*see* **Note 10**).

4.14 Efficacy of rAdMETase/SeMET on Bcl-2-Overexpressing Apoptosis-Resistant Lung Cancer Cells

4.14.1 Bcl-2 Overproducing Cell Lines

The A549 human lung cancer cell line has very low endogenous Bcl-2 levels and was transduced with a Bcl-2-containing retrovirus vector [34]. Two new clones, which showed elevated expression levels of Bcl-2, were selected. Bcl-2 expression was confirmed by Western blotting and ELISA. The high Bcl-2-expressing clone (B1S) had almost twice the Bcl-2 expression of clone BB [16].

Staurosporine induces apoptosis via a mitochondrial pathway [35]. The A549 parental line entered apoptosis within 3 h after incubation with 3 μM staurosporine. Hoechst 33258 staining showed that 20% of the cells had extensive nuclear condensation with the other cells showing moderate condensation. In contrast, when the BB and B1S clones were similarly treated with staurosporine, none of the cells showed nuclear condensation. Therefore, the clones that express elevated levels of Bcl-2 protein were resistant to a standard apoptosis-inducing agent [16].

4.14.2 Comparison of Efficacy of rAdMETase/SeMET Gene Therapy on A549, BB, and B1S

A549, BB, and B1S equally showed nuclear condensation 24 h after rAdMET/SeMET gene therapy as seen by Hoechst 33258 staining. In all, 20% of each clone showed extensive nuclear condensation and the rest showed moderate nuclear condensation. This result showed that rAdMETase/SeMET gene therapy caused

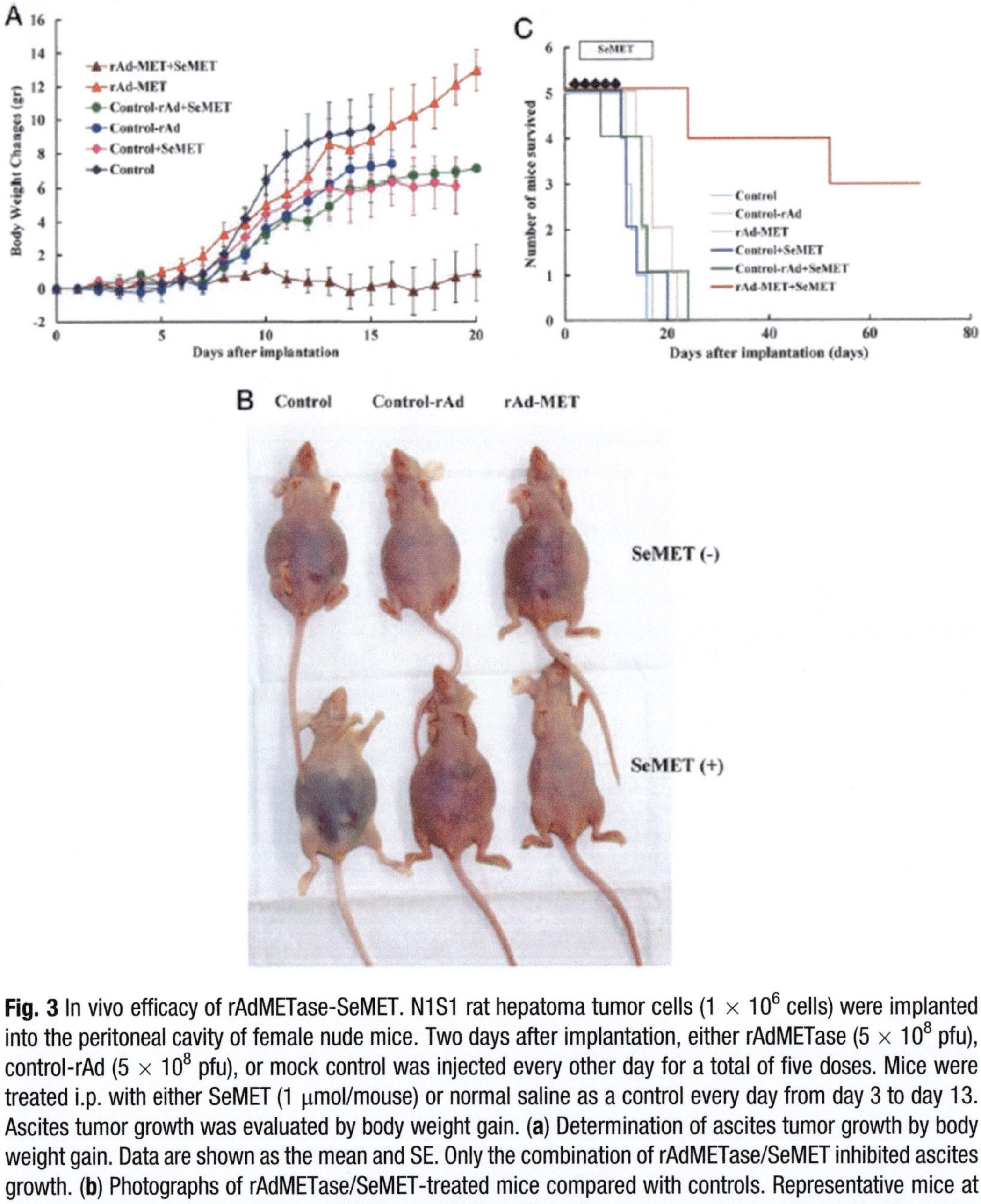

Fig. 3 In vivo efficacy of rAdMETase-SeMET. N1S1 rat hepatoma tumor cells (1×10^6 cells) were implanted into the peritoneal cavity of female nude mice. Two days after implantation, either rAdMETase (5×10^8 pfu), control-rAd (5×10^8 pfu), or mock control was injected every other day for a total of five doses. Mice were treated i.p. with either SeMET (1 μmol/mouse) or normal saline as a control every day from day 3 to day 13. Ascites tumor growth was evaluated by body weight gain. (**a**) Determination of ascites tumor growth by body weight gain. Data are shown as the mean and SE. Only the combination of rAdMETase/SeMET inhibited ascites growth. (**b**) Photographs of rAdMETase/SeMET-treated mice compared with controls. Representative mice at day 10 after tumor implantation. rAdMETase/SeMET-treated mice had no ascites. In contrast, other mice developed significant ascites. (**c**) Survival efficacy of rAdMET/SeMET-treated mice compared with controls [14]

apoptosis in the Bcl-2-overexpressing BB and B1S clones as well as the parental clone [16].

The Bcl-2-overexpressing clones were selected in high levels of G418 in which the parental cells died. The clones were shown by Western blotting to highly express Bcl-2 with B1S expressing more than BB. Bcl-2 was almost undetectable in the parental cells. ELISA testing confirmed the high levels of Bcl-2 in BB and B1S and very low levels in the parental cells. Bcl-2 overexpression also correlates with staurosporine resistance. Therefore, the properties of the clones are due to the high Bcl-2 expression and not due to the clonal variation [16].

The MTT assay showed that the rAdMETase/SeMET gene therapy killed the BB and B1S clones as efficiently as it killed the parental A549 cells. Cell survival curves were almost identical for each clone. The SeMET IC_{50} values for the parental and Bcl-2-overexpressing clones were similar in the range of 3.8–5.3 μM. Thus, rAdMETase/SeMET gene therapy is effective against Bcl-2-overexpressing cells [16].

Western blotting of the cytosolic fractions of the cells on rAdMETase/SeMET showed cytochrome c release into the cytosol in both parental A549 cells and the Bcl-2-overexpressing clones, BB and B1S. ELISA also showed that cytochrome *c* release occurred in each clone after rAdMETase/SeMET treatment. To confirm that the fractionation technique itself did not damage the mitochondria and cause cytochrome *c* release, we also prepared samples from untreated cells in the same way. No cytochrome *c* release was seen in these preparations from any of the clones [16].

Hamel et al. [36] reported that Bcl-2 significantly reduced the bystander effect in HSV-tk/GCV therapy. To evaluate the bystander effect of the rAdMETase/SeMET gene therapy, we co-cultured nontransduced cells with rAdMETase-transduced cells of each clone. rAdMETase/SeMET gene therapy showed a strong bystander effect even against Bcl-2-overexpressing BB and B1S clones. Cell survival curves of each clone were essentially identical. This strong bystander effect was thought to be caused by the diffusion to the nontransduced cells of gaseous methylselenol produced from SeMET in the METase-gene-transduced cells. Thus, methylselenol seems to induce apoptosis even in the presence of high levels of Bcl-2 [16] (*see* **Notes 11–13**).

SeMET itself is relatively nontoxic to mammalian cells since it cannot be converted to selenol [37, 38]. Methylselenol catalyzes oxidation of thiols [39] at ambient pO_2 to generate toxic reactive oxygen species such as superoxide [29, 40] and induces apoptosis. These oxidants are thought to activate the mitochondrial permeability transition and cause mitochondrial swelling and loss of membrane potential [30, 31]. Subsequently, cytochrome *c* is released into the cytosol and binds to Apaf-1 and activates caspase [32, 36], which in turn activates downstream caspases and induces apoptosis as we showed in rAdMETase/SeMET-treated cells [14, 16, 33] (*see* **Notes 12** and **14**).

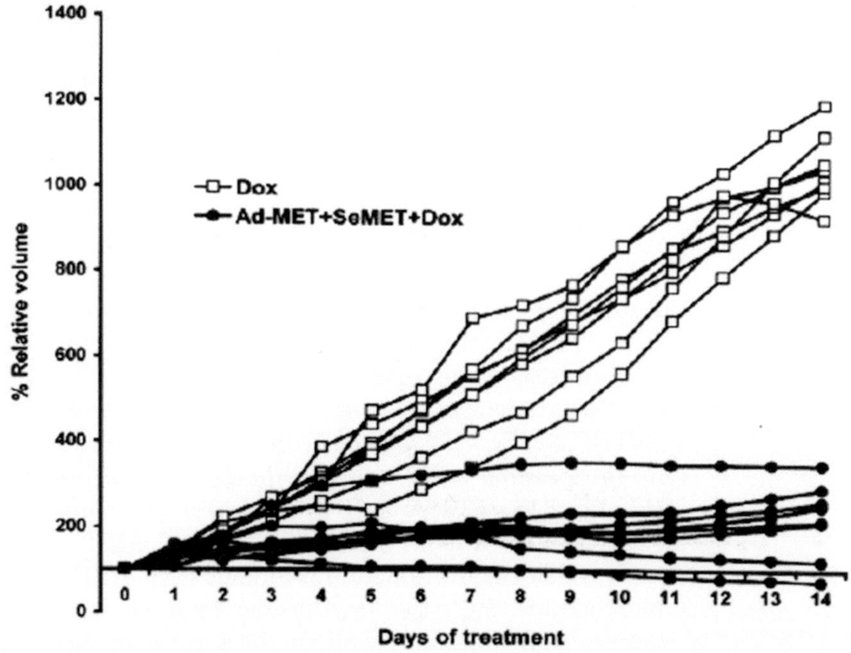

Fig. 4 A comparison of percent relative H460 tumor volume changes in the treatment and control groups. The percent relative volumes of individual tumors in various treatment groups have been plotted against the days of treatment with each graph comparing the outcome in two different groups. The tumor volumes increased about 8–12 times in 2 weeks in the untreated group. Tumor growth was only 1–2.5 times in the mice treated with the combination of Ad-METase/SeMET+DOX. SeMET, DOX, or Ad-METase individually were unable to inhibit the tumor growth at the doses used [15]

4.15 Efficacy of Doxorubicin (DOX) in Combination with Ad-METase/SeMET

The untreated group showed a 10-fold increase in the tumor volume after 2 weeks, and the increase was only 2.5-fold in the DOX + Ad-METase/SeMET group. H460 treatment with DOX alone at the low-dose used showed no difference as compared to the control group. There was a 5.8-fold increase in tumor volume in mice treated with Ad-METase/SeMET gene therapy alone. The tumor doubling time was increased to approximately 10 days with the combination therapy of Ad-MET+SeMET+DOX as opposed to 2–3 days in all other treatment groups [15].

The comparison of individual mice with H460 tumors showed the efficacy of the combination therapy of Ad-METase/SeMET and DOX compared to the untreated control. Whereas the tumor volumes increased 8–12-fold in 2 weeks in the untreated group, tumor growth was only 1- to 2.5-fold in the mice treated with the combination of Ad-METase/SeMET+DOX (Fig. 4) [15].

SeMET, DOX, or Ad-METase individually were unable to inhibit the tumor growth at the low doses they were used [15].

Similarly, the combination of Ad-METase+DOX and the combination of SeMET+DOX with control-Ad instead of Ad-METase were also ineffective when compared with the Ad-METase/SMET-DOX combination [15] (*see* **Note 10**).

Ad-METase/SeMET gene therapy alone did show efficacy when compared to the untreated control. The tumor growth was about three- to eightfold in the individual mice at the end of 2 weeks as opposed to eight- to tenfold in the untreated group [15].

A mutated cystathionine γ lyase (mCTH) was shown to be able to convert SeMET into methylselenol and cancer cell death [41].

Another study has shown that a lentivirus vector carrying methioninase increased the sensitivity of gastric cancer cells to cisplatinum [42]. Transfer of the gene P1K3Ca to normal mammary epithelial cells was sufficient to confer MET dependence to these cells [43]. Future studies will determine rAdMETase-SeMET+DOX efficacy of such cells as well as in patient-derived mouse models of cancer [44].

5 Notes

1. The GFP-METase fusion gene has the following advantages: (a) the expression levels of METase can be monitored by fluorescence in living cells and tissues and (b) the transduced cancer cell behavior in vivo can be easily visualized by GFP fluorescence such as metastasis formation [13].
2. The rAdMETase/SeMET combination is a novel approach to cancer gene therapy exploiting the production of the apoptosis-inducing methylselenol from SeMET in rAdMETase-transduced cancer cells. This approach is thus a new paradigm for cancer gene therapy. Selective expression and delivery systems can now be developed with the goal of clinical application [14].
3. There were no significant differences in the mean CIs between the two combinations on normal fibroblasts, again suggesting relative resistance of the normal fibroblasts to the *METase* gene.
4. We have thus demonstrated a new strategy of combination cancer therapy with the METase gene and its gene product. Future experiments will involve direct in vivo administration of the METase gene both with and without rMETase to tumor-bearing animals [13].
5. rAd-*METase* cancer gene therapy combined with rMETase treatment has many powerful features including (*a*) the high efficiency of transduction and the high expression of the rAd-*METase* gene in the cancer cells compared with retroviral gene delivery; (*b*) the ability to deplete both intracellular and extracellular MET, which strongly targets the increased MET

requirement of cancer cells; (*c*) the potential to target growing and resting cancer cells, which can be rendered more selective in the future using cancer-specific promoters to drive the *METase* gene; (*d*) the strong synergy of rAd-METase and rMETase, allowed reduced levels of each agent to be used, thus decreasing potential side effects; and (*e*) the relative resistance of the normal fibroblasts to the *METase* gene [13].

6. rMETase protein therapy degrades extracellular MET but cannot block the synthesis of MET inside the cells, whereas *METase* gene delivery via rAd-METase degrades intracellular MET but cannot block the uptake of MET. Perhaps MET depletion in both the extracellular space and within the cell accounts for the synergy in the cancer cells. Tisdale [45] has speculated that exogenous MET and intracellularly biosynthesized MET may be differentially used in cancer cells. Future experiments will attempt to elucidate the synergistic mechanism by determining the differential effects of rMETase and rAd-METase on cellular MET and methylation metabolism in tumors [13].
7. This strong bystander effect was thought to be caused by the diffusion to the nontransduced cells of gaseous methylselenol produced from SeMET in the METase-gene-transduced cells. Thus, methylselenol seems to induce apoptosis even in the presence of high levels of Bcl-2 [16].
8. SeMET itself is relatively nontoxic to mammalian cells since it cannot be converted to selenol [37, 38]. Methylselenol catalyzes oxidation of thiols [39] at ambient pO_2 to generate toxic reactive oxygen species such as superoxide [29, 40] and induces apoptosis. These oxidants are thought to activate the mitochondrial permeability transition and cause mitochondrial swelling and loss of membrane potential [30, 31]. Subsequently, cytochrome *c* is released into the cytosol and binds to Apaf-1 and activates caspase [32, 36], which in turn activates downstream caspases and induces apoptosis as we previously showed in rAdMETase/SeMET-treated cells [14, 16, 33].
9. METase gene transfer in combination with rMETase prolonged the survival time of tumor-bearing mice. Because we selected surviving cells after transduction of the GFP-METase gene, the extent of the METase expression in these cells may be limited. Thus the efficacy of the METase gene was enhanced by exogenous rMETase [13].
10. The overall survival of rMETase-treated animals with H460-GFP-METase tumors was significantly longer than either rMETase-treated or -untreated animals with H460-GFP tumors (*P*, *0*.05 in log-rank test).

11. A comparison of Ad-METase/SeMET with Ad-METase/SeMET+DOX indicates that the addition of DOX to Ad-METase/ScMET provides a stronger efficacy against the H460 tumor [15].
12. These results suggested that induction of apoptosis by *METase* gene/SeMET is caused by ROS generation from methylselenol, resulting in mitochondrial damage to release cytochrome *c* and activate the apoptotic cascade [14].
13. Methionine α,γ lyase (methioninase) from *Pseudomonas putida* catalyzes α,γ-elimination reactions of L-methionine and can degrade SeMET to methylselenol, α-ketobutyrate, and ammonia. We have taken advantage of this feature of the METase gene to design a gene-directed enzyme prodrug therapy system for cancer therapy [16].
14. rAdMETase/SeMET gene therapy could overcome Bcl-2 overexpression and induce apoptosis. We believe that the powerful advantages of rAdMETase/SeMET treatment are promising for future development of this gene therapy strategy [16].

References

1. Goseki N, Yamazaki S, Endo M, Onodera T, Kosaki G, Hibino Y, Kuwahata T (1992) Antitumor effect of methionine-depleting total parenteral nutrition with doxorubicin administration on Yoshida sarcoma-bearing rats. Cancer 69:1865–1872
2. Hoshiya Y, Guo H, Kubota T, Asanuma F, Yamada Y, Koh J, Kitajima M, Hoffman RM (1995) Human tumors are methionine dependent in vivo. Anticancer Res 15:717–718
3. Guo H, Tan Y, Kubota T, Moossa AR, Hoffman RM (1996) Methionine depletion modulates the antitumor and antimetastatic efficacy of ethionine. Anticancer Res 16:2719–2723
4. Goseki N, Yamazaki S, Shimojyo K, Kando F, Maruyama M, Endo M, Koike M, Takahashi H (1995) Synergistic effect of methionine-depleting total parenteral nutrition with 5-fluouracil on human gastric cancer: a randomized prospective clinical trial. Jpn J Cancer Res 86:484–489
5. Tan Y, Xu M, Tan XZ, Tan XY, Wang X, Saikawa S, Nagashima T, Sun X, Lenz M, Hoffman RM (1997) Overexpression and large-scale production of recombinant L-methionine-α-deamino-γ-mercaptomethane-lyase for novel anticancer therapy. Protein Expr Purif 9:233–245
6. Hori H, Takabayashi K, Orvis L, Carson DA, Nobori T (1996) Gene cloning and characterization of Pseudomonas putida L-methionine-α-deamino-γ-mercaptomethane-lyase. Cancer 56:2116–2122
7. Yoshioka T, Wada T, Uchida N, Maki H, Yoshida H, Ide N, Kasai H, Hojo K, Shono K, Maekawa R, Yagi S, Hoffman RM, Sugita K (1998) Anticancer efficacy in vivo and in vitro, synergy with 5-fluorouracil, and safety of recombinant methioninase. Cancer Res 58:2583–2587
8. Tan Y, Sun X, Xu M, Tan X-Z, Sasson A, Rashidi B, Han Q, Tan X-Y, Wang X, An Z, Sun F-X, Hoffman RM (1999) Efficacy of recombinant methioninase in combination with cisplatin on human colon tumors in nude mice. Clin Cancer Res 5:2157–2163
9. Kokkinakis DM, Hoffman RM, Frenkel EP, Wick JB, Han Q, Xu M, Tan Y, Schold SC (2001) Synergy between methionine stress and chemotherapy in the treatment of brain tumor xenografts in athymic mice. Cancer Res 61:4017–4023
10. Murakami T, Li S, Han Q, Tan Y, Kiyuna T, Igarashi K, Kawaguchi K, Hwang HK, Miyaki K, Singh AS, Hiroshima Y, Lwin TM, DeLong JC, Chishima T, Tanaka K, Bouvet M, Endo I, Eilber FC, Hoffman RM (2017) Recombinant methioninase effectively targets a Ewing's sarcoma in a patient-derived

orthotopic xenograft (PDOX) nude-mouse model. Oncotarget 8:35630–35638

11. Kawaguchi K, Igarashi K, Li S, Han Q, Tan Y, Kiyuna T, Miyake Y, Murakami T, Chmielowski B, Nelson SD, Russell TA, Dry SM, Li Y, Unno M, Eilber FC, Hoffman RM (2017) Combination treatment with recombinant methioninase enables temozolomide to arrest a BRAF V600E melanoma growth in a patient-derived orthotopic xenograft. Oncotarget 8:85516–85525
12. Igarashi K, Kawaguchi K, Li S, Han Q, Tan Y, Murakami T, Kiyuna T, Miyake K, Miyake M, Singh AS, Eckhadt MA, Nelson SD, Russell TA, Dry SM, Li Y, Yamamoto N, Hayashi K, Kimura H, Miwa S, Tsuchiya H, Singh RS, Eilber FC, Hoffman RM (2018) Recombinant methioninase in combination with DOX overcomes first-line DOX resistance in a patient-derived orthotopic xenograft nude-mouse model of undifferentiated spindle-cell sarcoma. Cancer Lett 417:168–173
13. Miki K, Xu M, An Z, Wang X, Yang M, Al-Refaie W, Sun X, Baranov E, Tan Y, Chishima T, Shimada H, Moossa AR, Hoffman RM (2000) Survival efficacy of the combination of the methioninase gene and methioninase in a lung cancer orthotopic model. Cancer Gene Ther 7:332–338
14. Miki K, Xu M, Gupta A, Ba Y, Tan Y, Al-Refaie W, Bouvet M, Makuuchi M, Moossa AR, Hoffman RM (2001) Methioninase cancer gene therapy with selenomethionine as suicide prodrug substrate. Cancer Res 61:6805–6810
15. Gupta A, Miki K, Xu M, Yamamoto N, Moossa AR, Hoffman RM (2003) Combination efficacy of doxorubicin and adenoviral methioninase gene therapy with prodrug selenomethionine. Anticancer Res 23:1181–1188
16. Yamamoto N, Gupta A, Xu M, Miki K, Tsujimoto Y, Tsuchiya H, Tomita K, Moossa AR, Hoffman RM (2003) Methioninase gene therapy with selenomethionine induces apoptosis in Bcl-2-overproducing lung cancer cells. Cancer Gene Ther 10:445–450
17. Tan Y, Sun X, Xu M, An Z, Tan X, Han Q, Miljkovic DA, Yang M, Hoffman RM (1998) Polyethylene glycol conjugation of recombinant methioninase for cancer therapy. Protein Expr Purif 12:45–52
18. Jones BN, Gilligan JP (1983) O-pthaldialdehyde pre-column derivatization and reversed-phase high-performance liquid chromatography of polypeptide hydrolysates and physiological fluids. J Chromatogr 266:471–482
19. Alley MC, Scudiero DA, Monks A, Hursey ML, Czerwinski MJ, Fine DL, Abbott BJ, Mayo JG, Shoemaker RH, Boyd MR (1988) Feasibility of drug screening with panels of human tumor cell lines using a microculture tetrazolium assay. Cancer Res 48:589–601
20. Wang X, Fu X, Hoffman RM (1992) A new patient-like metastatic model of human lung cancer constructed orthotopically with intact tissue via thoracotomy in immunodeficient mice. Int J Cancer 5:992–995
21. Wang W, Fu X, Hoffman RM (1992) A patient-like metastasizing model of human lung adenocarcinoma constructed via thoracotomy in nude mice. Anticancer Res 12:1399–1402
22. Tanaka H, Esaki N, Soda K (1977) Properties of L-methionine-g-lyase from *Pseudomonas ovalis*. Biochemistry 16:100–106
23. Keown WA, Campbell CR, Kucherlapati RS (1991) Methods for introducing DNA in mammalian cells. In: Goeddel DV (ed) Methods in enzymology, gene expression technology, vol 185. Academic Press, Inc., San Diego, pp 527–537
24. Schilder RJ, Hall L, Monks A, Handel LM, Fornace AJ Jr, Ozols RF, Fojo AT, Hamilton TC (1990) Metallothionine in gene expression and resistance to cisplatin in human ovarian cancer. Int J Cancer 45:416–422
25. Rasheed S, Nelson-Rees WA, Toth EM, Arnstein P, Gardner MB (1974) Characterization of newly derived human sarcoma cell line (HT-1080). Cancer 33:1027–1033
26. Chou TC, Talalay P (1987) Applications of the effect principle for the assessment of low-dose risk of carcinogens and for the quantitation of synergism, antagonism or chemotherapeutic agents. In: New avenues in development cancer chemotherapy, Bristol Myers symposium series. Academic Press, New York, pp 37–64
27. Wills KN, Maneval DC, Menzel P, Harris MP, Sutjipto S, Vaillancourt MT, Huang WM, Johnson DE, Anderson SC, Wen SF et al (1994) Development and characterization of recombinant adenoviruses encoding human p53 for gene therapy of cancer. Hum Gene Ther 5:1079–1088
28. Ganther HE (1990) Activity of methylated forms of selenium in cancer prevention. Cancer Res 50:1206–1211
29. Yan L, Spallholz JE (1993) Generation of reactive oxygen species from the reaction of selenium compounds with thiols and mammary tumor cells. Biochem Pharmacol 45:429–437
30. Green DR, Reed JC (1998) Mitochondria and apoptosis. Science 281:1309–1312

31. Cai J, Yang J, Jones DP (1998) Mitochondrial control of apoptosis: the role of cytochrome c. Biochim Biophys Acta 1366:139–149
32. Li P, Nijhawan D, Budihardjo I, Srinivasula SM, Ahmad M, Alnemri ES, Wang X (1997) Cytochrome c and dATP-dependent formation of Apaf-1/caspase-9 complex initiates an apoptotic protease cascade. Cell 91:479–489
33. Thornberry NA, Lazebnik Y (1998) Caspases: enemies within. Science 281:1312–1316
34. Iwahashi H, Eguchi Y, Yasuhara N, Hanafusa T, Matsuzawa Y, Tsujimoto Y (1997) Synergistic anti-apoptotic activity between Bcl-2 and SMN implicated in spinal atrophy. Nature 390:413–417
35. Nutt LK, Chandra J, Pataer A, Fang B, Roth JA, Swisher SG, O'Neil RG, McConkey DJ (2002) Bax-mediated Ca^{2+} mobilization promotes cytochrome c release during apoptosis. J Biol Chem 277:20301–20308
36. Hamel W, Magnelli L, Chiarugi VP, Israel MA (1996) Herpes simplex virus thymidine kinase/ganciclovir-mediated apoptosis death of bystander cells. Cancer Res 56:2697–2702
37. Spallholz JE (1994) On the nature of selenium toxicity and carcinostatic activity. Free Radic Biol Med 17:45–64
38. Stewart MS, Spallholz JE, Nelder KH, Pence BC (1999) Selenium compounds have disparate abilities to impose oxidative stress and induce apoptosis. Free Radic Biol Med 26:42–48
39. Clark LC, Combs GF, Turnbull BW, Slate EH, Chalker DK, Chow J, Davis LS, Glover RA, Graham GF, Gross EG, Krongrad A, Lesher JL Jr, Park HK, Sanders BB Jr, Smith CL, Taylor JR (1996) Effects of selenium supplementation for cancer prevention in patients with carcinoma of the skin. A randomized controlled trial. JAMA 276:1957–1963
40. Chaudiere J, Courtin O, Leclaire J (1992) Glutathione oxidase activity of selenocystamine: a mechanistic study. Arch Biochem Biophys 296:328–336
41. Virani NA, Thavathiru E, McKernan P, Moore K, Benbrook DM, Harrison RG (2018) Anti-CD73 and Anti-OX40 immunotherapy coupled with a novel biocompatible enzyme prodrug system for the treatment of recurrent, metastatic ovarian cancer. Cancer Lett 425:174–182. https://doi.org/10.1016/j.canlet.2018.03.027
42. Xin L, Yang WF, Zhang HT, Li YF, Liu C (2018) The mechanism study of lentiviral vector carrying methioninase enhances the sensitivity of drug-resistant gastric cancer cells to cisplatin. Br J Cancer 118:1189. https://doi.org/10.1038/s41416-018-0043-8
43. Lien EC, Ghisolfi L, Geck RC, Asara JM, Toker A (2017) Oncogenic PI3K promotes methionine dependency in breast cancer cells through the cystine-glutamate antiporter xCT. Sci Signal 10(510):eaao6604. https://doi.org/10.1126/scisignal.aao6604
44. Hoffman RM (2017) Patient-derived mouse models of cancer. In: Coleman WB, Tsongalis GJ (eds) Molecular and translational medicine. Humana Press, New Jersey
45. Tisdale MT (1980) Changes in tRNA methyltransferase activity and cellular S-adenosylmethionine content following methionine deprivation. Biochim Biophys Acta 609:296–305

Chapter 15

Selenomethionine and Methioninase: Selenium Free Radical Anticancer Activity

Julian E. Spallholz

Abstract

Colloidal selenium, was first used to treat cancer as early as 1911 in both humans and mice. Selenium was identified as the toxic component in forage plants of sheep, cattle, and horses in the 1930s. The animal toxicity of selenium compounds was determined to be from the metabolism by animals of the elevated concentrations of Se-methylselenocysteine and selenomethionine in plants. The metabolism of both Se-methylselenocysteine and selenomethionine by animals gives rise to the metabolite, methylselenide (CH_3Se-), which if in sufficient concentration oxidizes thiols and generates superoxide and other reactive oxygen species. Cancer cells that may overly express methionine gamma-lyase, or beta-lyase (methioninase), by induced viral genomic expression, are susceptible to free radical-induced apoptosis from selenomethionine or Se-methylselenocysteine supplementation.

Key words Selenium, Selenide, Selenomethionnic, Cancer, Prevention, Therapy

1 Introduction

1.1 Selenium Metabolism in Plants: Selenomethionine and Se-Methylselenocysteine

Sulfur (S) and selenium (Se) are sister elements along with oxygen in the VIA Chalcogen Period of the Periodic Table. In the greater biological systems of plants and animals, organic compounds formed with S or Se can and do elementally replace one another [1–4]. From soils, sulfates give rise to the synthesis of methionine by plants, one of the nine essential dietary amino acids for animals and humans [5]. Its sister element selenium, arising from soils as mostly selenates, tracks sulfate metabolism in plants giving rise to the amino acid selenomethionine. The amount of selenomethionine made by plants is determined by the species of plant and the Se content of the soil upon which the plant is growing.

Robert M. Hoffman (ed.), *Methionine Dependence of Cancer and Aging: Methods and Protocols*, Methods in Molecular Biology, vol. 1866, https://doi.org/10.1007/978-1-4939-8796-2_15,

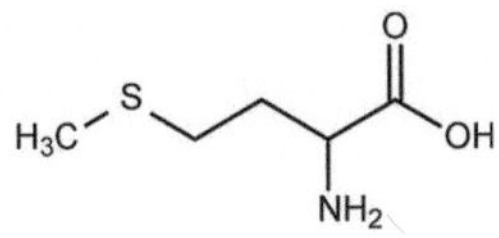

Methionine

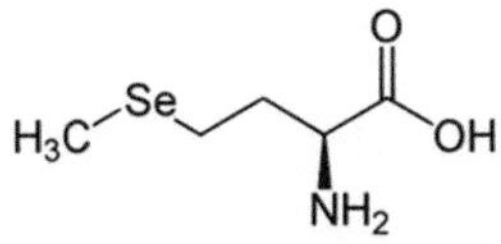

Selenomethionine

Most plant species do not require Se from soils[1], but however, trace amounts of selenomethionine is synthesized and incorporated into bacterial, yeast, and plant proteins in place of methionine [6]. Cereal-grain-producing plants, i.e., wheat and oats, along with brewer's yeast, predominately synthesize selenomethionine from inorganic selenium. Cruciferous vegetables, i.e., broccoli and garlics, predominately synthesize Se-methylselenocysteine, which is not incorporated into protein. This latter amino acid is highly concentrated by selenium-accumulator plants, i.e., species of Astragalus and others, growing on highly concentrated Se shale soils. Selenate, similar to sulfate from soils, is assimilated and the more toxic form of Se, selenite, analogues to sulfite, is formed by the plant's reduction of selenate. Thus, the occurrence of predominately selenomethionine in cereal food plants, and Se-methylselenocysteine in cruciferous and selenium-accumulator plants, may be viewed as a selenium detoxification process of the more toxic plant bio-reduced selenate, selenium, selenite [7, 8].

Ingested by animals and humans, selenomethionine serves as the primary dietary source of the most recently-discovered dietary-essential element, selenium. As methionine from plants is the essential amino acid precursor of the amino acid cysteine, selenomethionine is the predominate amino acid in providing ~85% of the selenium to Nature's 21st protein amino acid, selenocysteine [9]. The remaining 15% of dietary Se for selenocysteine can be met by numerous other natural dietary selenium compounds or dietary supplements. Selenocysteine is genetically encoded by UGA and incorporated into 25 different human selenium-containing proteins, noted over time, including glutathione peroxidase (EC 1.11.1.9), first recognized as an antioxidant selenium-containing enzyme in 1973 [10].

[1] Controlled experiments of the growth of the selenium-accumulator plants with varied concentrations of soil selenium have suggested that Se may be required by the selenium-accumulator but not the non-accumulator plants. Absorbed selenium is rapidly transported to the leaves and their organelles. I. Rosenfeld, Biochemical and Chemical Studies of Astragalus Leaves and Roots. Agricultural Experiment Station; University of Wyoming, Laramie, WY Bulletin #385 April 1962.

1.2 Selenium Toxicity

Prior to the recognition that selenium was an essential nutrient in 1958 [11] and component of selenocysteine within Glutathione peroxidase in 1973 [10], selenium was known only as a toxicant found in selenium-accumulator plants. Selenium toxicity is manifested mostly in range livestock, horses, cattle, and sheep principally, affecting growth, loss of hair and mane, ill thrift, low fertility, and neurotoxicity. Encountered by range animals, Se-methylselenocysteine was first identified as being the primary toxic compound from within the leaves of selenium-accumulator plants. Later, selenomethionine and other selenium compounds were also recognized for their toxicity in experimental animals. Selenium was to become known as the "Essential Poison" [12], and all selenium compounds, depending on their chemical composition and administered dosage, were to be found toxic to either animals or people. The underlying reason for its toxicity to plants, animals, and humans would not be accurately recognized until 1988 when Seko et al. [13–15] first showed that selenite in the presence of reduced glutathione (GSH) generated superoxide ($O_2^{\cdot -}$) as presented in Fig. 1.

In 1992, Chaudière et al. [16] showed that a diselenide, selenocystamine, upon reduction was also capable of generating superoxide in the presence of GSH, as shown in Fig. 2.

With the recognition that selenite and other diselenides could oxidize GSH and other thiols generating superoxide, over time it became clear that selenide anions (RSe^{-}) were redox catalysts generating superoxide and that oxidative stress accounted for selenium toxicity [17, 18]. Interestingly, the predominant natural food plants forming selenoamino acids, selenomethionine, and Se-methylselenocysteine were not very toxic in animals and did not by themselves readily form selenides. Consequently, neither of these two selenoamino acids generated superoxide in an experimental in vitro chemiluminescent assay for superoxide generation. Both amino acids were almost equally toxic to animals in vivo, but at highly elevated selenium concentrations of 100× or more of the dietary selenium requirement of rodents being 0.10–0.20 mgSe/kg of diet [19]. For humans the tolerable upper level TUL of unspecified selenium ingestion is 400 μg/Se/day. Metabolism of these selenoamino acids was to be the key in unlocking their inherent but naturally sequestered selenium toxicity.

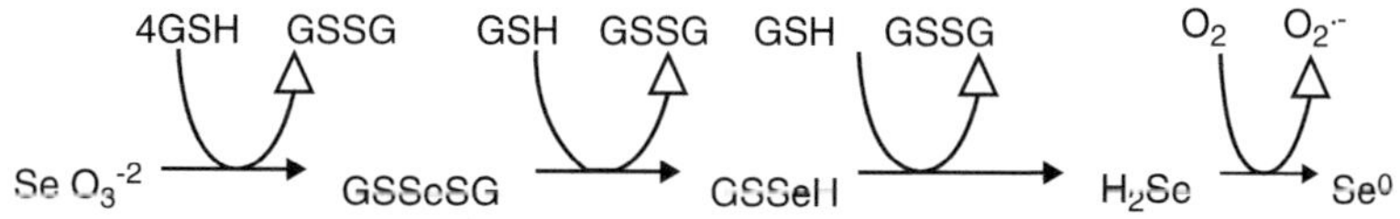

Fig. 1 Selenium Redox of Selenite Schematic by Seko et al., a 1988 Poster

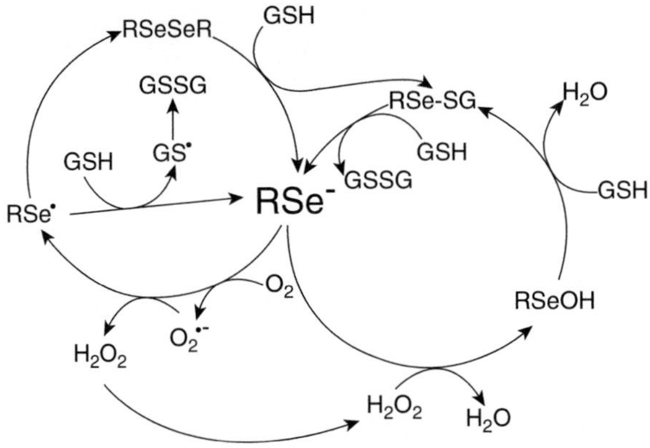

Fig. 2 Selenium Redox Schematic of Diselenide Reduction by Chaudière et al., 1992

2 Primer on Selenium and Cancer Prevention

Selenium, Element 34, was discovered in Gripsholm, Sweden, as a red deposit formed during the production of sulfuric acid. It was identified in 1817 by JJ Berzelius in his laboratory at the Karolinska Institute in Stockholm where Berzelius recognized its chemical properties to be similar to sulfur and tellurium [20]. Soon known to be toxic, in 1912 it was reported in a respected French Journal, *Le Province Medicale*, that injection of colloidal selenium was without human systemic toxicity but provided for the reduction and disappearance of a patient's lingual tumor [21]. Colloidal selenium was also used with an eosin carrier to treat tumors in mice as reported by A. Wasserman and F. Keysser in the preceding year, 1911. As reported, the Se-eosin cancer treatment was successful in mice, but further research was not fully convincing of the initial reports of colloidal selenium cancer-treatment success [22].

In the 1960s after Schwarz and Foltz showed that selenium was an essential mineral (nutrient) for the prevention of dietary liver necrosis in rats [23], Shamberger and Frost [24] and Frost and Lish [25] began to report an epidemiological inverse relationship between levels of Se in blood, serum, and plasma and the incidence of cancer in human populations. This relationship seemingly held to be true among humans where selenium was shown to be low in soils, foods, and blood [26]. This epidemiological association culminated in the highly cited 1996 research paper of Clark et al. where a significant reduction, ~50% in cancers of the prostate, colon, and lung tissues, was reported [27]. In the cohort of ~1300 male patients with a low selenium intake as measured by selenium in blood, the subjects were given a 200 μgSe/day supplement of yeast fortified with selenite selenium. The selenium yeast "supplemental product," then as now, is mostly comprised of the selenoamino acids selenomethionine, ~80–90%; 7–10% Se-methylselenocysteine; <2–3% other organic selenium compounds, and traces of selenite in which the yeast is grown [28].

The 1996 study by Clark et al. had lasted about 7 years and its primary focus was the effect of selenium supplementation, using supplemental Se-yeast or placebo, for the prevention of melanoma. Overall mortality and risk of reduced cancer from the prostate, colon, and lung tissues were the secondary observations of the study. The results from this 1996 selenium supplementation study of Clark et al. evoked additional "cancer prevention" studies in animals and surveys of selenium-associated "cancer reductions" in human populations where selenomethionine was predominantly from plant foods and selenomethionine and selenocysteine were predominant in animal foods. Such efforts culminated in the SELECT Trial, a Selenium and Vitamin E Cancer Prevention Trial, involving ~35,000 men over the age of 50 years to see if selenium would again reduce prostate cancer [29–31]. The SELECT Trial, a Phase 3 research trial, primarily sponsored by the National Cancer Institute (NCI), deviated from the Clark study in that the selenium yeast used as the selenium supplemental form by Clark et al. was replaced with an equal amount of pure supplemental synthetic selenomethionine equivalent to 200 μg Se/day. Added to the study were cohorts receiving selenomethionine and vitamin E together and vitamin E alone. The study was begun in 2001 and was planned to culminate in 2013. In 2008 however, the SELECT Trial was abruptly brought to an early halt due to the lack of evidence of any cancer-preventing effect of the selenomethionine and/or vitamin E supplementation over control subjects. The follow-up to the SELECT Trail in 2011 found no significant differences between subjects for prostate or other cancers. There was a trend in the data for the selenium-supplemented group to have a higher incidence of diabetes and the vitamin E-alone subjects, having a higher risk of prostate cancer.

The debate continues to this day about the possible reasons why the SELECT Trial failed in its attempt to replicate the 1996 study results of Clark et al. Reasons suggested include the following: the initial selenium status of the subjects was more "normal" in the SELECT Trial than that of the Clark cohort, and that the supplement was changed from a "fortified" Se-yeast in the Clark study to pure selenomethionine with and without vitamin E in the SELECT Trial. More recent Se-yeast speciation studies have shown that Se-yeast contains not just selenomethionine, but several other chemical forms of selenium that it is argued could have had a more ready impact on the final prostate-cancer outcome [32, 33].

3 Comparative Anticancer Chemistry of Selenium Compounds

Selenium compounds are all toxic to animals and humans, as well as viruses, bacteria, and plants, depending on chemical composition, dose, and exposure time. The commonly-employed experimental selenium compound to prevent skin cancer, such as in the Clark experiments and in the SELECT Trial for prostate cancer, is selenomethionine, the major component of Se-yeast. Its pure chemical form is not very toxic to cells in culture, animals, or people. A comparative dietary toxicity study between the more toxic selenite and relatively non-toxic selenomethionine in the rat showed 2 mg/Se/kg diet selenite is toxic whereas it takes 20–30 mg/Se/kg diet of selenomethionine to be toxic. The other major selenium component in Se-yeast, Se-methylselenocysteine, has similar toxicity in the rat to selenomethionine [19].

With cancer cells in vitro or experimental tumors in vivo; selenomethionine alone is never as toxic in preventing growth, as is selenite or the diselenides, selenocystine or selenocystamine [34]. The earliest comparative studies of the various forms of selenium on cancer were in 1979 and 1980 by Poirier and Milner [35] and Greeder and Milner [36], a full 8–9 years before selenium toxicity was beginning to be understood as a pro-oxidative chemistry generating superoxide [37]. In summary, the Poirier, Greeder, and Milner publications showed that selenite, selenium dioxide, and selenocystine were all toxic to Ehrlich ascites cancer cells (EATC) both in vitro and in vivo in mice. Selenate was less toxic than selenite and selenomethionine, at the comparable selenium concentrations experimentally tested and not significantly different from controls. The anticancer properties of the selenium compounds in vitro or in vivo as tested by these authors and later for human and canine breast cancer cells [38, 39] were congruent with the later-discovered property of selenium selenides as oxidants of thiols, thereby generating superoxide [18]. This redox chemistry thus explains selenium toxicity and selenium's anticancer property as shown by Seko et al. [13] for the intermediate perselenides formed from selenite and GSH, and Chaudière et al. [16] for the diselenides, as discussed above. The redox chemistry shown in Figs. 1 and 2 also explains why selenomethionine and the other major dietary selenoamino acid, Se-methylselenocysteine, are not by themselves normally toxic to cells in vitro or toxic to humans [40]. The answer to their lack of significant toxicity is that these selenoamino acids simply do not spontaneously form redox selenides in vitro or in vivo.

4 Selenomethionine: Anticancer Nutrient/Prodrug with Methioninase

The vitamin B6-dependent enzyme methionine-γ-lyase (EC 4.4.1.11) (methioninase), hydrolyzes the essential amino acid methionine as shown below:

Methionine + $H_2O \rightarrow NH_3$ + α-Ketoglutarate + Methanethiol (CH_3SH)

Methioninase has been the subject of an extensive 2017 review [41].

Methionine deficiency/starvation arrests numerous cancers, including cancers of the brain and neural system [42, 43]. Methioninase has been shown to be useful and nontoxic in the treatment of cancer when administered systemically by reducing the circulating levels of methionine [44, 45]. Because methionine is so important as an essential amino acid to the maintenance and sustainment of cancer cells, selenomethionine was discovered to be an alternate, but more toxic substrate of methioninase [46–48] to cancer cells by generating methaneselenol (methylselenol) [49].

Selenomethionine + $H_2O \rightarrow NH_3$ + α-Ketoglutarate + Methaneselenol (CH_3SeH)

In 2001 Miki et al. [50, 51] virally transfected cancer cells with the methioninase gene which had been cloned from *Pseudomonas putida*. When cancer cells expressing viral methioninase were exposed to selenomethionine the authors reported that cytotoxicity was increased over ~1000× compared to control cancer cells (please *see* Chap. 14 of the present volume). The release of methylselenol, actually methylselenide (CH_3Se^-) from the selenomethionine substrate by methioninase, generated oxidative stress by redox cycling [52] as shown in the schematics of Fig. 2 of Chaudière [16]. As shown for selenite in cells, the target organelle for selenium or the products of the selenium redox chemistry are the mitochondrion, causing "mitochondrial swelling" as described by Levander for selenite toxicity [53]. The oxidative stress from the methioninase/selenomethionine generation of methylselenide released mitochondrial cytochrome c, initiating the enzymatic caspase cascade resulting in apoptosis. Free radical selenium redox chemistry and selenium's anticancer properties with the predicted causes of cell death by selenium by apoptosis were reviewed by Spallholz in 1994 [18].

In 2003 Gupta et al. combined methioninase gene therapy with selenomethionine, generating methylselenide and the anthracycline doxorubicin [47], another redox-generating chemotherapeutic drug [55] to treat H460 human lung cancer in nude mice. The authors reported significantly reduced tumor growth in these mice with the combined therapy protocol than with either of the therapy regimens used alone (please *see* Chap. 14 of the present volume).

Mitochondrial membrane BCL-2 is a member of the BCL family of anti-apoptotic proteins. Elevated levels of BCL-2 impart resistance to various chemotherapeutic drugs among its other normal mitochondrial functions. Methioninase gene therapy combined with selenomethionine was shown by Yamamoto et al. in 2003 [51] to inhibit an apoptosis-resistant human lung cancer cell line overexpressing BCL-2 by targeting the mitochondrion. Redox selenium attached to a prostate-specific monoclonal antibody, B72.3 targeted mitochondria within LS174T prostate cancer cells visualized by transmission electron microscopy [57]. These results suggest that redox organic selenium compounds such as selenite, generating superoxide within cells, can disrupt mitochondria leading to apoptosis. Cancers with elevated mitochondrial BCL-2 may be effectively treated with redox selenium compounds in combination with regular chemotherapy.

5 Limits to Selenomethionine as a Cancer Prevention Prodrug

Spallholz et al. used an in vitro chemiluminescent assay capable of superoxide detection [52] to determine that recombinant methioninase and selenomethionine together generated superoxide in a concentration-dependent manner, while methioninase incubated with Se-methylselenocysteine or methionine did not generate any measurable superoxide. This experimental observation, along with the methioninase gene transfer/selenomethionine experimentations above, and experiments with selenium compounds known to directly generate methylselenide, dimethyldiselenide, and superoxide [17, 53], has led many researches to conclude that the cancer chemoprevention species from dietary sources is methylselenol [49–52], i.e., methylselenide, arresting cancer cell growth. Thus, the two major dietary sources of selenium that are and have been used for chemoprevention studies in animal and humans, selenomethionine and Se-methylselenocysteine, to be effective must encounter and be internalized by cancer cells that express methioninase [45] or in the case of Se-methylselenocysteine its β-lyase (EC 4.4.1.13) enzyme [54–58], both of which must be introduced into the cancer cells by gene therapy.

During the period of the ongoing SELECT Trial our laboratory screened DU-145 and PC-3 prostate cancer cell lines and a normal prostate epithelial cell line PZ-HPV-7 with selenomethionine (SeMET) and Se-methylselenocysteine (SeMC) for (1) toxicity and (2) presence of cytosolic enzyme extracts of the cells to generate methylselenide and superoxide in the in vitro chemiluminescent assay. The IC_{50} for the three cell lines using [^{3}H] thymidine was as follows: for DU-145, SeMC was 40 nM; for SeMet, 800 nM. For PC-3, the SeMC was 80 nM and for SeMet was 800 nM. The normal prostate epithelial cell line PZ-HPV-7 IC50 values were SeMC 3200 nM and SeMet 1000 nM. These in vitro IC_{50} cytotoxicity results correlated with the ability of the different cell line extracts to generate methylselenide from SeMet and SeMC as measured by the chemiluminescent monitoring of superoxide generation using lucigenin [59].

The inferences drawn from the comparative toxicity of the selenium compounds above and from the literature are that selenium selenides are likely to be much more toxic to cancer cells than selenomethionine or Se-methylselenocysteine in the absence of the lyases which generate methylselenide. When the lyases are introduced by viral gene transformation, as shown for the methioninase experiments, selenomethionine and Se-methylselenocysteine can be therapeutic. Se-methylselenocysteine has been recently reported to be the better chemoprevention dietary supplement than selenomethionine [60–62], in agreement with the in vitro experiments above.

6 Summary

Selenium compounds that chemically form selenides are toxic in vitro in a dose- and time-dependent manner and have anticancer or chemoprevention properties. Methylated selenium compounds such as selenomethionine and Se-methylselenocysteine are not toxic, but when exposed to their respective enzymes γ- and β-lyases, methylselenide (CH_3Se^-) is generated; oxidation of thiols commences, superoxide($O_2^{\cdot -}$) is generated, and if subsequent and sufficient oxidative stress is generated, cell death, usually by apoptosis, occurs. Sufficient amounts of these two enzymes genetically introduced into cancer cells determine the therapeutic potential of selenomethionine or Se-methylselenocysteine.

Dedication/Acknowledgments

This chapter is dedicated to *Edgar N. Drake, PhD* (1937–2017). Dr. Ed Drake was Chair and Professor of Chemistry at Angelo State University for many years. As an analytical chemist, he became interested in selenium analyses, and selenium as a chemoprevention dietary supplement. In 2001 he authored a book, "Selenium: Are You Getting Enough to Reduce Your Risk of Cancer?" He was thoroughly versed in selenium biochemistry and one of the early selenium scientists to recognize the pro-oxidant properties of selenium compounds (*see* Ref. 37). Following retirement, Ed and his wife Nina lived for many years in Estes Park, Colorado, and had a "Million-Dollar View" of Long's Peak in Rocky Mountain

National Park. The author and his wife visited Ed and Nina in Estes Park both in summer and winter, where selenium was always a major conversation topic. He will be missed by the selenium community and the people that knew him.

References

1. Dingwall D (1962) Selenium analogues of biologically active sulphur compounds. Pharm Pharmacol 14:765–778
2. Hurd-Karrer AM (1933) Inhibition of selenium injury to wheat pants by sulfur. Science 78:560
3. Ochoa-Solano A, Gitler C (1968) Incorporation of ^{75}Se-selenomethionine and ^{35}S-methionine into chicken egg white proteins. J Nutr 94:243–248
4. Mackowiak CL, Amacher MC (2008) Soil sulfur amendments suppress selenium uptake by alfalfa and western wheatgrass. J Environ Qual 37:772–779
5. Milner JA (1979) Assessment of the essentiality of methionine, threonine, tryptophan, histidine and isoleucine in immature dogs. J Nutr 109:1351–1357
6. McConnell KP, Hoffman JL (1972) Methionine-selenomethionine parallels in rat liver polypeptide chain synthesis. FEBS Lett 24:60–62
7. Franke KW (1934) A new toxicant occurring naturally in certain samples of plant foodstuffs. J Nutrition 8:597–608
8. Whanger PD (2002) Selenocompounds in plants and animals and their biological significance. J Am Coll Nutr 21:223–232
9. Böck A, Forchhammer K, Heider J et al (1991) Selenocysteine: the 21st amino acid. Mol Microbiol 5:515–520
10. Rotruck JT, Pope AL, Ganther HE et al (1973) Selenium: biochemical role as a component of glutathione peroxidase. Science 179:588–590
11. Schwarz K, Foltz CM (1958) Factor 3 activity of selenium compounds. J Biol Chem 233:245–251
12. Jukes TH (1983) Selenium, an "essential poison". J Appl Biochem 5:233–234
13. Seko Y, Saito Y, Kitahara J, Imura N et al (1989) Active oxygen generation by the reaction of selenite with reduced glutathione *in vitro*. In: Wendel A (ed) Selenium in biology and medicine. Springer, Berlin Heidelberg; Tubingen, pp 70–73
14. Kitahara J, Seko Y, Imura N (1993) Possible involvement of active oxygen species in selenite toxicity in isolated rat hepatocytes. Arch Toxicol 67:497–501
15. Seko Y, Imura N (1997) Active oxygen generation as a possible mechanism of selenium toxicity. Biomed Environ Sci 10:333–339
16. Chaudière J, Courtin O, Leclaire J (1992) Glutathione oxidase activity of selenocystamine: a mechanistic study. Arch Biochem Biophys 296:328–336
17. Chen JJ, Boylan LM, Wu CK et al (2007) Oxidation of glutathione and superoxide generation by inorganic and organic selenium compounds. Biofactors 31:55–66
18. Spallholz JE (1994) On the nature of selenium toxicity and carcinostatic activity. Free Radic Biol Med 17:45–64
19. Shriver BJ, Praytor LM, Boylan LM et al (2000) Response of growing rats to supplemental selenium in the form of L-Se-methylselenocysteine or L-selenomethionine. FASEB J 14:A513
20. Berzelius JJ (1817) Sur deux metaux nouveaux (litium et selenium). Schweigger J 2:1818–1823
21. Letter May 6, 1912. In references to a publication to the use of selenium to treat a tongue epithelioma; Le Province Medicale; 13 April 1912 (Paris)
22. Sugiura K, Benedict SR (1929) The action of certain dyestuffs on the growth of transplantable tumors. J Cancer Res 13:340 Wasserman A, Keyser F
23. Schwarz K, Foltz CM (1957) Selenium as an integral part of factor 3 against dietary necrotic liver degeneration. J Am Chem Soc 79:3292–3293
24. Shamberger RJ, Frost DV (1969) Possible protective effect of selenium against human cancer. Can Med Assoc J 100:682
25. Frost DV, Lish PM (1975) Selenium in biology. Annu Rev Pharmacol 15:259–284
26. Clark LC, Cantor KP, Allaway WH (1991) Selenium in forage crops and cancer mortality in U.S. counties. Arch Environ Health 46:37–42
27. Clark LC, Combs GF Jr, Turnbull BW et al (1996) Effects of selenium supplementation

for cancer prevention in patients with carcinoma of the skin. A randomized controlled trial. Nutritional Prevention of Cancer Study Group. JAMA 276:1957–1963

28. Uden PC, Boakye HT, Kahakachchi C et al (2004) Element selective characterization of stability and reactivity of selenium species in selenized yeast. J Anal At Spectrom 19:65–73
29. Klein EA, Thompson IM, Lippman SM et al (2001) SELECT: the next prostate cancer prevention trial. Selenium and Vitamin E cancer prevention trial. J Urol 166:1311–1315
30. Cook ED (2002) Selenium and vitamin e cancer prevention trial--this one's for us. J Natl Med Assoc 94:856–858
31. Lippman SM, Klein E, Goodman PJ et al (2009) Effect of selenium and vitamin E on risk of prostate cancer and other cancers: the selenium and vitamin e cancer prevention trial (SELECT). JAMA 301:39–51
32. Sharma AK, Amin S (2013) Post SELECT: selenium on trial. Future Med Chem 5:163–174
33. Lü J, Zhang J, Jiang C et al (2016) Cancer chemoprevention research with selenium in the post-SELECT era: promises and challenges. Nutr Cancer 268:1–17
34. Stewart M, Neldner K, Spallholz JE et al (1999) Selenite, selenocystamine, and selenomethionine have disparate abilities to impose oxidative stress and induce apoptosis in mouse keratinocytes. Free Radic Biol Med 26:42–48
35. Poirier KA, Milner JA (1979) The effect of various seleno-compounds on Erlich ascites tumor cells. Bio Trace Elem Res 1:25–34
36. Greeder GA, Milner JA (1980) Factors influencing the inhibitory effect of selenium on mice inoculated with Erlich ascites tumor cells. Science 209:825–827
37. Drake EN (2006) Cancer chemoprevention: selenium as a prooxidant, not an antioxidant. Med Hypotheses 67:318–322
38. Watrach AM, Milner JA, Watrach MA et al (1984) Inhibition of human breast cancer cells by selenium. Cancer Lett 25:41–47
39. Fico ME, Poirier KA, Watrach AM, Watrach MA, Milner JA (1986) Differential effects of selenium on normal and neoplastic canine mammary cells. Cancer Res 46:3384–3388
40. Marshall JR, Burk RF, Payne OR et al (2017) Selenomethionine and methyl selenocysteine: multiple-dose pharmacokinetics in selenium-replete men. Oncotarget 8:26312–26322
41. Suganya K, Govindan K, Prabha P et al (2017) An extensive review on L-methioninase and its potential applications. Biocatal Agric Biotechnol 12:104–115
42. Hoshiya Y, Guo H, Kubota T et al (1995) Human tumors are methionine dependent in vivo. Anticancer Res 15:717–718
43. Cavuoto P, Fenech MF (2012) A review of methionine dependency and the role of methionine restriction in cancer growth control and life-span extension. Cancer Treat Rev 38:726–736
44. Cellarier E, Durando X, Vasson MP et al (2003) Methionine dependency and cancer treatment. Cancer Treat Rev 29:489–499
45. Hoffman RM (2015) Development of recombinant methioninase to target the general cancer-specific metabolic defect of methionine dependence: a 40-year odyssey. Expert Opin Biol Ther 15:21–31
46. Tan Y, Xu M, Guo H, Sun X, Kubota T, Hoffman RM (1996) Anticancer efficacy of methioninase in vivo. Anticancer Res 16:3931–3936
47. Gupta A, Miki K, Xu M, Yamamoto N, Moossa AR, Hoffman RM (2003) Combination efficacy of doxorubicin and adenoviral methioninase gene therapy with prodrug selenomethionine. Anticancer Res 23:1181–1188
48. Sato D, Nozaki T (2009) Methionine gamma-lyase: the unique reaction mechanism, physiological roles, and therapeutic applications against infectious diseases and cancers. IUBMB Life 61:1019–1028
49. Ip C, Thompson HJ, Zhu Z et al (2000) In vitro and in vivo studies of methylseleninic acid: evidence that a monomethylated selenium metabolite is critical for cancer chemoprevention. Cancer Res 60:2882–2886
50. Miki K, Xu M, Gupta A et al (2001) Methioninase cancer gene therapy with selenomethionine as suicide prodrug substrate. Cancer Res 61:6805–6810
51. Yamamoto N, Gupta A, Xu M et al (2003) Methioninase gene therapy with selenomethionine induces apoptosis in bcl-2-overproducing lung cancer cells. Cancer Gene Ther 10:445–450
52. Spallholz JE, Palace VP, Reid TW (2004) Methioninase and selenomethionine but not Se-methylselenocysteine generates methylselenol and superoxide in an in vitro chemiluminescent assay: implications for the nutritional carcinostatic activity of selenoamino acids. Biochem Pharmacol 67:47–554
53. Levander OA, Morris VC, Higgs DJ (1973) Acceleration of thiol-induced swelling of rat liver mitochondria by selenium. Biochemistry 12:4586–4590
54. Cooper AJL, Bruschi SA, Irirarte-Marino A et al (2002) Mitochondrial aspartate

aminotransferase catalysis cysteine S-conjugate β-lyase reactions. Biochem J 368:253–261

55. Keizer HG, Pinedo HM, Schuurhuis GJ et al (1990) Doxorubicin (adriamycin): a critical review of free radical-dependent mechanisms of cytotoxicity. Pharmacol Ther 47:219–231
56. Suzuki KT, Kurasaki K, Suzuki N (2007) Selenocysteine beta-lyase and methylselenol demethylase in the metabolism of e-methylated selenocompounds into selenide. Biochim Biophys Acta 1770:1053–1061
57. Chen L (1997) Cytotoxicity of antibody-selenium immunoconjugates against erythrocytes and cancer cells. Doctoral Dissertation, Texas Tech University
58. Cooper AJ, Krasnikov BF, Niatsetskaya ZV et al (2011) Cysteine S-conjugate β-lyases: important roles in the metabolism of naturally occurring sulfur and selenium-containing compounds, xenobiotics and anticancer agents. Amino Acids 41:7–27
59. Reid TW, Grey T, Spallholz JE (2003) A comparison of the ability of se-methylselenocysteine and selenomethionine to kill human prostate cancer cells in vitro. NIH Symposium on Selenium Proteins, Abstract/Poster; Bethesda, MD
60. Medina D, Thompson H, Ganther H et al (2001) Se-methylselenocysteine: a new compound for chemoprevention of breast cancer. Nutr Cancer 40(1):12–17
61. Jiang C, Wang Z, Ganther H et al (2001) Caspases as key executors of methyl selenium-induced apoptosis (anoikis) of DU-145 prostate cancer cells. Cancer Res 61:3062–3070
62. Lu Z, Qi L, Li GX et al (2015) Se-methylselenocysteine suppresses the growth of prostate cancer cell DU145 through annexin 43-induced apoptosis. J Cancer Res Ther 11:840–845

Chapter 16

Safety and Toxicity of Recombinant Methioninase and Polyethylene Glycol (PEG) Recombinant Methioninase in Primates

Robert M. Hoffman, Zhijian Yang, Yuying Tan, Qinghong Han, Shukuan Li, and Shigeo Yagi

Abstract

Methionine (MET) is a general metabolic therapeutic target in cancer, whereby cancer cells have an elevated requirement for MET, termed MET dependence. We have developed recombinant L-methionine α-deamino-γ-mercaptomethane lyase (recombinant methioninase [rMETase, EC 4.4.1.11]) as targeted therapy of all cancer types. Pharmacokinetics, MET depletion, antigenicity, and toxicity of rMETase were examined in macaque monkeys. Pharmacokinetic analysis showed that rMETase was eliminated with a $T_{1/2}$ of 2.49 h. A 2-week i.v. administration of 4000 units/kg every 8 h/day for 2 weeks resulted in a steady-state depletion of plasma MET to less than 2 μM. The only manifest toxicity was decreased food intake and slight weight loss. Serum albumin and red-cell values declined transiently during treatment. Rechallenge on day 28 resulted in anaphylactic shock and death in one animal. Pretreatment with hydrocortisone prevented the anaphylactic reaction. Anti-rMETase antibodies (at 10^{-3}) were found after the first challenge, increased to 10^{-6} after the fourth challenge, and decreased to 10^{-2} by 2 months post-therapy. Therefore, the therapeutic potential of rMETase is limited by its short plasma half-life and immunologic effects, including high antibody production in mice and anaphylactic reactions in monkeys. To overcome these limits, rMETase has been coupled to methoxypolyethylene glycol succinimidyl glutarate polyethylene glycol (MEGC-PEG-5000). The pharmacokinetics, antigenicity, and toxicity of MEGC-PEG-rMETase in macaque monkeys were evaluated using an escalating-dose strategy. In pharmacokinetic studies, a single 4000 units/kg dose showed that MEGC-PEG-rMETase holoenzyme activity was eliminated with a biological half-life of 1.3 h, and the MEGC-PEG-rMETase apoenzyme was eliminated with a biological half-life of 90 h, a 36-fold increase compared with non-PEGylated rMETase. The disparity in the $T_{½}$ of the apoenzyme and the holoenzyme reflects the loss of co-factor pyridoxal-L-phosphate of the circulating MEGC-PEG-rMETase. A 7-day i.v. administration of 4000 units/kg every 12 h resulted in a steady-state depletion of plasma MET to <5 μmol/L. The only manifest toxicity was decreased food intake and slight weight loss. Red cell values and hemoglobin declined transiently. Subsequent challenges did not result in any immunologic reactions. Anti-MEGC-PEG-rMETase antibodies were 100- to 1000-fold less than antibodies elicited by naked rMETase, thereby suggesting clinical potential of MEGC-PEG-rMETase as a broad anticancer agent.

Key words Recombinant methioninase, rMETase, Polyethylene glycol, PEG, PEG-rMEtase, Macaque monkeys, Safety, Antigenicity, Anaphylaxis, Anemia, Half-life, Holoenzyme, Apoenzyme, Pyridoxal-L-Phosphate

Robert M. Hoffman (ed.), *Methionine Dependence of Cancer and Aging: Methods and Protocols*, Methods in Molecular Biology, vol. 1866, https://doi.org/10.1007/978-1-4939-8796-2_16,

1 Introduction

Methionine (MET) dependence has been observed in many human cancer cell lines and patient cancer xenografts in animal models, including patient-derived orthotopic xenograft (PDOX) mouse models [1–4]. MET dependence is a metabolic defect seen only in cancer cells and precludes the cells from growing under MET restriction (MR) [1] (*see* **Note 1**) (Table 1).

L-Methionine α-deamino-γ-mercaptomethane lyase (recombinant methioninase [rMETase, EC 4.4.1.11]) is a pyridoxal-L-phosphate (PLP)-dependent enzyme that targets MET dependence of cancer cells. Kreis and Hession [5] were the first to use a METase for cancer treatment. Their Clostridium METase could deplete MET in vivo but was unstable.

rMETase has been cloned from *Pseudomona putida* [6] and produced in *Escherichia coli* [7, 8].

rMETase alone or in combination with chemotherapeutic agents such as cisplatinum (CDDP), 5-fluorouracil (5-FU), 1,3-bis(2-chloroethyl)-1-nitrosourea (BCNU), and temozolomide (TEM) has shown efficacy and synergy, respectively, in mouse models of colon cancer, lung cancer, and brain cancer [9–12] and PDOX models of sarcoma and melanoma [2–4, 13, 14] (Table 1).

Table 1
Efficacy of recombinant methioninase on patient-derived orthotopic xenograft (PDOX) mouse models

Cancer type	Route	rMETase-alone effect	rMETase combination	Arrest/regress	Publication
Melanoma (BRAF +)	i.p.	Sensitive	+Temozolomide	Arrests tumor	[15]
Melanoma (BRAF -)	i.p.	Sensitive	+Temozolomide	Arrests tumor	[2]
Pancreatic cancer	i.p.	Sensitive	+Gemcitabine	Regresses tumor	[42]
Osteosarcoma	i.p.	Arrests tumor	+Cisplatinum and *S. typhimurium* A1-R	Regresses tumor	[45]
Undifferentiated spindle-cell sarcoma	i.p.	Arrests tumor	+Doxorubicin	Regresses tumor	[41]
Ewing's sarcoma	i.p.	Sensitive	--	--	[14]
Ewing's sarcoma	Oral	Arrests tumor	+*S. typhimurium* A1-R	Regresses tumor	[43]
Synovial sarcoma	i.p.	Sensitive		Arrests tumor	[44]
Melanoma (BRAF +)	Oral	Arrests tumor	+ip-rMETase	Arrests tumor	[3]
Pancreatic cancer	Oral	Arrests tumor	+ip-rMETase	Regresses tumor	[42]

rMETase in combination with gemcitabine (GEM) is active in PDOX models of pancreatic cancer [41, 42] (Table 1).

The findings from a pilot Phase I clinical trial showed that rMETase depleted plasma MET levels without observed clinical toxicity over a period up to ~24 h in patients with advanced cancer [15, 16] (*see* **Note 2**).

rMETase has been tested for safety in macaque monkeys [17]. rMETase could deplete plasma MET to <2 μmol/L with a *T*½ of 2.49 h, but a subsequent challenge with rMETase resulted in severe anaphylactic shock in one animal and high anti-rMETase antibody titers after the fourth challenge. Thus, rMETase is limited by its short plasma circulating half-life and potentially severe immunologic reactions [18].

Conjugation of protein therapeutics with polyethylene glycol (PEG) reduces antigenicity [19]. PEGylated forms of several proteins are used in the clinic including adenosine deaminase, asparaginase, α-interferon, and a growth hormone antagonist [20–24].

rMETase was coupled to methoxypolyethylene glycol succinimidyl glutarate-5000 (MEGC-PEG-5000) [25]. MEGC-PEG-rMETase increased the serum half-life of the apoenzyme up to 20-fold and increased MET depletion time up to 12-fold compared with unmodified rMETase. No anaphylaxis reactions were found and only low levels of anti-rMETase antibodies were detected. A further prolongation of MET depletion by MEGC-PEG-rMETase was achieved by supplementation with pyridoxal-5′-phosphate (PLP) [25] administration.

In an unexpected breakthrough, we have recently found that oral administration of rMETase is highly effective with PDOX models [41–43].

This chapter reviews the comparison of rMETase with and without MEGC-PEGrMETase for the pharmacokinetics, antigenicity, and systemic toxicity with repeated administration in macaque monkeys [18] (*see* **Note 3**).

2 Materials

1. rMETase (Shionogi & Co. Ltd., Osaka, Japan): The rMETase was more then 95% pure by high-performance liquid chromatography and a single band of M_r 43,000 on SDS-PAGE with a tetramer:oligomer ratio of 96.7:3.3. The specific enzyme activity of rMETase was 55 units/mg. The endotoxin level was 0.06 EU/mg [26–29].

2. Male *Macaca fascicularis* monkeys, aged 5–7 years, and weighing 6–8 kg (Suzhou West Hill Experimental Animal Co., Ltd., Suzhou, China).
3. Pyridoxal-5′-phosphate (PLP).
4. EDTA-coated tubes.
5. DTT.
6. $EDTA_2Na$.
7. 50% Trichloroacetic acid.
8. 3-Methyl-2-benzothiazolinone hydrazone solution containing 0.1% 3-methyl-2-benzothiazolinone hydrazone hydrochloride monohydrate (Wako, Osaka, Japan).
9. Acetonitrile.
10. Fluoraldehyde derivative reagent.
11. *O*-phthaldialdehyde (OPA).
12. Sodium acetate (pH 7.0).
13. Supelcosil LC-18DB column (25 cm × 4.8 cm, particle size 5 μm, Supelco, Bellefonte, PA).
14. Methanol.
15. Tetrahydrofuran methanol sodium acetate (pH 7.2).
16. Fluorescence spectrophotometer.
17. MEGC-PEG (NOF corporation, Kawasaki, JAPAN).

3 Methods

3.1 rMETase

3.1.1 Dose Ranging

1. Randomly assign six *Macaca fascicularis* monkeys to three dose levels of 1000 units/kg, 2000 units/kg, and 4000 units/kg.
2. Administer single doses of 1000, 2000, or 4000 units/kg rMETase solution to groups of three via the saphenous vein of the hind limbs under anesthesia consisting of 15 mg/kg ketamine hydrochloride administered i.m.
3. Fast all monkeys 8 h before and after dosing.
4. Administer rMETase by bolus injection over 1–2 min [17].

3.1.2 Repeated Dose Administration

1. Based on the dose-ranging study, administer a dose of 4000 units/kg rMETase to each of the four naive monkeys three times per day at 8-h intervals for 14 consecutive days.
2. As controls, administer two monkeys the same volume of vehicle solution in the same manner as the rMETase-treated monkeys.
3. Fast all animals 2 h before and after each injection [17].

3.1.3 Challenge Doses

1. On day 28 after administration of rMETase, administer two rMETase-treated monkeys challenge injections of rMETase at the same dose used in the repeated-dose studies.
2. Administer another two rMETase-treated monkeys monthly challenge injections of rMETase for 4 months with hydrocortisone (50 mg) pretreatment i.v. 10 min before each challenge injection [17].

3.2 MEGC-PEG-rMETase

1. Couple MEGC-PEG-5000 to rMETase using molar ratios of PEG/rMETase of 60:1. Analyze with matrix-assisted desorption ionization (MALDI)-time-of-flight/mass spectrometry to show that the MEGC-PEG-rMETase subunit has a 59.8–81.0 kDa molecular mass, corresponding to 3–7 PEG molecules per subunit. Thaw frozen MEGC-PEG-rMETase and warm to 37 °C just before use. Constitute the vehicle solution with 10 mmol/l sodium phosphate buffer containing 0.1 mmol/l PLP (pH 7.9) [18].
2. Use male *Macaca fascicularis* monkeys, aged 5–7 years, and weighing 6–8 kg. Individually house the monkeys in stainless steel cages in a controlled environment (12 h/day artificial lighting; 12 times/h ventilation; 20–25 °C room temperature; 40–60% humidity). Feed the monkeys monkey chow, fruit, and water at scheduled times. Acclimatize all the monkeys in their cages for a 2-week period before the initiation of treatment. During this period, observe the monkeys for clinical signs and examine for food consumption, body weight, hematology, and blood chemistry [18].
3. Use dose-escalating of 1000 units/kg, 4000 units/kg, and 8000 units/kg MEGC-PEG-rMETase. Administer i.v. to the same monkeys via the saphenous veins of the hind limbs.
4. Observe at 2-week intervals between each dose. Fast the monkeys 8 h before and after dosing.
5. Collect blood samples at different time points after each dosing and measure for plasma rMETase activity and MET levels [18].

3.3 Dose and Challenge Schedule

1. On the basis of the dose-ranging study, administer naïve monkeys MEGC-PEG-rMETase at a dose of 4000 units/kg each, twice daily at 12-h intervals for 7 consecutive days.
2. On days 29, 50, and 71 after administration of MEGC-PEGrMETase, give MEGC-PEG-rMETase-treated monkeys challenge injections of MEGC-PEG-rMETase at a dose of 4000 units/kg.
3. Fast all animals 2 h before and after each injection [18].

3.4 Determination of Plasma rMETase Activity

1. Repeat dosing during 7 days and challenge injections of MEGC-PEG-rMETase or rMETase.
2. Draw blood samples, collect all of the blood samples in EDTA-coated tubes, and centrifuge at 13,000 rpm for 2 min at 4 °C to obtain plasma.
3. Aliquot plasma samples and freeze at −70 °C [18].
4. Measure 50 μl of sample diluted in 100 mmol/L potassium phosphate buffer (pH 8.0) containing 0.01% DTT, 1 mmol/L $EDTA_2Na$, 10 μmol/L PLP, and 0.05% Tween 80, and mix with 1 mL of substrate solution (100 mmol/L potassium phosphate buffer [pH 8.0] containing 25 mmol/L MET and 10 μmol/L PLP) in a glass test tube.
5. Vortex the reaction mixture immediately and incubate at 37 °C without shaking for precisely 10 min.
6. Stop the reaction by adding 100 μL 50% trichloroacetic acid.
7. Centrifuge the suspension at 13,000 rpm for 2 min.
8. Collect the supernatant (0.8 mL) in a glass tube containing 1.6 mL of 1 mol/l acetate buffer (pH 5.0).
9. Add 0.6 mL of 3-methyl-2-benzothiazolinone hydrazone solution containing 0.1% 3-methyl-2-benzothiazolinone hydrazone hydrochloride monohydrate to the tube, mix well, and incubate at 50 °C for 40 min.
10. Measure the absorbance of the reaction mixture at 320 nm.
11. Carry out the assay in triplicate.
12. Calculate the ΔE by subtracting the average absorbance of blanks from the average absorbance of the reaction mixture.
13. Calculate the enzyme activity by the following formula: Activity (units/mL) = $0.548\ (1.07 + 2.2\Delta E)\ \Delta E$. One unit of enzyme is defined as the amount of enzyme that produces 1 μmol/L α-ketobutyrate per minute at a non-limiting concentration of L-methionine [18].
14. Determine the amount of MEGC-PEG-rMETase holoenzyme in the absence of PLP in the substrate solution.
15. All of the procedures are the same as the rMETase enzyme assay except that 5 μL of the sample in 45 μL of distilled water is mixed with 1 mL of substrate solution in the first reaction step.
16. Due to the change of sample volume, calculate the enzyme activity from the following formula: Activity (units/mL) = $27.4\ (1.07 + 2.2\Delta E)\ \Delta E$ [18].

3.5 Determination of Plasma MET

1. Measure the plasma MET concentration after treatment with rMETase or MEGC-PEGrMETase using a pre-column

derivatization, followed by high-performance liquid chromatography separation based on a method described previously with modification [30].

2. Use 10 μL of plasma sample or MET standard.
3. Identify plasma MET by the retention time of a MET standard solution and quantify according to a MET standard curve. The limit of detection is 0.5 μmol/L MET.
4. Precipitate 10 μL of plasma sample or MET standard with 30 μL of acetonitrile, followed by centrifugation at 10,000 rpm for 5 min.
5. Mix 10 μL of the supernatant with 5 μL of a fluoraldehyde derivative reagent, *O*-phthaldialdehyde, for 1 min at room temperature, followed by addition of 150 μL of 0.1 mol/L sodium acetate (pH 7.0).
6. Load 20 μL of the reaction mixture on a reversed-phase Supelcosil LC-18DB column (25 cm × 4.8 cm, particle size 5 μm, Supelco, Bellefonte, PA).
7. Separate the amino acid derivatives by using a gradient elution of 40–60% solution B (methanol) in solution A [tetrahydrofuran/methanol/0.1 mol/L sodium acetate (pH 7.2), 5:95:900] at a flow rate of 1.5 mL/min.
8. Use a fluorescence spectrophotometer for detection, with excitation at 350 nm and emission at 450 nm.
9. Identify plasma MET by the retention time of a MET standard solution and quantitate according to a MET standard curve [18].

3.6 Pharmacokinetic Analysis

1. Generate the concentration-time curves for plasma MEGC-PEG-rMETase or rMETase apoenzyme and holoenzyme as the plasma enzyme activity (units/mL) versus time after a single MEGC-PEGrMETase or rMETase administration at doses of 2000 and 4000 units/kg.
2. Choose an appropriate pharmacokinetic model on the basis of the profile of the concentration–time curve.
3. Calculate the pharmacokinetics parameters including initial drug concentration, elimination constant, apparent volume of distribution, $T_{1/2}$, area under (concentration–time) curve (AUC), and total body clearance (CL) for a one-compartment model.
4. Calculate the parameters including apparent volume of distribution, distributive-phase half-life, elimination-phase half-life, rate constant for exchange between the peripheral and central compartment, rate constant for exchange between the central

and peripheral compartment, total elimination rate constant, AUC, and CLs for a two-compartment model.

5. Carry out the pharmacokinetic modeling and pharmacokinetic parameter estimations using pharmacokinetic software 3P97 (Mathematics Institute, Academy of Science, Beijing, China) [18].

3.7 Systemic Toxicity Studies

1. Observe the clinical parameters daily including vital signs, gastrointestinal symptoms, infections, and overall activity and behavior after MEGC-PEGrMETase or rMETase treatment.
2. Record daily the food consumption and body weights during the treatment period.
3. Calculate the average daily food consumption weekly [18].

3.8 Hematology and Blood Chemistry

1. Collect blood samples for hematology and blood chemistry examinations, 2 mL blood samples via the saphenous vein from each animal after MEGC-PEGrMETase or rMETase treatment.
2. Make the collections on days 3, 6, 11, 22, 29, 33, 50, 54, 71, and 75 during the experimental period.
3. Collect approximately 1 ml of the blood sample into EDTA-coated tubes.
4. Analyze the blood with an automated hematology analyzer for the following hematologic parameters: red blood cells, white blood cells, platelets, hemoglobin, hematocrit, mean corpuscular hemoglobin, mean corpuscular volume, and mean corpuscular hemoglobin concentration.
5. Collect approximately 1 ml of the blood sample into serum-separator tubes and centrifuge.
6. Analyze the resulting sera samples with an automated chemistry analyzer for the following blood chemistry parameters: aspartate aminotransferase, alanine aminotransferase, alkaline phosphatase, total protein, albumin, total bilirubin, cholesterol, glucose, blood urea nitrogen, creatinine, Ca^{2+}, NA^{+}, K^{+}, and Cl^{-} [18].

3.9 Histopathology

1. Sacrifice one monkey from the MEGC-PEG-rMETase- or rMETase-treated group and the control monkey at the end of the study.
2. Perform gross necropsy and weigh the brain, lung, liver, adrenals, kidneys, and spleen.
3. Collected immediately the tissues from the heart, aorta, lungs, liver, and kidneys and fix in 10% neutral-buffered formalin for histopathology examinations [18].

3.10 Determination of Plasma Anti-rMETase Antibody

1. Collect blood samples on days 3, 6, 29, 33, 50, 54, 71, and 75 after administration of MEGC-PEG-rMETase or rMETase for determination of plasma anti-rMETase antibody.
2. Prepare plasma and store at −70 °C. Perform plasma anti-PEG-rMETase IgG antibody measurements using a sandwich ELISA as described previously [25].
3. Add 100 μL rMETase (200 μg/mL) in 0.1 mol/L carbonate-coating buffer (pH 9.5) to each well of a 96-well microplate and incubate at 4 °C overnight.
4. Wash the plate three times with PBS (pH 7.4) containing 0.05% Tween 20, blocked for 2 h at room temperature with 200 μL PBS assay buffer (pH 7.4) containing 10% FBS.
5. After washing three times, add 100 μL of tenfold serial dilutions of the plasma samples in PBS to appropriate wells, incubate for 2 h at room temperature, and then wash again.
6. Add 100 μl of optimally diluted anti-monkey IgG immunoglobulin and horseradish peroxidase conjugate (Sigma, St. Louis, MO) to each well.
7. Incubate the plate for 1 h at room temperature and wash three times.
8. Add 100 μL of substrate solution containing *O*-phenylenediamine dihydrochloride and hydrogen peroxide to each well, followed by 30-min incubation at room temperature.
9. Add 50 μL of 2 N sulfuric acid to each well to stop the color reaction. Measure the absorbance of each well at 492 nm.
10. Examine the presence of neutralizing antibody in plasma (0.2 mL) obtained from rMETase-treated monkeys.
11. Mix the plasma with 0.2 mL of various concentrations of rMETase solution.
12. Use the saline and plasma obtained from a vehicle-treated monkey as blank and negative control, respectively.
13. After incubation at 37 °C in a water bath for 30 min, measure the reaction mixtures for rMETase enzyme activity [18].

4 Results

4.1 rMETase

4.1.1 Dose-Ranging Study of rMETase for Plasma MET Depletion

Plasma MET in the monkeys after three single doses of rMETase was determined: Plasma MET concentration decreased from pre-treatment levels of 11–26 μM to the limit of detection level by 30 min and remained at the limit of detection for 4 h in all monkeys receiving three single doses of rMETase. It was found that plasma MET could be depleted below 5 μM for 8 h using rMETase doses of

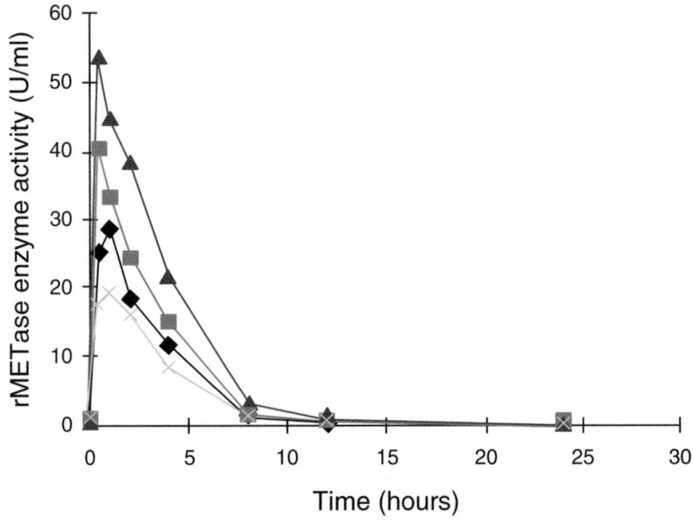

Fig. 1 Plasma rMETase concentration–time profiles in monkeys after 2000 and 4000 units/kg doses of rMETase at time 0. Monkeys 962,147 and 960,427 were dosed with 2000 units/kg. Monkeys 970,475 and 970,985 were dosed with 4000 units/kg. Blood was sampled at the times indicated. rMETase activity was measured. A $T_{1/2}$ of 2.49 h for rMETase was calculated from these data. Diamond, 962,147; Square, 960,427; Triangle, 970,475; Cross, 970,985 [17]

1000, 2000, and 4000 units/kg. The 4000 units/kg rMETase dose was found to be sufficient to deplete plasma MET to approximately 1 μM for 8 h [17] (*see* **Note 3**).

4.1.2 Pharmacokinetics

Pharmacokinetics was examined in the monkeys receiving a single i.v. injection of rMETase at a dose of 2000 or 4000 units/kg. The plasma rMETase concentration–time profiles of the monkeys are presented in Fig. 1. The i.v. injection of rMETase showed a rapid reduction of plasma enzyme activity with a $T_{1/2}$ of 2.49 h. Total systemic body clearance of rMETase was 11.28 and 30.77 mL/h for the 2000 and 4000 units/kg doses, respectively [17].

4.1.3 Plasma rMETase Activity in Monkeys Receiving Repeated Doses of rMETase

In all four monkeys treated with 4000 units/kg rMETase three times per day for 2 weeks, plasma rMETase enzyme activity could be continually maintained at greater than 18.3 ± 10.6 units/mL, with highest observed plasma enzyme activity of 125.5 ± 54.7 units/mL during the 2-week treatment period. The plasma 8-h rMETase concentration–time profiles showed no statistically-significant differences on days 1, 5, 9, 14, and 66 [17].

4.1.4 MET Depletion in Monkeys Receiving Repeated Doses of rMETase

During the 2-week, three-times-per-day treatment period, plasma MET in the rMETase-treated monkeys was depleted effectively by repeated doses of rMETase. The plasma MET was depleted to the limit of detection for at least 4 h after each i.v. injection of rMETase.

At 8 h after each injection, the plasma MET level ranged from 0.9 ± 0.6 to 2.2 ± 1.2 μM. By day 66, the MET levels returned to day-1 pretreatment levels [17] (*see* **Note 3**).

4.1.5 Effect of rMETase on Food Intake and Body Weight

All monkeys treated with rMETase or vehicle tolerated the 2-week treatment period. Two monkeys had mild vomiting reaction after each injection of rMETase within the first 6 days of treatment. From days 7 to 14, vomiting and faintness were observed in all rMETase-treated monkeys. Mild diarrhea occurred in two rMETase-treated monkeys on days 11 and 12. These reactions disappeared after the termination of the 2-week treatment [17].

Reduced food intake and body weight loss occurred in all rMETase-treated monkeys during the 2-week treatment period. The mean daily feed consumption value (g/day) in rMETase-treated monkeys was reduced from the pretreatment level of 265 ± 26 to 168 ± 15 g/day in the first week and 1.8 ± 3.6 g/day in the second week of treatment. Food consumption recovered after the 2-week treatment (38 ± 15 g/day in third week) and returned to normal in the fourth week. The mean body weight loss in the rMETase-treated monkeys was 9.3 ± 3.3% (range from 4.7 to 12.5%) in the first week of treatment and 18.2 ± 5.2% (range from 11.8 to 25%) in the second week of treatment. Body weight gain after the 2-week treatment period was found to be slow (16.3 ± 3.8% in the fourth week) [17].

4.1.6 Immunological Reactions to rMETase

Anaphylactic shock occurred in two monkeys immediately after the first challenge injection of rMETase on day 28. Both monkeys were immediately given i.v. injections of hydrocortisone at a dose of 50 mg/monkey. One monkey recovered 1 h later and survived, whereas the other monkey did not recover and was sacrificed for necropsy. To prevent anaphylactic shock in the remaining two monkeys, hydrocortisone was given 10 min before each challenge injection of rMETase. A total of four challenge injections were given to these two monkeys at an interval of 1 month. Only vomiting, face flushing, and piloerection were observed after each challenge injection. Anaphylactic shock did not occur in any other animal regardless of challenges given [17].

4.1.7 Anti-rMETase Antibody

The measurement of plasma antibody during rMETase treatment period demonstrated that anti-rMETase antibodies were induced. The anti-rMETase antibodies were detected 26 days after the initiation of the 2-week rMETase treatment period and increased with each monthly challenge injection. The antibody titer decreased rapidly after termination of the rMETase challenge. The detection of antibody subtypes indicated that IgG was the dominant anti-rMETase antibody, although a low titer of IgM antibody was also observed [17].

The anti-rMETase antibodies appeared to be neutralizing in vitro. However, we found that both plasma rMETase enzyme activity and MET depletion in the rMETase-treated monkeys were not influenced when the anti-rMETase antibody was induced. Although plasma rMETase activity on day 66 seemed to be lower after the challenge dose of 4000 units/kg was given than that on days 1, 5, 9, and 14, similar plasma MET depletion profiles on days 1 and 66 indicated that anti-rMETase antibodies produced in the monkey plasma were not sufficient to reduce the MET depletion efficacy of rMETase. These data indicated that the anti-rMETase antibodies produced in the plasma of the monkeys were not sufficient to reduce the MET depletion efficacy of rMETase; rMETase antibodies, therefore, did not have a significant neutralizing effect [17].

4.1.8 Effect of rMETase on Hematological and Blood Chemical Parameters

All hematology parameters were normal during the 2-week treatment except red blood cells (RBC) and hemoglobin (Hgb), which were found to decrease from day 9 of rMETase treatment. White blood cells (WBC) and Hgb were reduced to 34% and 40% of pretreatment level, respectively, by the end of the treatment period, indicating a mild anemia. The blood chemistry examinations revealed no abnormalities in most liver function tests, renal function, glucose, lipids, and electrolytes in the rMETase-treated monkeys compared with the controls and pretreatment values. However, decreased albumin/globulin and higher total bilirubin and indirect bilirubin values were noted from day 5 of rMETase treatment [17].

4.1.9 Histopathological Effects of rMETase

There were no obvious gross lesions observed in the major organs of the rMETase-treated monkey at necropsy except for ascites with a light yellow color. The organ weights, including heart, liver, kidney, lung, spleen, brain, and adrenal glands, were in the normal range. No histological changes were observed in the heart, kidney, trachea, lung, and thoracic aorta. In the kidney, a small fraction of epithelial cells of the proximal convoluted tubules showed slightly fine granular vacuolization. In the liver, the structures of the lobules, sinusoids, hepatocyte plates, and hepatocytes were normal. However, scattered spotty necrosis infiltrated with acute and chronic inflammatory cells was observed. Some of the hepatocytes showed cloudy degeneration and fatty metamorphosis [17].

4.2 MEG-PEG-rMETase

4.2.1 Dose-Ranging Study for Optimal MEGC-PEG-rMETase-Mediated MET Depletion

Plasma MET depletion was determined in the monkeys after three single doses of MEGC-PEG-rMETase of 1000, 4000, and 8000 units/kg. Plasma MET concentration decreased from pretreatment levels of ~9 and 15 μmol/L to the limit of detection level by 30 min and remained at the limit of detection for 8 h and <5 μmol/l for 12 h in the monkeys receiving doses of 4000 and 8000 units/kg MEGC-PEG-rMETase. Therefore, 4000 units/kg MEGCPEG-rMETase was found to be sufficient to deplete plasma MET for at least 8 h (*see* **Note 3**) [18].

4.2.2 Pharmacokinetics of MEGC-PEG-rMETase

Pharmacokinetics were determined after a single i.v. injection of MEGC-PEG-rMETase at doses of 2000 and 4000 units/kg. MEGC-PEG-rMETase showed a rapid reduction of plasma holoenzyme activity with a $T_{1/2}$ of 1.3 h. AUC and CLs (total body clearance) were 63.1 units/mL/h and 63.4 mL/h for 4000 units/kg, respectively. For 2000 units/kg, the holoenzyme $T_{1/2}$ was 1.7 h with a AUC and CLs of 45.8 units/ml/h and 43.6 ml/h, respectively. A one-compartment model adequately described the disposition of the MEGC-PEG-rMETase holoenzyme activity. However, the plasma concentration–time curve of MEGC-PEGrMETase apoenzyme activity was biexponential with an initial rapid distributive phase, followed by an elimination phase with an extended half-life of 90 h for 4000 units/kg and 143.3 h for 2000 units/kg. Apoenzyme AUC and CLs were 7437 units/mL/h and 0.54 mL/h, respectively, for 4000 units/kg, and 5814 units/mL/h and 0.34 mL/h, respectively, for 2000 units/kg. A two-compartment model consisting of a central and peripheral compartment was fitted to the plasma concentration–time profile of MEGC-PEGrMETase plasma apoenzyme activity. The data suggest that PLP was rapidly lost from MEGC-PEG-rMETase after injection, which is consistent with observations made previously in mice [25]. The extended half-life of MEGC-PEG-rMETase apoenzyme activity indicates that PEGylation of rMETase has more effect on clearance of the apoenzyme than PLP stabilization in vivo [18].

4.2.3 Plasma MEGC-PEG-rMETase Activity in Monkeys Receiving Repeated Doses of MEGC-PEG-rMETase

In the monkeys treated with 4000 units/kg MEGC-PEG-rMETase twice daily for 7 days, plasma MEGC-PEG-rMETase holoenzyme activity maintained the same concentration–time profile during the 7-day treatment and subsequent challenge period. The plasma MEGC-PEGrMETase apoenzyme concentration–time profiles increased on days 4 and 7 due to accumulation of the apoenzyme after repeated dosing [18].

4.2.4 MET Depletion in Monkeys Receiving Repeated Doses of MEGC-PEG-rMETase

During the 7-day treatment period, plasma MET in the MEGC-PEG-rMETase-treated monkeys was effectively depleted by 4000 units/kg bolus twice daily i.v. Plasma MET was maintained at <5 μmol/L for at least 12 h after each dose of MEGC-PEG-rMETase. At 12 h after each dose of MEGC-PEG-rMETase, the average plasma MET levels on days 1, 4, and 7 were 3 μmol/L, 3.9 μmol/L, and 4.3 μmol/L, respectively. During the following challenge period, the average plasma MET levels at 12-h time points were slightly increased. Because no neutralizing antibody was identified, the reason for this reduced MET depletion efficiency needs to be additionally investigated (Fig. 2) [18].

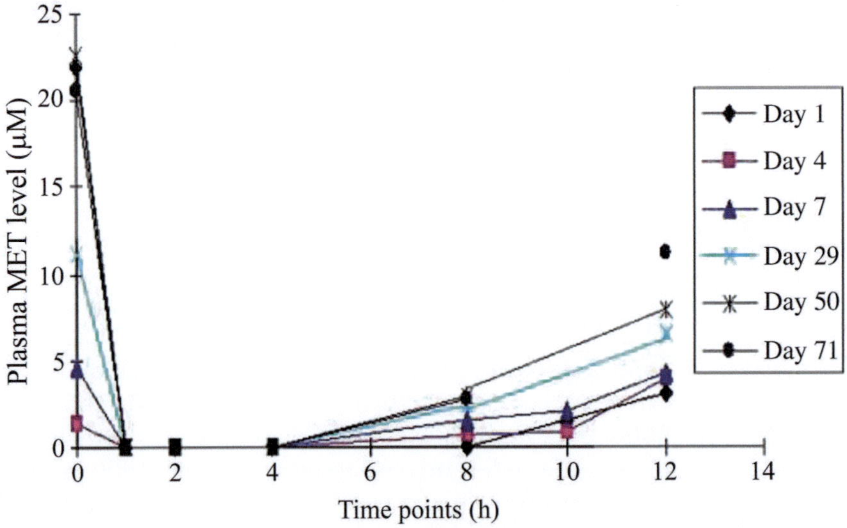

Fig. 2 Plasma MET depletion by MEGC-PEG-rMETase. Monkeys ($n = 2$) were treated with 4000 units/kg MEGC-PEG-rMETase i.v. twice daily for 7 days and three challenges on days 29, 50, and 71. Blood was sampled at the indicated times. Plasma MET concentration was measured as described in the Methods. The data of each time point are presented as mean values from two monkeys [18]

4.2.5 Effect of MEGC-PEG-rMETase on Food Intake and Body Weight

All of the monkeys treated with MEGC-PEG-rMETase or vehicle tolerated the 7-day treatment period. Reduced food intake and slight body weight loss occurred in both MEGC-PEG-rMETase-treated monkeys during the 7-day treatment period. Food consumption recovered after the end of the 7-day treatment period. The body weight loss in the two MEGC-PEG-rMETase-treated monkeys was 7 and 7.8% on day 7. Body weight gain occurred after the 7-day treatment ended [18].

4.2.6 Effect of MEGC-PEG-rMETase on Hematologic and Blood Chemical Parameters

All of the hematology parameters were normal during the 7-day treatment except red blood cells and hemoglobin, which were found to decrease from day 3 of MEGC-PEG-rMETase treatment. RBC and Hgb were reduced to 45% and 41% of pretreatment level, respectively, by the end of the 7-day treatment period indicating anemia. Blood chemistry determinations revealed no abnormalities in most liver function tests, renal function, glucose, lipids, and electrolytes in the MEGC-PEGrMETase-treated monkeys compared with the controls and pretreatment values [18].

4.2.7 Immunologic Reactions to MEGC-PEG-rMETase

No anaphylactic shock or other immunologic reactions occurred in the two monkeys given the three challenge injections on days 29, 50, and 71 of MEGC-PEG-rMETase after the 7-day repeated treatment [18].

4.2.8 Determination of Plasma Anti-MEGC-PEG-rMETase Antibodies

Plasma-specific anti-MEGC-PEG-rMETase IgG antibodies were not detected until day 29 at which point a 10^{-2} plasma antibody titer was detected in the MEGC-PEG-rMETase-treated monkeys. The challenge injections of MEGC-PEG-rMETase on days 29, 50, and 71 resulted in slightly increased plasma antibody titers up to 10^{-3} to 10^{-4} on day 71. The antibody levels elicited by MEGC-PEG-rMETase were much less than those elicited by naked rMETase described above. Plasma anti-MEGC-PEG-rMETase antibody was not identified as a neutralizing antibody, because no significant enzyme activity losses were observed when 2 units/mL MEGC-PEG-rMETase were incubated in vitro with anti-MEGC-PEG-rMETase antibody-positive serum [18] (*see* **Notes 3** and **4**).

4.2.9 Histopathological Effects of MEGC-PEG-rMETase

One monkey from the MEGC-PEG-rMETase-treated and one from the control group were sacrificed at the end of the study. There were no obvious gross lesions observed in the major organs of the MEGC-PEG-rMETase-treated monkey at necropsy. The organ weights, including heart, liver, kidney, lung, spleen, brain, and adrenal glands, were in the normal range. No gross histologic changes were observed in the tissues examined [18].

5 Notes

1. MET dependence, the elevated minimal MET requirement for cell growth relative to normal cells, has been observed in many human cancer cell lines and cancer xenografts in mouse models, including patient-derived orthotopic xenograft (PDOX) mouse models [1–5, 13, 14] (Table 1). MET dependence is a metabolic defect seen only in cancer cells and precludes the cells from growing when MET is restricted. MET dependence is thought to be due to increased rates of transmethylation in

Table 2
Comparison of MEGC-PEG-rMETase and naked rMETase in primates

	MEGC-PEG-rMETase	Naked rMETase [15]
$T_{1/2}$	90–143 h	2.5 h
Plasma MET depletion (<5 μM)	12 h	8 h
ASA	None	Shock and death
Maximum plasma antibody titers	10^{-4}	10^{-6}
Neutralizing antibody	Not detected	Present

MEGC-PEG-rMETase was administered i.v. at a dose of 4000 U/kg for 7 days twice a day with challenges on days 29, 50, and 71. Naked rMETase was administered i.v. at a dose of 4000 U/kg for 14 days three times a day with challenges on days 28, 66, 86, and 116. Abbreviations: $T_{1/2}$ biological half-life, *ASA* active systemic anaphylaxis [18] cancer cells compared with normal cells [31, 32]. It has been demonstrated that MET restriction inhibits the growth of cancer cells by causing them to arrest predominantly in the S/G_2 phase of the cell cycle and to eventually undergo apoptosis [33–37], as well as make cancer cells sensitive to S/G_2 drugs [36–38].

2. The efficacy of MET depletion by rMETase to reduce tumor growth has now been documented with a variety of tumors that include Lewis lung carcinoma [10], several human colon cancer lines [9], and glioblastoma [11, 12, 35]. An even more important observation is the growing evidence that a variety of chemotherapeutic agents appear to be synergistically enhanced by plasma MET depletion; these include doxorubicin [36], 5-fluorouracil and mitomycin C [39, 40], CDDP [9], and nitrosoureas [11, 12, 35]. rMETase has recently found to be effective in patient-derived orthotopic xenograft (PDOX) mouse models (Table 1) [2–4, 13, 14].
3. The effectiveness of antitumor activity of rMETase or PEG-rMETase is dependent on its ability to deplete MET in the plasma and subsequently in the tumor. A plasma MET level of approximately 1 μM at 8 h could be achieved by 4000 units/kg dose. Therefore, 4000 units/kg doses were used to achieve a constantly lowered plasma MET level and for antigenicity and toxicity determination [17]. The hematology studies demonstrated that mild anemia occurred in rMETase- or PEG-rMETase-treated monkeys [10, 17].
4. Comparison of MEGC-PEG-rMETase and rMETase in primates. Two significant differences have been observed between MEGC-PEG-rMETase and naked rMETase [17]. The most important is the lack of any immunologic reaction in the MEGC-PEG-rMETase-treated monkeys. In contrast, rMETase elicited anaphylactic shock in monkeys, unless they were pretreated with hydrocortisone. The second important result was the 90–143-h half-life of MEGC-PEG-rMETase apoenzyme activity, compared with 2.5 h for naked rMETase, indicating that the apoenzyme form of MEGC-PEG-rMETase persisted for very long periods in the monkey plasma. As we have observed previously in mice [25], PLP supplementation greatly extends the MEGC-PEG-rMETase holoenzyme activity. Such studies will also be performed in primates to determine whether PLP supplementation can extend the half-life of holoenzyme activity of MEGC-PEG-rMETase (Table 2) [18].

References

1. Hoffman RM (2015) Development of recombinant methioninase to target the general cancer-specific metabolic defect of methionine dependence: a 40-year odyssey. Expert Opin Biol Ther 15:21–31
2. Kawaguchi K, Igarashi K, Li S, Han Q, Tan Y, Miyake K, Kiyuna T, Miyake M, Murakami T, Chmielowski S, Nelson SD, Russell TA, Dry SM, Li Y, Unno M, Eilber FC, Hoffman RM (2018) Recombinant methioninase (rMETase) is an effective therapeutic for BRAF-V600E-negative as well as -positive melanoma in patient-derived orthotopic xenograft (PDOX) mouse models. Oncotarget 9:915–923
3. Kawaguchi K, Han Q, Li S, Tan Y, Igarashi K, Kiyuna T, Miyake K, Miyake M, Chmielowski B, Nelson SD, Russell TA, Dry SM, Li Y, Eckhardt MA, Unno M, Eilber FC, Hoffman RM (2018) Targeting methionine with oral recombinant methioninase (o-rMETase) arrests a patient-derived orthotopic xenograft (PDOX) model of BRAF-V600E mutant melanoma: implications for clinical cancer therapy and prevention. Cell Cycle 17 (3):356–361
4. Kawaguchi K, Miyake K, Han Q, Li S, Tan Y, Igarashi K, Lwin TM, Higuchi T, Kiyuna T, Miyake M, Oshiro H, Bouvet M, Unno M, Hoffman RM (2018) Targeting altered cancer methionine metabolism with recombinant methioninase (rMETase) overcomes partial gemcitabine-resistance and regresses a patient-derived orthotopic xenograft (PDOX) nude mouse model of pancreatic cancer. Cell Cycle 21:1–6
5. Kreis W, Hession C (1973) Isolation and purification of L-methionine-alpha-deamino-gamma-mercaptomethane-lyase (L-methioninase) from Clostridium sporogenes. Cancer Res 33:1862–1865
6. Tanaka H, Esaki N, Soda K (1977) Properties of L-methionine g-lyase from *Pseudomonas ovalis*. Biochemistry 16:100–106
7. Hori H, Takabayashi K, Orvis L, Carson DA, Nobori T (1996) Gene cloning and characterization of Pseudomonas putida L-methionine α-deamino-γ-mercaptomethanelyase. Cancer Res 56:2116–2122
8. Tan Y, Xu M, Tan X-Z, Tan X-Y, Wang X, Saikawa Y, Nagahama T, Sun X, Lenz M, Hoffman RM (1997) Overexpression and large-scale production of recombinant L-methionine-α-deamino-γ-mercaptomethane-lyase for novel anticancer therapy. Protein Expr Purif 9:233–245
9. Tan Y, Sun X, Xu M, Tan X-Z, Sasson A, Rashidi B, Han Q, Tan X-Y, Wang X, An Z, Sun F-X, Hoffman RM (1999) Efficacy of recombinant methioninase in combination with cisplatin on human colon tumors in nude mice. Clin Cancer Res 5:2157–2163
10. Yoshioka T, Wada T, Uchida N, Maki H, Yoshida H, Ide N, Kasai H, Hojo K, Shono K, Maekawa R, Yagi S, Hoffman RM, Sugita K (1998) Anticancer efficacy *in vivo* and *in vitro*, synergy with 5-fluorouracil, and safety of recombinant methioninase. Cancer Res 58:2583–2587
11. Kokkinakis DM, Schold SC Jr, Hori H, Nobori T (1997) Effect of long-term depletion of plasma methionine on the growth and survival of human brain tumor xenografts in athymic mice. Nutr Cancer 29:195–204
12. Kokkinakis DM, Wick JB, Zhou Q-X (2002) Metabolic response of normal and malignant tissue to acute and chronic methionine stress in athymic mice bearing human glial tumor xenografts. Chem Res Toxicol 15:1472–1479
13. Murakami T, Li S, Han Q, Tan Y, Kiyuna T, Igarashi K, Kawaguchi K, Hwang HK, Miyaki K, Singh AS, Nelson SD, Dry SM, Li Y, Hiroshima Y, Lwin TM, DeLong JC, Chishima T, Tanaka K, Bouvet M, Endo I, Eilber FC, Hoffman RM (2017) Recombinant methioninase effectively targets a Ewing's sarcoma in a patient-derived orthotopic xenograft (PDOX) nude-mouse model. Oncotarget 8:35630–35638
14. Kawaguchi K, Igarashi K, Li S, Han Q, Tan Y, Kiyuna T, Miyake Y, Murakami T, Chmielowski B, Nelson SD, Russell TA, Dry SM, Li Y, Unno M, Eilber FC, Hoffman RM (2017) Combination treatment with recombinant methioninase enables temozolomide to arrest a BRAF V600E melanoma growth in a patient-derived orthotopic xenograft. Oncotarget 8:85516–85525
15. Tan Y, Zavala J Sr, Xu M, Zavala J Jr, Hoffman RM (1996) Serum methionine depletion without side effects by methioninase in metastatic breast cancer patients. Anticancer Res 16:3937–3942
16. Tan Y, Zavala J Sr, Han Q, Xu M, Sun X, Tan X-Z, Tan X-Y, Magana R, Geller J, Hoffman RM (1997) Recombinant methioninase infusion reduces the biochemical endpoint of serum methionine with minimal toxicity in high-stage cancer patients. Anticancer Res 17:3857–3860

17. Yang Z, Wang J, Yoshioka T, Li B, Lu Q, Li S, Sun X, Tan Y, Yagi S, Frenkel EP, Hoffman RM (2004) Pharmacokinetics, methionine depletion, and antigenicity of recombinant methioninase in primates. Clin Cancer Res 10:2131–2138
18. Yang Z, Wang J, Lu Q, Xu J, Kobayashi Y, Takakura T, Takimoto A, Yoshioka T, Lian C, Chen C, Zhang D, Zhang Y, Li S, Sun X, Tan Y, Yagi S, Frenkel EP, Hoffman RM (2004) PEGylation confers greatly extended half-life and attenuated immunogenicity to recombinant methioninase in primates. Cancer Res 64:6673–6678
19. Kozlowski A, Harris JM (2001) Improvements in protein PEGylation: pegylated interferons for treatment of hepatitis C. J Control Release 72:217–224
20. Maeda H, Kabanov A, Kataska K, Okano T (2003) Advances in experimental medicine and biology: polymer drugs in the clinical stage, vol 519. Kluwer Academic/Plenum Publishers, Dordrecht
21. Park CWG, Chuo M Interferon polymer conjugates. United States Patent 5,951,974, September 14, 1999
22. Aguayo A, Cortes J, Thomas D, Pierce S, Keating M, Kantarjian H (1999) Combination therapy with methotrexate, vincristine, polyethylene-glycol conjugated-asparaginase, and prednisone in the treatment of patients with refractory or recurrent acute lymphoblastic leukemia. Cancer 86:1203–1209
23. Pool R (1990) "Hairy enzymes" stay in the blood. Science 248:305
24. Hershfield MS (1995) PEG-ADA replacement therapy for adenosine deaminase deficiency: an update after 8.5 years. Clin Immunol Immunopathol 76:S228–S232
25. Sun X, Yang Z, Li S, Tan Y, Zhang N, Wang X, Yagi S, Yoshioka T, Takimoto A, Mitsushima K, Suginaka A, Frenkel EP, Hoffman RM (2003) *In vivo* efficacy of recombinant methioninase is enhanced by the combination of polyethylene glycol conjugation and pyridoxal 5′ phosphate supplementation. Cancer Res 63:8377–8383
26. Takakura T, Ito T, Yagi S, Notsu Y, Itakura T, Nakamura T, Inagaki K, Esaki N, Hoffman RM, Takimoto A (2006) High-level expression and bulk crystallization of recombinant L-methionine γ-lyase, an anticancer agent. Appl Microbiol Biotechnol 70:183–192
27. Takakura T, Takimoto A, Notsu Y, Yoshida H, Ito T, Nagatome H, Ohno M, Kobayashi Y, Yoshioka T, Inagaki K, Yagi S, Hoffman RM, Esaki N (2006) Physicochemical and pharmacokinetic characterization of highly potent recombinant L-methionine γ-lyase conjugated with polyethylene glycol as an antitumor agent. Cancer Res 66:2807–2814
28. Kudou D, Misaki S, Yamashita M, Tamura T, Takakura T, Yoshioka T, Yagi S, Hoffman RM, Takimoto A, Esaki N, Inagaki K et al (2007) J Biochem 141:535–544
29. Takakura T, Mitsushima K, Yagi S, Inagaki K, Tanaka H, Esaki N, Soda K, Takimoto A et al (2004) Anal Biochem 327:233–240
30. Jones BN, Gilligan JP (1983) O-Phthaldialdehyde precolumn derivatization and reversed-phase high-performance liquid chromatography of polypeptide hydrolysates and physiological fluids. J Chromatogr 266:471–482
31. Judde JG, Ellis M, Frost P (1989) Biochemical analysis of the role of transmethylation in the methionine dependence of tumor cells. Cancer Res 49:4859–4865
32. Tisdale MJ (1980) Effect of methionine deprivation on methylation and synthesis of macromolecules. Br J Cancer 42:121–128
33. Guo H, Lishko V, Herrera H, Groce A, Kubota T, Hoffman RM (1993) Therapeutic tumor-specific cell-cycle block induced by methionine starvation *in vivo*. Cancer Res 53:5676–5679
34. Hoffman RM, Jacobsen SJ (1980) Reversible growth arrest in simian virus 40-transformed human fibroblasts. Proc Natl Acad Sci U S A 77:7306–7310
35. Kokkinakis DM, von Wronski MA, Vuong TH, Brent TP, Schold SC Jr (1997) Regulation of O6-methylguanine-DNA methyltransferase by methionine in human tumour cells. Br J Cancer 75:779–788
36. Stern PH, Hoffman RM (1986) Enhanced *in vitro* selective toxicity of chemotherapeutic agents for human cancer cells based on a metabolic defect. J Natl Cancer Inst 76:629–639
37. Yano S, Takehara K, Zhao M, Tan Y, Han Q, Li S, Bouvet M, Fujiwara T, Hoffman RM (2016) Tumor-specific cell-cycle decoy by *Salmonella typhimurium* A1-R combined with tumor-selective cell-cycle trap by methioninase overcome tumor intrinsic chemoresistance as visualized by FUCCI imaging. Cell Cycle 15:1715–1723
38. Yano S, Li S, Han Q, Tan Y, Bouvet M, Fujiwara T, Hoffman RM (2014) Selective methioninase-induced trap of cancer cells in S/G_2 phase visualized by FUCCI imaging confers chemosensitivity. Oncotarget 5:8729–8736
39. Goseki N, Yamazaki S, Shimojyu K, Kando F, Maruyama M, Endo M, Koike M, Takahashi H

(1995) Synergistic effect of methionine-depleting total parenteral nutrition with 5-fluorouracil on human gastric cancer: a randomized, prospective clinical trial. Jpn J Cancer Res 86:484–489
40. Miki K, Xu M, Gupta A, Ba Y, Tan Y, Al-Refaie W, Bouvet M, Makuuchi M, Moossa AR, Hoffman RM (2001) Methioninase cancer gene therapy with selenomethionine as suicide prodrug substrate. Cancer Res 61:6805–6810
41. Igarashi K, Kawaguchi K, Li S, Han Q, Tan Y, Murakami T, Kiyuna T, Miyake K, Miyake M, Singh AS, Eckhadt MA, Nelson SD, Russell TA, Dry SM, Li Y, Yamamoto N, Hayashi K, Kimura H, Miwa S, Tsuchiya H, Singh RS, Eilber FC, Hoffman RM (2018) Recombinant methioninase in combination with DOX overcomes first-line DOX resistance in a patient-derived orthotopic xenograft nude-mouse model of undifferentiated spindle-cell sarcoma. Cancer Lett 417:168–173
42. Kawaguchi K, Miyake K, Han Q, Li S, Tan Y, Igarashi K, Kiyuna T, Miyake M, Higuchi T, Oshiro H, Zhang Z, Razmjooei S, Wangsiricharoens S, Bowet M, Singh SR, Unnu M, Hoffman RM (2018) Oral recombinant methioninase (o-rMETase) is superior to injectable rMETase and overcomes acquired gemcitabine resistance in pancreatic cancer. Cancer Lett 432:251–259
43. Miyake K, Kiyuna T, Li S, Han Q, Tan Y, Zhao M, Oshiro H, Kawaguchi K, Higuchi T, Zhang Z, Razmjooei S, Barangi M, Wangsiricharoen S, Murakami T, Singh AS, Li Y, Nelson SD, Eilber FC, Bouvet M, Hiroshima Y, Chishima T, Matsuyama R, Singh SR, Endo I, Hoffman RM (in press) Combining tumor-selective bacterial therapy with *Salmonella typhimurium* A1-R and cancer metabolism targeting with oral recombinant methioninase (o-rMETase) regressed a Ewing's sarcoma in a PDOX model. Chemotherapy. https://doi.org/10.1159/000495574
44. Igarashi K, Kawaguchi K, Li S, Han Q, Tan Y, Gainor E, Kiyuna T, Miyake K, Miyake M, Higuchi T, Oshiro H, Singh AS, Eckardt MA, Nelson SD, Russell TA, Dry SM, Li Y, Yamamoto N, Hayashi K, Kimura H, Miwa S, Tsuchiya H, Eilber FC, Hoffman RM (2018) Recombinant methioninase combined with doxorubicin (DOX) regresses a DOX-resistant Dynovial sarcoma in a patient-derived orthotopic xenograft (PDOX) mouse model. Oncotarget 9:19263–19272
45. Igarashi K, Kawaguchi K, Kiyuna T, Miyake K, Miyake M, Li S, Han Q, Tan Y, Zhao M, Li Y, Nelson SD, Dry SM, Singh AS, Elliott IA, Russell TA, Eckardt MA, Yamamoto N, Hayashi K, Kimura H, Miwa S, Tsuchiya H, Eilber FC, Hoffman RM (2019) Tumor-targeting *Salmonella typhimurium* A1-R combined with recombinant methioninase and cisplatinum eradicates an osteosarcoma cisplatinum-resistant lung metastasis in a patient-derived ortho topic xenograft (PDOX) mouse model: decoy, trap and kill chemotherapy moves toward the clinic. Cell Cycle 17:801 809

Chapter 17

Pilot Phase I Clinical Trial of Methioninase on High-Stage Cancer Patients: Rapid Depletion of Circulating Methionine

Robert M. Hoffman, Yuying Tan, Shukuan Li, Qinghong Han, Jorge Zavala Sr, and Jorge Zavala Jr

Abstract

Methionine (MET) has been shown to be a tumor-selective therapeutic target for cancer, since cancer cells require higher amounts of MET to divide and survive than normal cells. This phenomena is known as MET dependence and is probably due to MET overuse by cancer cells. A pilot clinical trial was initially carried out with non-recombinant METase (METase) produced from *Pseudomonas putida* and subsequently highly purified. No acute clinical toxicity was observed for any criteria measured in the three patients. The depletion of serum MET started within 30 min of the infusion and was maintained for 4 h after the infusion was completed in patient 1 and patient 2. The lowest serum MET levels were 35% and 19% of the pretreatment level, respectively, in patient 1 and patient 2. Patient 3 received a 10 h i.v. infusion of METase without any sign of side effects. MET was depleted over 200-fold from 23.1 to 0.1 μM by the 10-h infusion of patient 3. No clinical toxicity was observed in any criteria measured in patient 3. Subsequently, another pilot Phase I clinical trial was carried out of serum MET depletion in cancer patients by recombinant METase (rMETase) cloned from *Pseudomonas putida* and produced in *E. coli*. Patients with advanced breast cancer, lung cancer, renal cancer, and lymphoma were given a single rMETase treatment at doses ranging from 5000 to 20,000 units by i.v. infusion over 6–24 h. No clinical toxicity was observed in any patient after rMETase treatment. rMETase levels were measured at 0.1 to 0.4 units per ml of serum in the patients which correspond to therapeutic levels in vitro. The lowest serum MET levels in rMETase-treated patients were 0.1% of the pretreatment levels corresponding to approximately 0.1 μM, which also correlates to therapeutic levels in vitro as well as in vivo. The results of the METase and rMETase pilot Phase I clinical trials therefore indicate that i.v. infusion of rMETase is safe and effectively depletes its biochemical target of serum MET, suggesting potential efficacy in future clinical trials.

Key words Methionine (MET) dependence, Methioninase, Advanced cancer patient, High-stage, Clinical trial, MET restriction

1 Introduction

Many laboratories have identified the elevated methionine (MET) requirement of tumors as a highly selective tumor target [1]. Unlike normal cells, many cancer cells will not grow when MET is restricted (MR) due to an elevated requirement for MET, a

Robert M. Hoffman (ed.), *Methionine Dependence of Cancer and Aging: Methods and Protocols*, Methods in Molecular Biology, vol. 1866, https://doi.org/10.1007/978-1-4939-8796-2_17,

condition that allows normal cells to survive for long periods. When cancer cells stop growing due to MET restriction, they specifically arrest in the late S/G_2 phase of the cell cycle, effecting selective synchrony of cancer cells for cell cycle-specific chemotherapy [2–4].

Goseki et al. have demonstrated the principle of clinical efficacy of MR in Phase II clinical trials with a MR total parenteral solution (TPN) given to high-stage gastric cancer patients. The MR TPN solutions doubled the response and survival rate of cancer patients when administered in combination with 5-fluorouracil (5-FU) and mitomycin C (MMC), compared to the latter two drugs given with MET-replete TPN [5–7].

We initially purified endotoxin-free METase from *Pseudomonas putida* in order to develop anti-MET chemotherapy targeting the MET dependence of tumors in vivo [4, 8]. The early in vivo studies carried out in our laboratory have shown that METase effectively inhibited the growth of the Yoshida sarcoma and the human lung tumor H460 in nude mouse xenograft models [9]. Clinical pharmacokinetics studies showed that native METase depleted serum MET levels more than 100-fold without toxicity [4, 7].

Our laboratory cloned the *Pseudomonas putida* METase gene into a high-expression vector which was transformed into *E. coli*. With this high-expression clone, we have established scale-up protocols which produce high-purity, low-endotoxin recombinant METase (rMETase) [10]. Preclinical studies have shown that rMETase has high potential as an effective broad-spectrum tumor-selective agent without acute toxicity in nude mice with human tumor xenografts [11]. In vitro studies with rMETase demonstrated universally lower IC_{50} values, by approximately an order of magnitude, in a broad range of human cancer cells compared to five types of normal cells [12]. Pilot clinical Phase I trials of advanced cancer patients demonstrated that rMETase restricted serum MET levels to 0.1% of untreated levels without any clinical toxicity. This depleted level of serum MET also corresponds to a potential therapeutic level [4, 7].

2 Materials

1. pAC-1 rMETase high-expression clone (AntiCancer Inc. San Diego, CA).
2. *E. coli*.
3. pT7–7 vector containing the T7 RNA polymerase promotor.
4. *Pseudomonas putida*.
5. Terrific Broth.
6. Cavitator-type homogenizer (Microfluidics Corp., Newton, MA, model #HC 8000).
7. DEAE Sepharose FF (pH 7.2) (Pharmacia, Uppsala, Sweden).

8. Potassium chloride.
9. Potassium phosphate buffer pH 7.2.
10. DEAE Sepharose FF (pH 8.3) (Pharmacia).
11. ActiClean Etox (Sterogene, Arcadia, CA).
12. Sodium chloride.
13. Sodium phosphate (pH 7.2).
14. HPLC with L-6200A Intelligent pump (Hitachi, Ltd., Tokyo, Japan).
15. Supelco Progel™ TSK column (G3000 SW_{XL}, 30 cm × 7.8 mm) column (Supelco, Bellefonte, PA).
16. Spectrophotometer (Hitachi U2000).
17. Polyacrylamide-precast plates.
18. Tris-glycine buffer (pH 8.3).
19. 3-Methyl-2-benzothiazolinone hydrazine.
20. α-Ketobutyrate.
21. Limulus amebocyte lysate (LAL) test (Biowhittaker, Walkersville, MD).
22. o-Phthaldialdehyde (OPA) (sigma).
23. Acetonitrile (75 μL).
24. Sodium acetate (pH 7.0).
25. Tetrahydrofuran.
26. Methanol.
27. Fluorescence spectrophotometer (Hitachi, F1000).

Patients and treatment. Nine patients with advanced-stage breast cancer, lung cancer, kidney cancer, and lymphoma participated in a pilot Phase I trial of rMETase (Table 1). Patient selection requirements included no chemotherapy or radiotherapy in the four previous months before this study. The diagnosis of the original cancer and the metastases was confirmed by pathologic analysis. There were no other coexistent medical problems of sufficient magnitude to jeopardize full compliance with this study. Informed consent forms followed IRB approval guidelines [7].

Table 1
Patient characteristics and rMETase toxicity [4]

	Patient #1	Patient #2	Patient #3
Primary cancer	Breast cancer	Breast cancer	Breast cancer
Metastasis	lung and axillary lumph nodes	Axillary lumph nodes	Axillary lumph nodes
Sex	Female	Female	Female
Age	46	54	45
Dose of methioninase	5000 units	10,000 units	20,000 units
Hours i.v. infusion	2 h	2 h	10 h
Sample collection	Before treatment, during treatment every hour, 10 h after treatment	Before treatment, during treatment every hour, 10 h after treatment	Before treatment, during treatment every hour, 10 h after treatment

3 Methods

3.1 High-Expression Clone of rMETase and Fermentation Conditions [10]

1. Establish the pAC-1 rMETase high-expression clone and use for the production of rMETase.
2. Use the previously-described fermentation procedure for host *E. coli* cells and the purification protocol for rMETase [10].
3. Construct pAC-1 with the pT7–7 vector containing the T7 RNA polymerase promotor for high expression of the rMETase gene cloned from *Pseudomonas putida* [10].
4. Grow the host *E. coli* in Terrific Broth and harvest when the OD_{600} reaches 20.
5. Produce rMETase at approximately 1 g/L of fermentation broth [7].

3.2 Purification of rMETase [10]

3.2.1 Precolumn Treatment

1. Disrupt the bacterial pellet with a cavitator-type homogenizer.
2. Carry out heat treatment of the homogenate out at 50 °C for 1 min [7].

3.2.2 First Column

1. Use a DEAE Sepharose FF column (pH 7.2)
2. Elute rMETase with a linear gradient of 40–200 mM potassium chloride in 10 mM potassium phosphate buffer pH 7.2.
3. Identify the fractions containing rMETase by yellow color and activity assay [7].

3.2.3 Second Column

1. Use a DEAE Sepharose column (pH 8.3)
2. Elute rMETase with a linear gradient of 80–200 mM potassium chloride in 10 mM potassium phosphate buffer (pH 8.3).
3. Identify the fractions containing rMETase by yellow color and activity assay [7].

3.2.4 Third Column

1. To eliminate endotoxin, apply purified rMETase (10–20 mg protein/ml) on an ActiClean Etox column.
2. Elute the protein with elution buffer (0.12 M sodium chloride in 10 mM sodium phosphate pH 7.2).
3. Identify the fractions containing rMETase by yellow color and activity assay [7].

3.3 Analysis of rMETase [10]

3.3.1 HPLC

1. Use an Hitachi L-6200A Intelligent pump with a Supelco Progel™ TSK column (G3000 SW_{XL}, 30 cm × 7.8 mm) for HPLC analysis of rMETase purity.
2. Load a sample and elute with elution buffer (0.12 M sodium chloride in 10 mM sodium phosphate buffer, pH 7.2).
3. Identify the protein-containing fractions with a spectrophotometer (Hitachi U2000) at a wavelength of 280 nm [7].

3.3.2 Electrophoresis [10]

1. Carry out electrophoresis in 7.5% polyacrylamide-precast plates in 0.2 M Tris-glycine buffer, pH 8.3, both with and without 0.1% SDS [7].

3.3.3 rMETase Activity Assay [10]

1. Carry out the assay out in a 1 ml volume of 50 mM phosphate buffer pH 8.0, containing 10 μM pyridoxal phosphate and 10 mM MET, for 10 min at 37°C with varying amounts of enzyme and detect with 3-methyl-2-benzothiazolinone hydrazone at OD335.
2. Calculate the specific activity as units/mg protein.
3. Define one unit of enzyme as the amount that catalyzes the formation of 1 mmol of α-ketobutyrate per minute [10].

3.3.4 Endotoxin Assay [10]

1. Measure the endotoxin level with the limulus amebocyte lysate (LAL) test.
2. Measure the concentration of endotoxin at a wavelength of 410 nm [7].

3.3.5 Serum MET Measurement

1. Perform serum MET measurement by HPLC after derivatization of serum amino acids with a fluoraldehyde reagent, o-phthaldialdehyde (OPA) [13].
2. Derivatize a MET standard by OPA.
3. Precipitate serum samples (25 μL) with acetonitrile (75 μL).
4. Mix 10 μL supernatant with 5 μL OPA.

5. After 1 min, add 50 μL of 0.1 M sodium acetate (pH 7.0) and load a 20 μL sample on a reversed-phase Supelcosil LC-18DB HPLC column (particle size 5 μm, 25 cm × 4.8 mm) at room temperature.
6. Accomplish resolution of the amino acid derivatives with solution A (tetrahydrofuran/methanol/0.1 M sodium acetate pH 7.2; 5/95/900) and solution B (methanol).
7. Run a gradient from 20 to 60% solution B at a flow rate of 1.5 ml/min.
8. Read the eluate with a fluorescence spectrophotometer (Hitachi, F1000) at a wavelength of 350–450 nm.
9. The limit of detection is approximately 0.1 μM MET [7].

3.3.6 Formulation for rMETase

1. Formulate rMETase at a concentration of 10–20 mg/mL in 0.12 M sodium chloride and 10 mM sodium phosphate buffer (pH 7) [7].
2. Administer rMETase to the patients using 99% pure enzyme with an endotoxin level of less than 2 EU/mg protein [7].

3.3.7 Infusion

1. Dilute rMETase with sterilized 0.9% sodium chloride solution in a total volume of 800–1200 ml just before infusion.
2. Administer to patients 5000 units (0.25 g) to 20,000 units (1.0 g) of rMETase by continuous i.v. infusion for 6–24 h [7].

3.3.8 Patient Observation and Sample Collection

1. Observe all patients carefully for vital signs.
2. Measure pulse, respiration rate, blood pressure, and temperature every 2 h.
3. Collect blood samples and urine samples before treatment, during treatment every 4 h, and at 24 h.
4. Use blood samples for rMETase pharmacokinetics (50 μL), serum MET measurement (25 μL), and laboratory analysis.
5. Laboratory tests and measurements should include a complete blood count with differential, prothrombin time, partial thromboplastin time, electrolytes, protein, albumin, blood urea nitrogen, creatinine lactic dehydrogenase, alkaline phosphatase, calcium, uric acid, total and direct bilirubin, serum alanine aminotransferase, and urinalysis.
6. Perform a chest X-ray, electrocardiogram, and pertinent radiographic studies for evaluable/measurable disease.
7. Determine toxicity according to WHO criteria [7].

4 Results

Patient characteristics. Characteristics of patients who were tested with METase are shown in Table 1. Vital signs are shown in Table 2. None of the three patients had any side effects during or after the i.v. infusion of METase. Pulse, respiration rates, temperature, and blood pressure had almost no change during and after the treatment [4].

A total of nine patients were evaluated with rMETase infusion. Of these nine patients, four had stage III or IV breast cancer. One had stage III renal cancer, one had stage IV lung cancer, two had stage III lymphoma, and one had stage IV gastric carcinoma. Their characteristics are listed in Table 3 [7].

Toxicity evaluation. None of the cases had any observable clinical toxicity during or after a single i.v. infusion of METase. Pulse, respiration rates, temperature, and blood pressure had almost no change during and after treatment [7].

Toxicity was evaluated according to standard WHO criteria [14]. The physical evaluation and the laboratory determination before and after treatment were compared. No acute clinical toxicity was observed in any of the criteria measured. The patients were treated as described in the protocol of Table 1. Blood and urine were collected before treatment, during treatment, and 24 h after the start of treatment. The results suggest that i.v. infusion of METase did not cause any functional damage to major organs.

Table 2
Vital parameters of patients treated with methioninase [4]

Patient	Treatment	Temperature	Pulse	Respiration rate	Blood pressure
	Before	36.7	134	21	110/70
# 1	During (Max)	36.8	138	22	120/80
	(Min)	36.4	125	24	110/70
	After	36.6	127	24	120/80
	Before	36.7	74	14	118/78
#2	During (Max)	36.6	74	12	120/80
	(Min)	36.6	70	14	110/70
	After	36.7	74	14	110/74
	Before	36.4	67	14	110/74
# 3	During (Max)	37.0	76	14	128/74
	(Min)	36.0	66	12	90/70
	After	36.3	65	12	114/88

Table 3
Patient characteristics and rMETase toxicity [7]

Diagnosis		Methionine (μM)		METase		Toxicity	
Cancer	Stage	Base	Lowest	Units	Hours	Symptom	Laboratory
Breast cancer	IV	28.6	0.5	10,000	8	–	–
Kidney cancer	III	N/A	N/A	20,000	24	–	–
Breast cancer	III	N/A	N/A	5,000	24	–	–
Lung cancer	IV	N/A	N/A	10,000	6	–	–
Lymphoma	III	N/A	N/A	10,000	8	–	–
Breast cancer	IV	35	0.28	10,000	8	–	–
Lymphoma	III	N/A	N/A	10,000	8	–	–
Gastric cancer	IV	34	1.27	10,000	8	–	–
Breast cancer	IV	34.7	0.1	20,000	8	–	–

There was no hematological, renal, neurological, or cardiac toxicity in any of the patients [4, 7] (*see* **Note 1**).

Pharmacokinetics results. Pharmacokinetic data of single infusion were obtained for METase levels in the serum. The half-life of METase in patient 1 and patient 2, who received i.v. infusions for 2 h, was 2 h (Figs. 1 and 2) and in patient 3, who received i.v. infusion for 10 h, it was 10 h (Fig. 3). The results suggested that the half-life of METase was related to the infusion time rather than the dose. The infusion time should be further studied in future trials [4].

Pharmacokinetic data of single infusions were obtained for rMETase levels in the serum. Typical pharmacokinetics data are shown in Fig. 4. Serum rMETase levels achieved were between 0.1 units/mL and 0.4 units/mL which correlate with the therapeutic doses of rMETase for cancer cells in vitro [1]. These data suggest that the i.v. infusion of rMETase in patients can reach effective doses without toxicity [7].

Depletion of MET in the serum. The depletion of serum MET started within 30 min of rMETase infusion, and was maintained for 4 h after the infusion was completed in patient 1 and patient 2. The lowest serum MET levels were 35% and 19% of the pretreatment level, respectively, in patient 1 and patient 2 (Figs. 1 and 2). Patient 3 received a 10-h i.v. infusion of 20,000 units of METase without any signs of side effects and maintained serum levels of METase as high as 50% of the maximum level for another 10 h after infusion. MET was depleted over 200-fold from 23.1 to 0.1 μM within 10 h of infusion. These results demonstrated that METase could deplete MET to a very low level within 1 h of i.v. infusion. MET could be

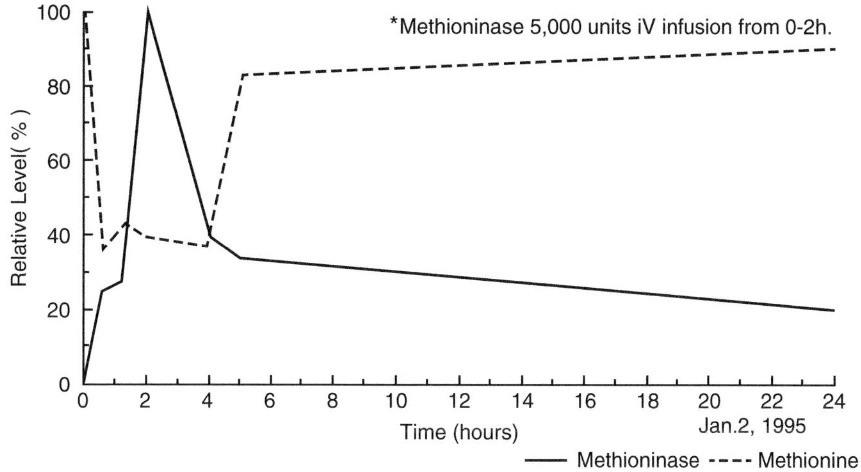

Fig. 1 Patient 1 received an i.v. infusion for 2 h with 5000 units of methioninase. The blood samples were collected before treatment, every hour during treatment, and every 2 h up to 20 h after treatment. The levels of MET and methioninase were measured by HPLC and activity assay respectively, and the relative levels were calculated [4]

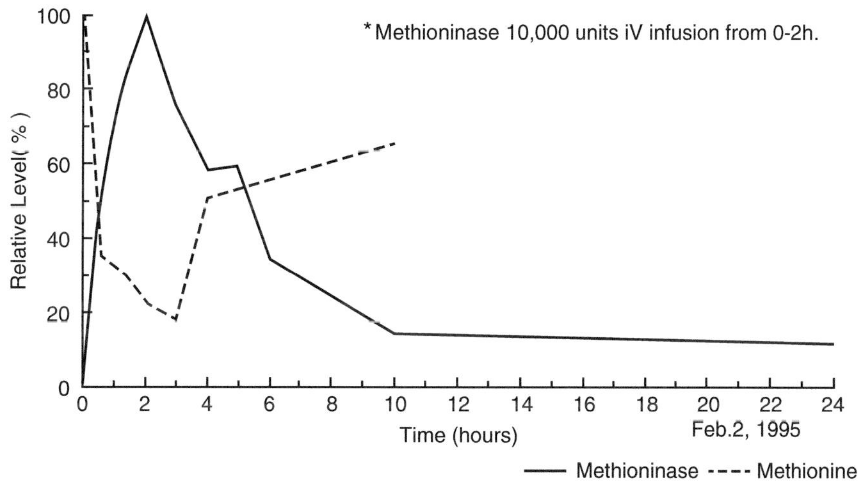

Fig. 2 Patient 2 received an i.v. infusion for 2 h with 10,000 units of methioninase. The blood samples were collected before treatment, every hour during treatment, and every 2 h up to 20 h after treatment. The levels of MET and methioninase were measured by HPLC and activity assay, respectively and the relative levels were calculated [4]

maintained at low levels after i.v. infusion for a long period without any observed side effects. This could be the basis for METase inhibition of tumor growth [15] (*see* **Note 2**).

The depletion of serum MET started within 60 min of the infusion of rMETase and reached maximum depletion after 2 h. MET depletion was maintained during the infusion and for at least 2 h after the infusion was completed. MET was depleted as low as

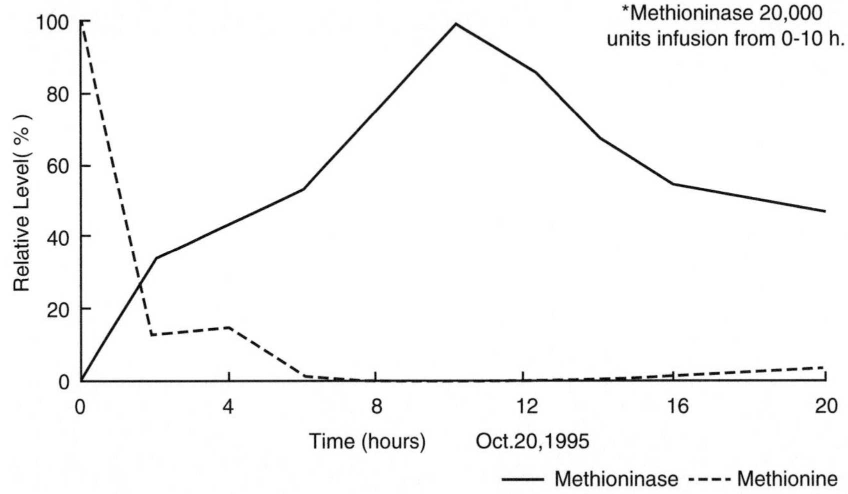

Fig. 3 Patient 3 received an i.v. infusion for 10 h with 20,000 units of methioninase. The blood samples were collected before treatment, every hour during treatment, and every 2 h up to 20 h after treatment. The levels of MET and methioninase, were measured by HPLC and activity assay, respectively and the relative levels were calculated [4]

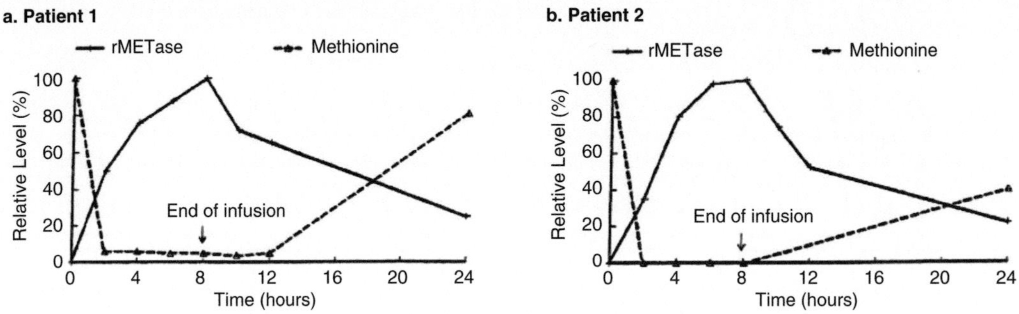

Fig. 4 rMETase pharmacokinetics and serum MET levels in patients **a** and **b**. rMETase was measured by activity assay (*see* text). MET levels were determined by HPLC (*see* text) [7].

approximately 0.1 μM within 2 h (Table 3, Fig. 5) in patients corresponding to more than a 500-fold depletion. These levels of depleted MET correspond to therapeutic levels for cancer cells in vitro [1, 7] (*see* **Note 3**).

5 Notes

1. Laboratory tests and measurements included a complete blood count with differential, prothrombin time, partial thromboplastin time, electrolytes, protein, albumin, blood urea nitrogen, creatinine lactic dehydrogenase, alkaline phosphatase, calcium, uric acid, total and direct bilirubin, serum alanine

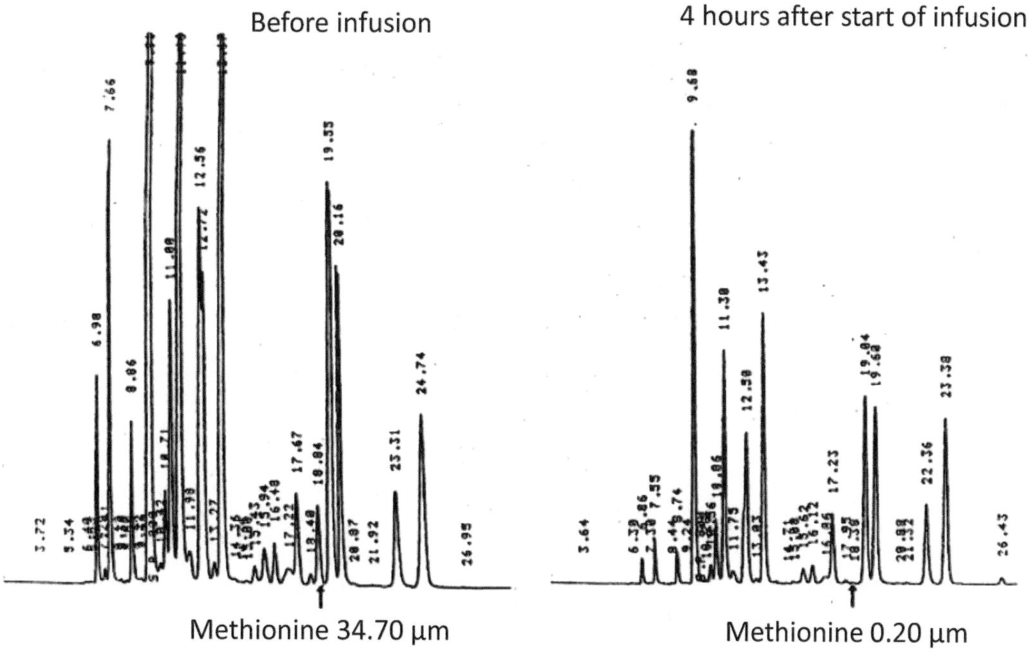

Fig. 5 Serum methionine measurement was performed by HPLC (Hitachi L-6200A Intelligent pump, Hitachi, Ltd., Tokyo, Japan) after derivation of serum amino acids with a fluoraldehyde reagent, o-phthaldialdehyde (OPA). A methionine standard (Sigma) was derivatized by OPA. The eluate was read by a fluorescence spectrophotometer (Hitachi F1000) at wavelengths of 350–450 nm. The limit of detection was approximately 0.1 μM MET [7]

aminotransferase, urinalysis, chest X-ray, electrocardiogram, and pertinent radiographic studies [7].

2. The results suggested that doses up to 20,000 units of METase (1.6 g) as i.v. infusion over 10 h were safe. The i.v. infusion of METase effectively depleted serum MET without any signs of side effects. The depletion of MET levels could be maintained after the 10-h i.v. infusion for an additional 10 h [4].
3. These results demonstrated that rMETase could essentially completely deplete MET without any observed clinical toxicity, which is the basis for inhibition of tumor growth. The results justify further clinical trials of this novel and promising agent [7].

References

1. Hoffman RM (2015) Development of recombinant methioninase to target the general cancer-specific metabolic defect of methionine dependence: a 40-year odyssey. Expert Opin Biol Ther 15:21–31
2. Hoffman RM, Jacobsen SJ (1980) Reversible growth arrest in SV40-transformed human fibroblasts. Proc Natl Acad Sci U S A 77:7306–7310
3. Guo H, Lishko K, Herrera H, Groce A, Kubota T, Hoffman RM (1993) Therapeutic tumor-specific cell cycle block induced by methioninase starvation in vivo. Cancer Res 53:5676–5679

4. Tan Y, Zavala J Sr, Xu M, Zavala J Jr, Hoffman RM (1996) Serum MET depletion without side effects by METase in metastatic breast cancer patients. Anticancer Res 16:3937–3942
5. Goseki N, Yamazaki S, Shimojyu K, Kando F, Maruyama M, Endo M, Koike M, Takahashi H (1995) Synergistic effect of methionine-depleting total parenteral nutrition with 5-fluorouracil on human gastric cancer. A randomized, prospective clinical trial. Jpn J Cancer Res 86:484–489
6. Goseki N, Yamazaki S, Endo M (1992) Antitumor effect of methionine-depleting total parenteral nutrition with doxorubicin administration on Yoshida sarcoma-bearing rate. Cancer 69:1865–1872
7. Tan Y, Zavala J Sr, Han Q, Xu M, Sun X, Tan X-Z, Tan X-Y, Magana R, Geller J, Hoffman RM (1997) Recombinant METase infusion reduces the biochemical endpoint of serum MET with minimal toxicity in high-stage cancer patients. Anticancer Res 17:3857–3860
8. Lishko VK, Lishko OV, Hoffman RM (1993) The preparation of endotoxin-free L-methionine-α-deamino-γ-mercaptomethane-lyase (L-methioninase) from Pseudomonas putida. Protein Expr Purif 4:529–533
9. Tan Y, Xu M, Sun X, Kubota T, Hoffman RM (1996) Anticancer efficacy of methioninase in vivo. Anticancer Res 16:3931–3936
10. Tan Y, Xu M, Tan XZ, Tan X, Wang X, Saikawa S, Nagahama T, Sun X, Lenz M, Hoffman RM (1997) Overexpression and large-scale production of recombinant L-methionine-α-deamino-γ-mercaptomethane-lyase for novel anticancer therapy. Protein Expr Purif 9:233–245
11. Tan Y, Sun X, Xu M, Tan X-Z, Sasson A, Rashidi B, Han Q, Tan X-Y, Wang X, An Z, Sun F-X, Hoffman RM (1999) Efficacy of recombinant methioninase in combination with cisplatin on human colon tumors in nude mice. Clin Cancer Res 5:2157–2163
12. Tan Y, Xu M, Hoffman RM (2010) Broad selective efficacy of recombinant methioninase and polyethylene glycol-modified recombinant methioninase on cancer cells in vitro. Anticancer Res 30:1041–1046
13. Jones BN, Gilligan JP (1983) α-Phthaldialdehyde precolumn derivatization and reversed-phase high-performance liquid chromatography of polypeptide hydrolysates and physiological fluids. J Chromatogr 266:471–482
14. Guidelines for reporting of adverse drug reactions (1985) Division of Cancer Treatment, National Cancer Institute, Bethesda, MD
15. Tan Y, Han O, An Z, Wang X, Hoffman RM (1995) Methioninase (AC 9301): a selective antitumor agent with a new mechanism of action. Proc Am Soc Clin Oncol 14:493

Chapter 18

Methionine Gamma Lyase from *Clostridium sporogenes* Increases the Anticancer Efficacy of Doxorubicin on A549 Cancer Cells In Vitro and Human Cancer Xenografts

V. S. Pokrovsky, N. Yu. Anisimova, D. Zh. Davydov, S. V. Bazhenov, N. V. Bulushova, G. B. Zavilgelsky, V. Y. Kotova, and I. V. Manukhov

Abstract

The anticancer efficacy of methionine γ-lyase (MGL) from *Clostridium sporogenes* (*C. sporogenes*) is described. MGL was active against cancer cells in vitro and in vivo. Doxorubicin (DOX) and MGL were more effective on A549 human lung-cancer growth inhibition than either agent alone in vitro and in vivo.

Key words Methioninase, *Clostridium sporogenes*, Anticancer efficacy, Doxorubicin, Lung cancer, Human tumor xenografts

1 Introduction

Methionine γ-lyase (MGL) [EC 4.4.1.11] is a pyridoxal 5′-phosphate-dependent enzyme, which catalyzes γ-elimination of L-methionine (MET) with the production of methyl mercaptan, α-ketobutyric acid, and ammonia. MGL is widely distributed in bacteria, and has been isolated from *Pseudomonas putida*, from the eukaryotic protozoa *Trichomonas vaginalis* and *Entamoeba histolytica*, from the fungus *Aspergillus flavipes* and several other microorganisms [1]. The enzyme is promising as an antitumor agent since MET is required in excess for the growth of malignant cells [2]. MGLs from diverse microorganisms that exhibit significant reduction of MET in vivo have shown efficacy against a wide spectrum of transplantable animal and human solid tumors [3] (*see* **Note 1**).

The first MGL was isolated from *Clostridium sporogenes* (*C. sporogenes*), by Kreis and Hession [4]. This MGL inhibited growth of P815 cells in vitro cultures and the Walker carcinosarcoma 256 of the rat in vivo. Compared with a MET-restricted (MR) diet, this enzyme had greater growth-inhibiting activity and

Robert M. Hoffman (ed.), *Methionine Dependence of Cancer and Aging: Methods and Protocols*, Methods in Molecular Biology, vol. 1866, https://doi.org/10.1007/978-1-4939-8796-2_18,

negligible toxicity when evaluated by weight loss of the host. Semipurified MGL reduced plasma MET to below 8% of the control [4].

MGL from *P. putida* is the most extensively studied MGL [3]. *P. putida* MGL, cloned in *E. coli* inhibited growth of the murine Lewis lung carcinoma in mice [5], human colon cancer xenografts [6], and glioblastoma [7] in many studies and in patient-derived orthotopic xenografts (PDOX) recently both as monotherapy [8–10]. Antitumor activity of the enzyme from *A. flavipes* with respect to several human tumors was observed in vivo [11]. MGL enhanced the efficacy of doxorubicin (DOX) [12], 5-fluorouracil (5-FU) [5], cisplatinum (CDDP) [6], and nitrosoureas [7, 13, 14]. MGL from *P. putida* was shown to be effective in combination with cisplatin, 5-fluorouracil (5-FU), and 1,3-bis(2-chloroethyl)-1-nitrosourea (BCNU) in mouse models of colon cancer, lung cancer, and brain cancer.

Recently the *MGL* gene from *C. sporogenes* was cloned, and the recombinant enzyme was purified and characterized [15]. Previous studies have evaluated the cytotoxic effect of the *C. sporogenes* MGL, in PC-3 prostate cancer and K562 human chronic erythroblastic leukemia cell cultures, with IC_{50} values 0.1–0.4 and 0.4–1.3 U/ml, respectively [15] (*see* **Note 1**).

2 Materials

- *Escherichia coli* strain BL21 (DE3) F- *ompT hsdS* B *gal dcm* (DE3) (Novagen).
- *C. sporogenes* MGL gene.
- *E. coli* strain K12 AB2463.
- L-broth.
- Agar medium.
- Kanamycin.
- KFK-2MP photocolorimeter.
- *E. coli* MDG1216 strain.
- Plasmid pET-mgl-Sporog.
- Glycerol.
- Tryptone (11.3 g/L).
- Yeast extract (5.6 g/L).
- ANCUM-2 M fermenter (Institute of Biological Instrumentation of RAS, Pushchino).
- Potassium-phosphate buffer with 0.001 M Na_4EDTA.
- DTT.

- Pyridoxal phosphate.
- APV-1000 disintegrator.
- PMSF solution.
- Q-Sepharose column.
- A VivaFlow ultrafiltration set.
- Phenyl-Sepharose FF.
- Amicon filters with UM-50 membrane.
- Sodium phosphate buffer.
- Sodium chloride.
- ALPHA 1–4 LD (freeze-dried).
- Trichloroacetic acid.
- Nessler's reagent.
- A549 cells (ATCC).
- RPMI 1640 medium (PanEco, Russia).
- Fetal bovine serum (PanEco, Russia).
- HEPES (PanEco, Russia).
- Sodium bicarbonate (PanEco, Russia).
- L Glutamine (PanEco, Russia).
- Streptomycin (PanEco, Russia).
- Penicillin (PanEco, Russia).
- Cisplatinum (CDDP) (Ebewe Pharma Ges.m.b.H.Nfg.KG, Austria).
- Doxorubicin (DOX) (Veropharm, Russia).
- Flasks (Nunc).
- Plates (Nunc).
- 3-(4,5-Dimethylthiazol-2-yl)-2,5-diphenyltetrazolium bromide (MTT) (Sigma-Aldrich).
- Pyridoxal-5-phosphate (PLP) (Sigma-Aldrich).
- Phosphate-buffered saline (PBS) (PanEco, Russia).
- Trypan blue (PanEco, Russia).
- Dimethyl sulfoxide (DMSO) (PanEco, Russia).
- Athymic mice (Balb/c nude, female; 18–20 g; 6–8 weeks old) (N.N. Blokhin Cancer Research Center).
- SPSS 21 software.

3 Methods

3.1 Bacterial Strains and Culture Conditions

1. Use *Escherichia coli* strain BL21 (DE3) F-*ompT hsdS* B *gal dcm* (DE3) (Novagen) to express the *C. sporogenes* MGL gene.
2. Grow bacteria in L-broth and on the agar medium at 37 °C.
3. Culture the transformed strains on media supplemented with kanamycin at a final concentration of 40 μg/mL.
4. Measure the optical density (OD) of the bacterial suspension at 590 nm using a KFK-2MP photocolorimeter.
5. Obtain the *E. coli* MDG1216 strain by the transformation of *E. coli* BL21 (DE3) cells with plasmid pET-mgl-Sporog [16].
6. After transformation, test *E. coli* MDG1216 clones for the ability to biosynthesize MGL and store in 40% glycerol in aliquots of 30 μL at −70 °C.
7. Use the working cell bank for growth of *E. coli* MDG1216.

3.2 MGL Production

1. Prepare inoculation medium containing tryptone (11.3 g/L), yeast extract (5.6 g/L), and glycerol (5.3 g/L). Grow *E. coli* MDG1216 strain in flasks (150 mL) at 37 °C and 200 rpm up to OD = 0.5 in this medium.
2. Carry out the production of MGL by growing the *E. coli* MDG1216 strain in an ANCUM-2 M fermenter (working volume 10 L; Institute of Biological Instrumentation of RAS, Pushchino) for a total fermentation time of 12.5 h.
3. Obtain 0.45–0.52 kg of wet biomass with an MGL content of up to 45% of the total protein.

3.3 Purification

1. Thaw harvested *E. coli* MDG1216 cells (200 g) (stored at −70 °C) and suspend in a 10 mM potassium-phosphate buffer with 0.001 M Na_4EDTA, 0.01% DTT, and 0.01 mM pyridoxal phosphate, pH 7.2 (buffer 1), at a ratio of 1:5.
2. Disrupt the cells using an APV-1000 disintegrator with the addition of a PMSF solution in dioxane up to a final concentration of 1 mM.
3. Centrifuge the cell lysate and subject the supernatant to a heat treatment in 20% (vol.) ethanol.
4. Precipitate the admixtures with PEG 6000.
5. Load the obtained supernatant on a Q-Sepharose column (300 mL) equilibrated with buffer 1.
6. Elute the main peak from the column with 0.3 M KCl in the same buffer.
7. Ultrafilter (VivaFlow set) the collected peak fractions using a membrane module with a cutoff threshold of 50 kDa.

8. Increase the KCl content in the retentate up to 1 M and add the load solution on a column of Phenyl-Sepharose FF (25 mL) equilibrated with buffer 1 containing 1 M KCl such that the MGL does not bind to the absorbent under the above conditions and flows through the column.
9. Concentrate the MGL-containing fraction with Amicon using the UM-50 membrane.
10. Enhance the content of KCl in the retentate up to 1.5 M and load the solution on a column of Phenyl-Sepharose FF (50 mL) equilibrated with buffer 1 containing 1.5 M KCl.
11. Elute the MGL from the column by decreasing the salt concentration up to 0.75 M in the buffer.
12. Desalinate the MGL solution and transfer to a 20 mM sodium phosphate buffer containing 0.15 M sodium chloride and 0.01 mM pyridoxal phosphate, pH 7.2, by ultra-diafiltration on the VivaFlow set using a membrane with a 50 kDa cutoff.
13. Add trehalose to the obtained protein solution at a ratio of 1.5:1 (vol./vol.).
14. Subject the final product to sterilizing filtration.
15. Bottle the sterile solution in dark-glass vials (2000 ± 200 MU per vial) and freeze-dry (ALPHA 1–4 LD).
16. Cap the ready-made vials for labeling and store at 2–8 °C.
17. Use SDS-PAGE for homogeneity and purity determination of the MGL (Fig. 1).

3.4 Enzymatic Assay

1. Constitute a reaction mixture of the 304 μL of working buffer (100 mM potassium phosphate buffer (pH 8.0), containing 0.01 mM pyridoxal phosphate and 0.01% dithiothreitol) and 76 μL 100 mM L-methionine.
2. Initiate the reaction by the addition of 20 μL of purified enzyme (2 mg/mL).

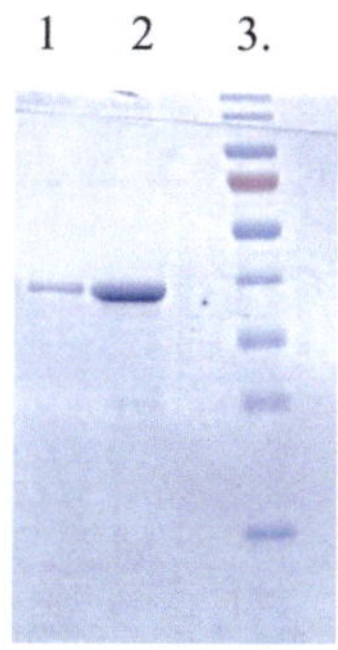

Fig. 1 SDS-PAGE for homogeneity and purity determination of MGL. (*lane 1*) 0.2 μg MGL; (*lane 2*) 4 μg MGL; (*lane 3*) protein markers (Fermentas, #SM0671)

3. Incubate the reaction mixture at 37 °C for 1 min and stop the reaction by adding 100 μL 1.5 M trichloroacetic acid.
4. Centrifuge the reaction mixture at 10,000 × *g* for 5 min at 4 °C to remove the precipitates.
5. Determine the ammonia released in supernatant using a colorimetric technique by adding 50 μl Nessler's reagent into the sample containing 50 μL supernatant and 1150 μL distilled water.
6. Vortex the contents in the sample and incubate at room temperature for 12 min and measure the OD at 450 nm.
7. Determine the ammonia produced in the reaction based on the standard curve obtained with ammonium sulfate.
8. Define 1 unit (U) of MGL activity as the amount of the enzyme that liberates 1 μmol of ammonia per min at 37 °C.
9. With this isolation and purification procedure, obtain an enzyme with a specific activity of 25.8–27.7 U/mg.

3.5 Cell Lines and Cell Viability Assay

1. Grow A549 human lung cancer cells in RPMI 1640 medium with supplements in flasks at 37 °C and 5% CO_2.
2. After 80% confluency, trypsinize the cells in exponential growth phase, suspend in fresh medium supplemented with 5×10^{-5} M pyridoxal-L-phosphate (PLP), and seed in 96-well plates in a concentration of 4×10^5 cell/ml.
3. Count the cells after treating with 0.4% trypan blue solution.
4. After 24 h, add different concentrations of tested drugs dissolved in PBS in wells.
5. Expose cells to different concentrations of CDDP, DOX, and MGL, alone and in combination, for 72 h.
6. Add PBS only in control wells with untreated cells.
7. Estimate the cell viability with the MTT assay as described in [17].
8. Measure the absorbance of DMSO with dissolved MTT–formazan crystals at 540 nm (Multiscan, Finland).
9. Express the results as (IC_{50}), the drug concentration that inhibited 50% cell growth.
10. Calculate the EC_{50} values from the concentration-effect relationships using Combenefit software.

3.6 Animal Experiments

1. Conduct all animal experiments in accordance with the internationally accepted principles for laboratory animal use and care, as described in the European Economic Community (EEC) guidelines (EEC Directive of 1986; 86/609/EEC),

and with approval from the Ethics Committee for Animal Experimentation of the N.N. Blokhin Cancer Research Center.

2. Subcutaneously inject A549, MCF7, or SKBR3 cells (2×10^6 cells) into the flank of mice for tumor growth.
3. Detect established tumors of ~100 mm^3 ± 10% in volume.
4. Randomly assign the mice to treatment arms and treat as follows: (a) 0.2 ml saline alone i.p. daily; (b) MGL at 1000 U/kg daily × 10 i.p., as determined by preliminary experiments (data not published); (c) DOX 2 mg/kg every other day × 5 i.p.; (d) CDDP 1.5 mg/kg every other day × 5 i.p.; (e) combination of (b and c); and (f) combination of (b and d).
5. Assess tumor volume three times a week using caliper measuring three perpendicular diameters, and measure the body weight every 4 days.
6. Calculate the tumor inhibitory ratio using the following formula: TGI (tumor growth inhibition, %) = $[(C - T)/C] \times 100$, where C is the mean tumor size of the vehicle control group and T is the mean tumor size of the treated group.

3.7 Analysis of Combined Drug Effect

1. Analyze the drug combination effect with the method of Chou and Talalay [15] with calculation of combination index (CI). The CI indicates antagonism (CI > 1), additivity (CI = 1), or synergism (CI < 1).
2. Calculate the modified coefficient of drug interaction (CDI) according to [18] where CDI < 1, = 1, or > 1 indicates that the drugs are synergistic, additive, or antagonistic, respectively. CDI <0.7 indicates that the drug is significantly synergistic.
3. Use average CDI to evaluate the total drug combination effect [19].

3.8 Statistical Analysis

1. Repeat experiments in vitro until three replicates yield coefficients $R > 0.9$ for all three median effect lines.
2. Make calculations of CI and average CDI values with Microsoft Office Excel 2010, EC50 values—with Combenefit software.
3. Use the Loewe and Bliss models for synergy/antagonism drug combination effect analysis.
4. Use SPSS 21 software for statistical analysis for in vivo experiments.
5. Use one-way ANOVA to compare efficacy of monotherapy and combined therapy.
6. Perform post hoc Dunnett's test to assess differences between the individual groups against one control.

7. Use the Dunnett's T3 test to assess differences between the individual groups. P values <0.05 are considered statistically significant.

4 Results

4.1 EC_{50} of MGL on A549, SK-BR3, SCOV3, and MCF7 Human Cancer Cell Lines

The calculated EC_{50} values for MGL were 4.4 U/mL for A549; 7.5 U/mL for SK-BR3; 2.4 U/mL for SKOV3; and 0.4 U/mL for MCF7.

4.2 MGL Synergistically Enhances the Cytotoxicity of CDDP on A549 Cells

Three different combinations, namely CDDP+MGL (5 U), CDDP +MGL (2.5 U), and CDDP+MGL (1.25 U), were used to compare MGL and CDDP alone (Fig. 2). The concentration of CDDP was varied from 0 to 50 μg/mL, whereas the amount of the enzyme was either (5 U or 2.5 U or 1.25 U).

As shown in Fig. 3 and Table 1 CDDP+MGL 5 U and CDDP +MGL 2.5 U combinations demonstrated higher cytotoxicity on A549 cells compared with CDDP alone at low concentration (0–0.5 μg/mL).

CI and average CDI values are shown in Table 1. The efficacy of CDDP+MGL 2.5 U and CDDP+MGL 1.25 U on A549 cells is synergistic (average CDI –0.74 and 0.78, respectively); CDDP +MGL 5 U are additive (average CDI –0.95). CDDP+MGL 2.5 U are more synergistic with a lower concentration of CDDP. Key results of this analysis are presented in Fig. 4.

4.3 MGL Synergistically Enhances the Cytotoxicity of DOX on A549 Cells

To investigate the effects of MGL and DOX on the proliferation of A549 cells, three different mixtures, namely DOX + MGL (5 U), DOX + MGL (2.5 U), and DOX + MGL (1.25 U), were used (Fig. 5). In each mixture the concentration of DOX ranged from 0 to 100 μg/ml, whereas the amount of the enzyme was constant (5 U or 2.5 U or 1.25 U).

As shown in Figs. 6 and 7 and Table 2, all combinations of DOX + MGL demonstrated higher cytotoxicity compared with DOX alone at 0–10 μg/ml concentrations.

Effect of DOX + MGL 1.25 U can be interpreted as synergistic when compared with DOX alone: CI corresponded to 0.74, average CDI –0.85. Effect of DOX + MGL 2.5 U and DOX + MGL 5 U was defined as additive.

4.4 MGL has Additive Cytotoxic Effect on SK-BR3 and SCOV-3 Cell Lines When Combined with CDDP and DOX

CDDP or DOX + MGL combinations were studied in SK-BR-3 and SCOV-3 cell lines. It was found that the DOX + MGL 5 or 2.5 U and CDDP + MGL 5 or 2.5 U combinations had a low synergistic effect against SK-BR3: average CDI values of DOX + MGL 5 U = 0.81; DOX + MGL 2.5 U = 0.79; CDDP + MGL 5 U = 0.71; and CDDP + MGL 2.5 U = 0.84.

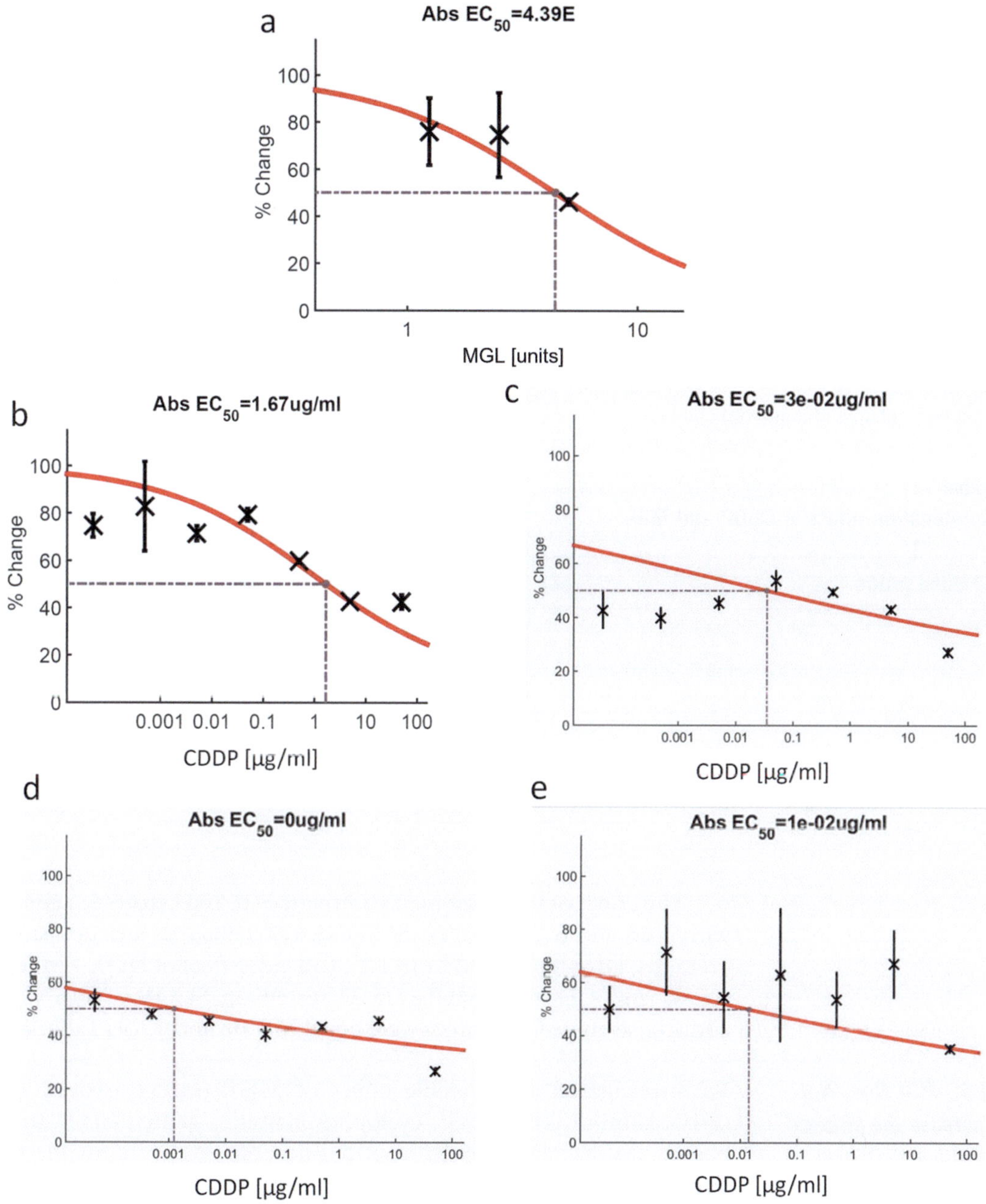

Fig. 2 EC_{50} values of MGL and CDDP, and CDDP+MGL combinations on A549 cells were calculated with Combenefit software for: (**a**) MGL; (**b**) CDDP alone; (**c**) CDDP+MGL 1.25 U; (**d**) CDDP+MGL 2.5 U; (**e**) CDDP +MGL 5 U

For SK-BR3, CDDP + MGL 1.25 U and DOX + MGL 1.25 U showed an additive effect: average CDI values were 1.02 and 1.16, respectively (Table 3).

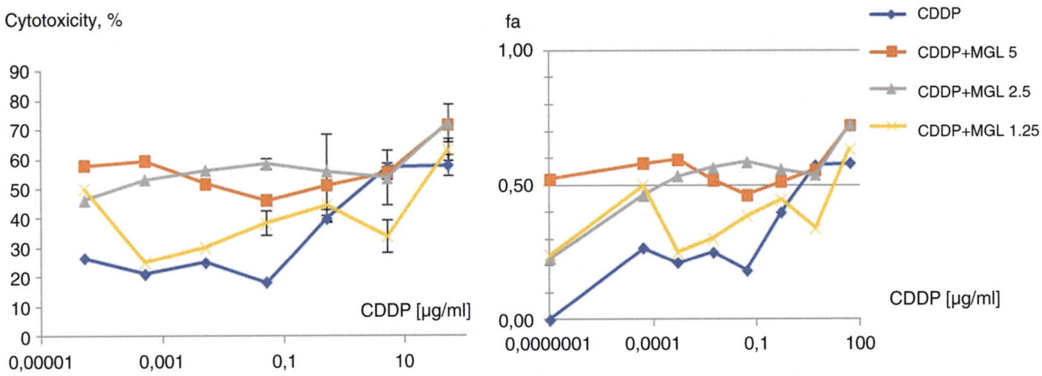

Fig. 3 Cytotoxic activity of CDDP+MGL combinations versus CDDP alone on A549 cells. (**a**) Cytotoxicity, %; (**b**) desired fractional affected (fa) cell kill

Table 1
Combination effect of CDDP and MGL

Tested drugs	EC_{50}	CI		Average CDI	
MGL	4.39 U	–	–	–	–
CDDP	1.67 μg/mL	–	–	–	–
CDDP+MGL 5 U	0.03 μg/mL	1.18	Additive or antagonistic	0.95	Additive
CDDP+MGL 2.5 U	0.002 μg/mL	0.68	Synergistic	0.74	Synergistic
CDDP+MGL 1.25 U	0.01 μg/mL	0.69	Synergistic	0.78	Synergistic

The effect of the combined treatment of tested cytotoxic agents with 1.25 and 5 U MGL on SCOV-3 was defined as antagonistic: average CDI values varied from 1.11 to 1.32. Effect of DOX + MGL 2.5 U and CDDP + MGL 2.5 U tested on SCOV-3 cells was additive: average CDI values were equal to 1.08 and 1.09 (Table 4).

4.5 MGL Does Not Increase the efficacy of Other Cytotoxic Agents In Vitro

We investigated the possible effect of MGL on cytotoxicity of carboplatinum, vincristine, cyclophosphamide, gemcitabine, etoposide, docetaxel, dacarbazine, and irinotecan. We were unable to detect a significant change of cytotoxicity of these agents when combined with MGL.

4.6 MGL Inhibits Growth of SK-BR3 Xenografts Similar to DOX and CDDP

Mice were transplanted with SK-BR-3 cells to establish subcutaneous xenografts. The initial tumor volume in each group was ~110 mm^3 ± 10% (range from 98.3 to 120.9 mm^3, day 1, treatment onset). At the end of the treatment (day 10), the average volume of the tumor reached 1172.3 ± 742.1 mm^3 in the control (vehicle) arm; 584.5 ± 215.1 mm^3 in the MGL arm (TGI 50%); 401.3 ± 179.7 mm^3 in the DOX arm (TGI 66%); 560.6 ± 162.1

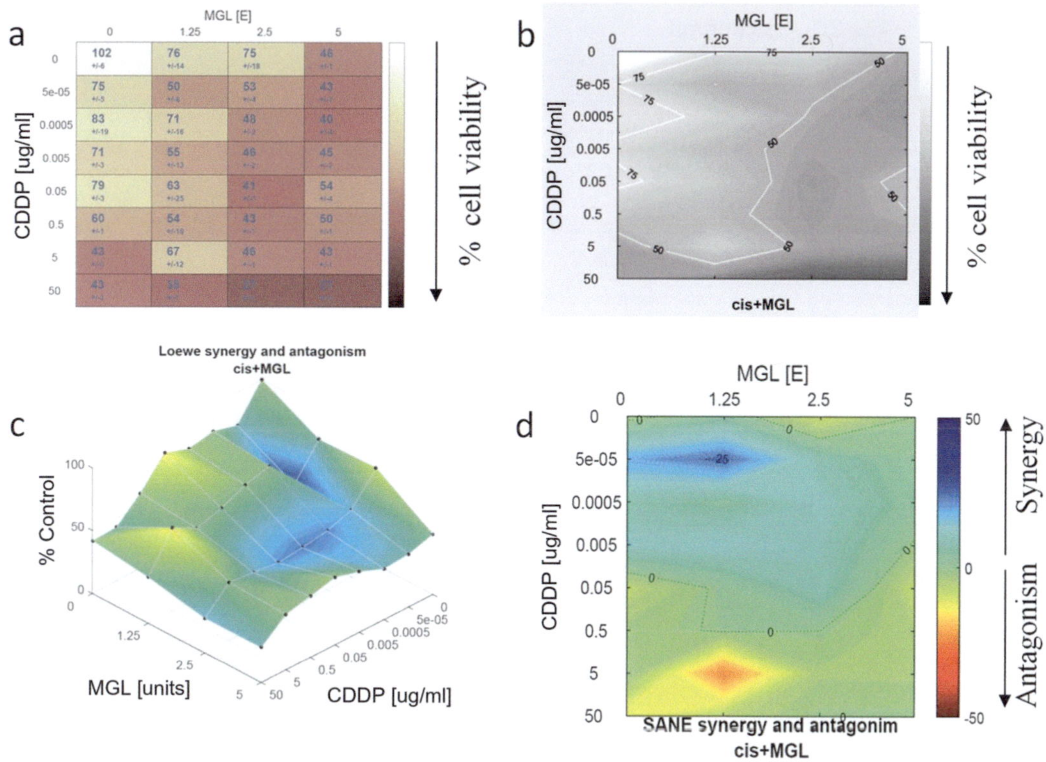

Fig. 4 Analysis of CDDP and MGL combination effect on % A549 cell viability: (**a**) Detailed analysis of cell survival after incubation with different concentrations of drugs; (**b**) contour Sane synergy and antagonism model of influence of CDDP and MGL to % cell viability; (**c**) Loewe mapped surface model for analysis of the influence concentration of components to effect of mixtures; (**d**) contour Loewe synergy and antagonism model of influence of CDDP and MGL to % cell viability

in the CDDP arm (TGI 52%); and 561.7 ± 247.0 mm^3 and 529.3 ± 144.9 in the combined DOX + MGL and CDDP + MGL arms (TGI 52 and 55%, respectively). No statistically-significant differences were observed between treatment arms (Fig. 8) (*see* **Note 2**).

4.7 MGL Inhibits Growth of MCF7 Xenografts Similar to CDDP or DOX

On day 1 (onset of treatment) initial xenograft volume reached ~100 mm^3, and mice were randomly assigned to six arms. At the end of the treatment (day 10), the volume of the tumor mass was 506.6 ± 269.4 mm^3 in the control (vehicle) arm; 134.5 ± 75.4 mm^3 in the MGL arm (TGI 74%, $p = 0.037$); 114.5 ± 55.3 mm^3 in the DOX arm (TGI 77%, $p = 0.029$); 162.6 ± 84.4 in the CDDP arm (TGI 68%, $p = 0.046$); and 125.7 ± 80.4 mm^3 and 219.4 ± 68.0 mm^3 in the combined DOX + MGL or CDDP + MGL arms (TGI 75%, $p - 0.033$ and 57%, $p = 0.118$, respectively). No statistically-

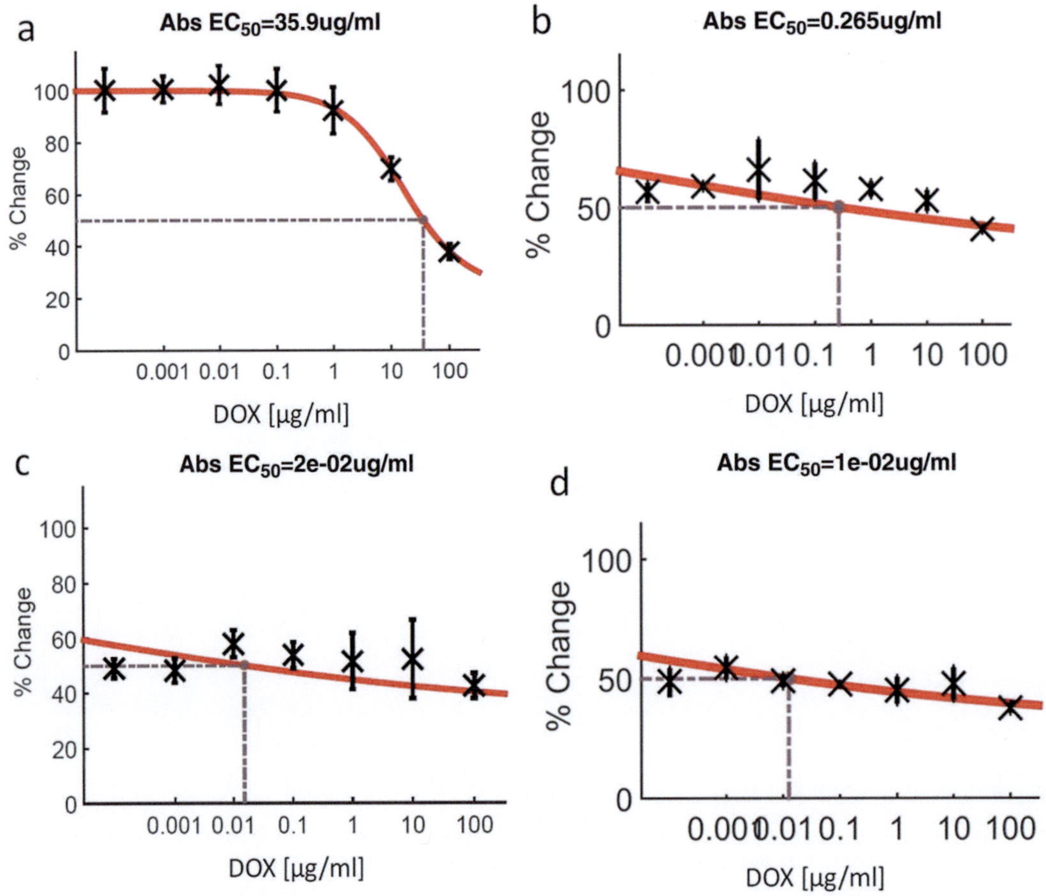

Fig. 5 EC_{50} values of DOX and DOX + MGL mixtures on A549 cells calculated using Combenefit software: (**a**) DOX alone; (**b**) DOX + MGL 1.25 U; (**c**) DOX + MGL 2.5 U; (**d**) DOX + MGL 5 U

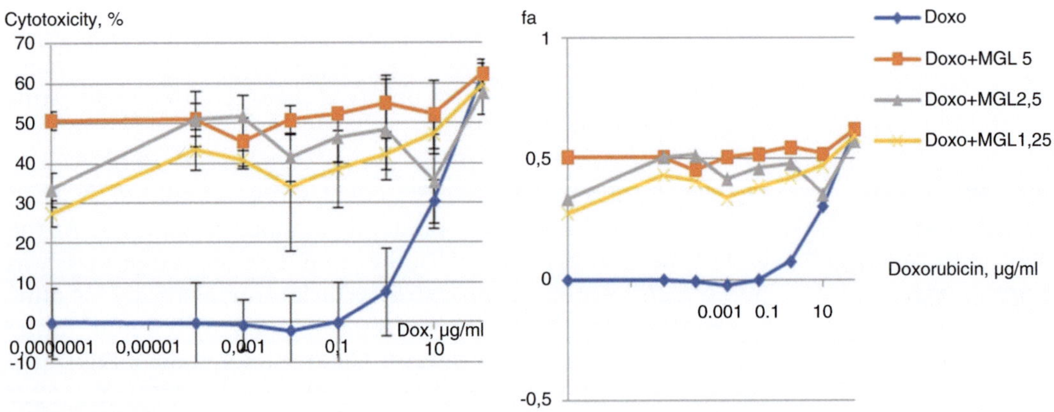

Fig. 6 Cytotoxic activity of DOX + MGL combinations versus DOX alone on A549 cells. (**a**) Cytotoxicity, %; (**b**) desired fractional affected (fa) cell kill

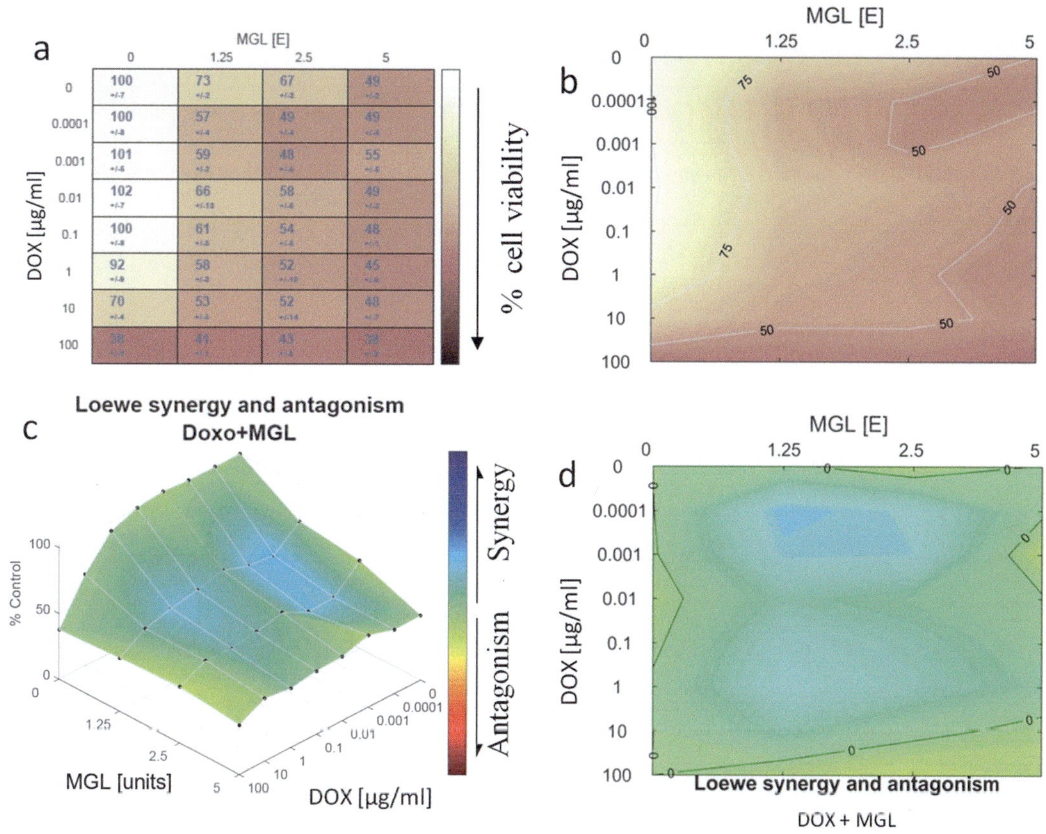

Fig. 7 Cell viability after co-incubation with MGL and DOX on A549 cells: (**a** and **b**) Analysis of cell survival with different concentrations of drugs; (**c**) contour Loewe synergy and antagonism model of influence of DOX and MGL on cell viability, %; (**d**) Loewe mapped surface model for analysis of the influence of concentration of components on mixtures

Table 2
Combination effect of DOX and MGL on A549 cells

Tested drugs	EC_{50}	CI		Average CDI	
DOX	35.9 μg/mL	–	–	–	–
DOX + MGL 5 U	0.01 μg/mL	1.011	Additive	0.97	Additive
DOX + MGL 2.5 U	0.02 μg/mL	1.002	Additive	0.89	Additive or synergistic
DOX + MGL 1.25 U	0.265 μg/mL	0.740	Synergistic	0.85	Synergistic

significant differences between treatment arms were observed (Fig. 9).

On day 1 (onset of treatment) initial xenograft volume was ~150 mm^3, and mice were randomly assigned to four arms. Four days after the end of the treatment (day 14), the volume of the

Table 3
Cytotoxicity of DOX or CDDP + MGL against SK-BR-3

Tested drugs	DOX + MGL		CDDP + MGL	
	EC_{50}	Average CDI	EC_{50}	Average CDI
MGL alone	2.4 U	–	–	–
Drug alone	2 μg/mL	–	0.59	–
Drug + MGL 5 U	0.06 μg/mL	0.81	0.41	0.71
Drug + MGL 2.5 U	0.07 μg/mL	0.79	1.87	0.84
Drug + MGL 1.25 U	0.29 μg/mL	1.02	2.53	1.16

Table 4
Cytotoxicity of DOX or CDDP + MGL against SCOV-3

Tested drugs	DOX + MGL		CDDP + MGL	
	EC_{50}	Average CDI	EC_{50}	Average CDI
MGL alone	4.4 U	–	–	–
Drug alone	0.07 μg/mL	–	1.5	–
Drug + MGL 5 U	0.07 μg/mL	1.27	1.7	1.32
Drug + MGL 2.5 U	0.31 μg/mL	1.08	0.6	1.09
Drug + MGL 1.25 U	1.0 μg/mL	1.11	0.5	1.28

4.8 MGL in Combination with DOX Significantly Decreases Tumor Growth in A549 Xenografts

tumor mass reached 1996.0 ± 200.0 mm^3 in the control (vehicle) arm; 1221.6 ± 177.3 mm^3 in the MGL arm (TGI 39%, $p = 0{,}045$, Dunnett T3); 1598.7 ± 202.5 mm^3 in the DOX arm (TGI 20%, $p = 0{,}660$); and 858.9 ± 123.0 mm^3 in the combined DOX + MGL arm (TGI 57%, $p < 0{,}001$). Combination treatment with MGL and DOX significantly decreased the tumor volume compared to monotherapy with MGL or DOX in A549 tumors. The inhibition rate of tumor growth in the combined arm was 57%, which was significantly greater than that in the DOX arm ($p = 0.033$), but not the MGL-alone arm ($p = 0.657$). None of the mice exhibited signs of physical discomfort during the treatment and follow-up periods. These results suggest that combination of MGL and DOX can significantly inhibit tumor growth in vivo (Fig. 10) (*see* **Notes 2** and **3**).

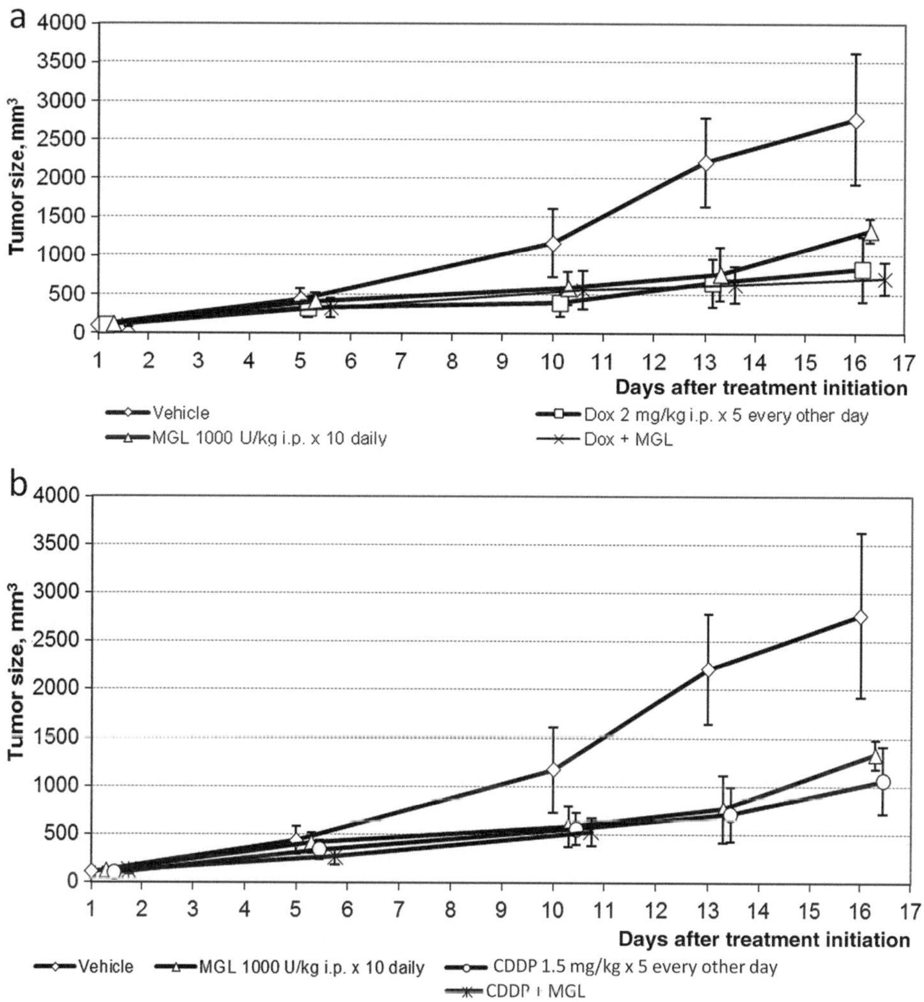

Fig. 8 Efficacy of MGL alone or in combination with DOX (**a**) or CDDP (**b**) on SK-BR3 xenografts. Breast cancer xenograft. SK-BR3 cells (7×10^6 cells) were injected subcutaneously into both flanks of nude mice (5 mice/group). After tumors were established, mice were treated with 2 mg/kg DOX or 1.5 mg/kg CDDP *i.p.* every other day $\times 5$, and 1000 U/kg MGL *i.p.* daily $\times 10$ as a single agent or in combination with the above drugs

5 Notes

1. A number of amino acid-cleaving enzymes have been studied in recent years, targeting amino-acid dependence as metabolic defects in cancer. These enzymes include asparaginase [19–21], lysine alpha-oxidase [22], phenylalanine ammonia-lyase [23], and MGL. Methionine dependence, the essential methionine requirement for cell growth, occurs frequently in many types of human cancer cell lines and animal models of cancer [24–28].

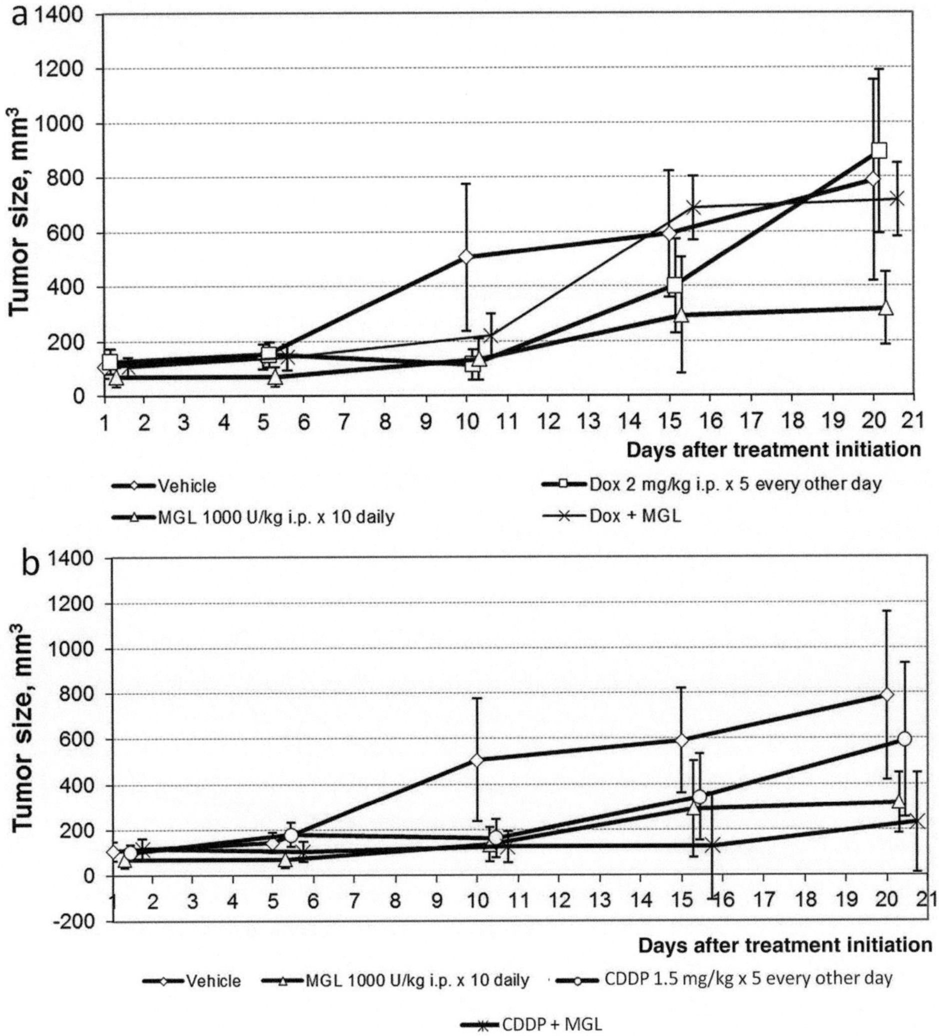

Fig. 9 Efficacy of MGL alone or with DOX (**a**) or CDDP (**b**) on MCF7 breast-cancer xenografts. MCF7 cells (7×10^6 cells) were injected subcutaneously into both flanks of nude mice (5 mice/group). After tumors were established, mice were treated with 2 mg/kg DOX or 1.5 mg/kg CDDP *i.p.* every other day $\times 5$, and 1000 U/kg MGL *i.p.* daily $\times 10$ as a single agent or in combination with the above drugs

2. Reduction of plasma MET below 5 mM arrests human xenograft growth in athymic mice [13], suggesting that a plasma MET level of <5 mM may be necessary to achieve significant anticancer effect in an animal model. We reported previously that $T_{1/2}$ of MGL from *C. sporogenes* after intravenous injection into mice is 1.31 ± 0.03 h. Mouse plasma MET decreased to an undetectable level 10 min after 1000 U/kg injection. This effect persisted for 6 h, indicating the feasibility of long-term reduction of MET to a negligible level (<5 μM) [29].

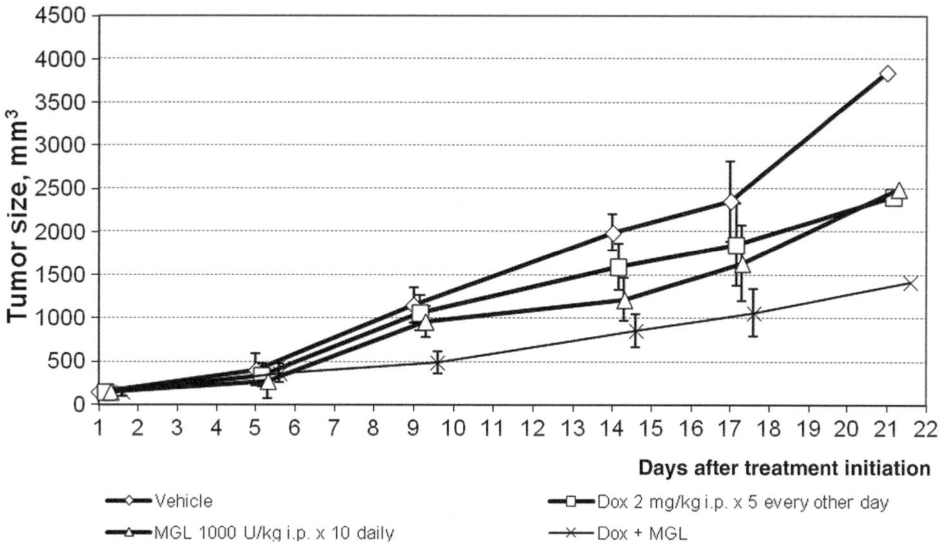

Fig. 10 Efficacy of the DOX + MGL combination on the A549 lung-cancer xenograft model. A549 cells (7×10^6 cells) were injected subcutaneously into both flanks of nude mice (5 mice/group). After tumors were established, mice were treated with 2 mg/kg DOX *i.p.* every other day $\times 5$, and 1000 U/kg MGL *i.p.* daily $\times 10$ as a single agent or in combination with the above drug

3. In our study, we found that combination of DOX and MGL is more effective in A549 tumor growth inhibition than either agent alone. The growth inhibitory effect of the DOX + MGL combination on the A549 xenograft was consistent with the results obtained in vitro. In contrast statistically-significant inhibition of tumor growth was not achieved with either MGL or DOX alone. Future studies are required to investigate cellular mechanisms of the potential of cytotoxic agents to increase MGL efficacy and to optimize the treatment schedule to achieve complete tumor regression.

References

1. El-Sayed AS (2010) Microbial L-methioninase: production, molecular characterization, and therapeutic applications. Appl Microbiol Biotechnol 86:445–467
2. Cellarier E, Durando X, Vasson MP et al (2003) Methionine dependency and cancer treatment. Cancer Treat Rev 29:488–489
3. Hoffman RM (2015) Development of recombinant methioninase to target the general cancer-specific metabolic defect of methionine dependence: a 40-year odyssey. Expert Opin Biol Ther 15:21–31
4. Kreis W, Hession C (1973) Biological effects of enzymatic deprivation of L-methionine in cell culture and an experimental tumor. Cancer Res 33:1866–1869
5. Yoshioka T, Wada T, Uchida N et al (1998) Anticancer efficacy in vivo and in vitro, synergy with 5-fluorouracil and safety of recombinant methioninase. Cancer Res 58:2583–2587
6. Tan Y, Sun X, Xu M et al (1999) Efficacy of recombinant methioninase in combination with cisplatin on human colon tumors in nude mice. Clin Cancer Res 5:2157–2163

7. Kokkinakis DM, Wick JB, Zhou Q-X (2002) Metabolic response of normal and malignant tissue to acute and chronic methionine stress in athymic mice bearing human glial tumor xenografts. Chem Res Toxicol 15:1472–1479
8. Murakami T, Li S, Han Q et al (2017) Recombinant methioninase effectively targets a Ewing's sarcoma in a patient-derived orthotopic xenograft (PDOX) nude-mouse model. Oncotarget 8:35630–35638
9. Kawaguchi K, Igarashi K, Li S et al (2017) Combination treatment with recombinant methioninase enables temozolomide to arrest a BRAF V600E melanoma growth in a patient-derived orthotopic xenograft. Oncotarget 8:85516–85525
10. Igarashi K, Kawaguchi K, Li S et al (2018) Recombinant methioninase in combination with DOX overcomes first-line DOX resistance in a patient-derived orthotopic xenograft nude-mouse model of undifferentiated spindle-cell sarcoma. Cancer Lett 417:168–173
11. El-Sayed AS, Shouman SA, Nassrat HM (2012) Pharmacokinetics, immunogenicity and anticancer efficiency of Aspergillus flavipes L-methioninase. Enzym Microb Technol 51 (4):200–210
12. Stern PH, Hoffman RM (1986) Enhanced in vitro selective toxicity of chemotherapeutic agents for human cancer cells based on a metabolic defect. J Natl Cancer Inst (Bethesda) 76:629–639
13. Kokkinakis DM, Schold SCJ, Hori H, Nobori T (1997) Effect of long-term depletion of plasma methionine on the growth and survival of human brain tumor xenografts in athymic mice. Nutr Cancer 29:195–204
14. Kokkinakis DM, Hoffman RM, Frenkel EP et al (2001) Synergy between methionine stress and chemotherapy in the treatment of brain tumor xenografts in athymic mice. Cancer Res 61:4017–4023
15. Morozova EA, Kulikova VV, Yashin DV et al (2013) Kinetic parameters and cytotoxic activity of recombinant methionine γ-Lyase from Clostridium tetani, Clostridium sporogenes, Porphyromonas gingivalis and Citrobacter freundii. Acta Nat 5(3):92–98
16. Anufrieva NV, Morozova EA, Kulikova VV et al (2015) Sulfoxides, analogues of L-methionine and L-cysteine as pro-drugs against gram-positive and gram-negative bacteria. Acta Nat 7(4):128–135
17. Pokrovskaya MV, Pokrovsky VS, Aleksandrova SS et al (2012) Recombinant intracellular Rhodospirillum rubrum L-asparaginase with low L-glutaminase activity and antiproliferative effect. Biochem (Moscow) Suppl B Biomed Chem 6(2):123–131
18. Wang WT, Zhao Y, Gao JL et al (2014) Cytotoxicity enhancement in MDA-MB-231 cells by the combination treatment of tetrahydropalmatine and berberine derived from *Corydalis yanhusuo* W. T. Wang. J Intercult Ethnopharmacol 3(2):68–72
19. Sidoruk KV, Pokrovsky VS, Borisova AA et al (2011) Creation of a producent, optimization of expression, and purification of recombinant Yersinia pseudotuberculosis L-asparaginase. Bull Exp Biol Med 152(2):219–223
20. Pokrovskaya MV, Aleksandrova SS, Pokrovsky VS et al (2015) Identification of functional regions in the Rhodospirillum rubrum L-asparaginase by site-directed mutagenesis. Mol Biotechnol 57(3):251–264
21. Pokrovsky VS, Kazanov MD, Dyakov IN et al (2016) Comparative immunogenicity and structural analysis of epitopes of different bacterial L-asparaginases. BMC Cancer 16:89
22. Sannikova EP, Bulushova NV, Cheperegin SE et al (2016) The modified heparin-binding L-Asparaginase of Wolinella succinogenes. Mol Biotechnol 58(8–9):528–539
23. Pokrovsky VS, Treshalina HM, Lukasheva EV et al (2013) Enzymatic properties and anticancer activity of L-lysine α-oxidase from Trichoderma cf. aureoviride Rifai BKMF-4268D. Anti-Cancer Drugs 24(8):846–851
24. Babich OO, Pokrovsky VS, Anisimova NY et al (2013) Recombinant l-phenylalanine ammonia lyase from Rhodosporidium toruloides as a potential anticancer agent. Biotechnol Appl Biochem 60(3):316–322
25. Mecham JO, Rowitch D, Wallace CD et al (1983) The metabolic defect of methionine dependence occurs frequently in human tumor cell lines. Biochem Biophys Res Commun 117:429–434
26. Hoffman RM, Erbe RW (1976) High in vivo rates of methionine biosynthesis in transformed human and malignant rat cells auxotrophic for methionine. Proc Natl Acad Sci U S A 73:1523–1527

27. Hoffman RM (1984) Altered methionine metabolism, DNA methylation, and oncogene expression in carcinogenesis: a review and symthesis. Biochim Biophys Acta 738:49–87
28. Guo H, Herrera H, Groce A, Hoffman RM (1993) Expression of the biochemical defect of methionine dependence in fresh patient tumors in primary histoculture. Cancer Res 53:2479–2483
29. Tisdale M, Eridani S (1981) Methionine requirement of normal and leukaemic haemopoietic cells in short term cultures. Leuk Res 5:385–394

Chapter 19

Methionine Restriction and Life-Span Extension

Robert M. Hoffman

Abstract

It has been known for almost a century that caloric restriction can extend the life span of rodents and many other types of animals. Approximately 25 years ago, it was found that a methionine-restricted (MR) diet could replace a caloric-restricted diet with the result of extending the life span of animals. This chapter summarizes the effects of MR on the reversal of diabetes, obesity, and other aspects of the metabolic syndrome, as well as extending the normal life span. The most effective way to restrict methionine in the body, using orally-delivered methioninase, is also explored.

Key words Aging, Methionine restriction, Life-span extension, Diabetes, Obesity, Methioninase, Oral delivery

1 Introduction

It has been known for almost a century that caloric restriction (CR) extends life span [1–3] in many animal species. Life-span extension by caloric restriction can reverse or delay many aspects of aging including immune senescence [4], cancer [5, 6], aberrant gene expression [7], anti-oxidant damage [8], DNA damage [9, 10], and insulin resistance [11]. Caloric restriction is effective in adult, as well as neonatal rats [10, 12].

Orentreich et al. discovered that restricting dietary methionine (MET) from 0.86 to 0.17% extended the life-span rats [10]. Removing cysteine as well as MET from diets increased longevity in rats by 30–40%, despite that they were fed ad libitum. MET restriction (MR) decreased mortality from all causes of death. Orentreich et al. observed that CR was not necessary for MR-mediated life-span extension. Orentreich showed that MR and not overall CR was responsible for the increase in longevity in the MR group [13].

MR in rats resulted in a 42% increase in mean and 44% increase in maximum life span, and in 43% lower body weight compared to

Robert M. Hoffman (ed.), *Methionine Dependence of Cancer and Aging: Methods and Protocols*, Methods in Molecular Biology, vol. 1866, https://doi.org/10.1007/978-1-4939-8796-2_19, © Springer Science+Business Media, LLC, part of Springer Nature 2019

controls. Increases in blood glutathione (GSH) levels of 81 and 164% were observed in mature and old MR rats, respectively [14].

MR rats had significantly reduced visceral fat; decreased basal insulin, glucose, and leptin; and increased adiponectin and triiodothyronine. Insulin responses of older MR animals were similar to young animals. MR prevented age-associated increases in serum lipids and reduction in insulin-like growth factor 1 (IGF-1) [15]. MR increased total energy expenditure and limited fat deposition despite increased food consumption in Fischer 344 rats [16], decreased body weight and adiposity, and improved insulin sensitivity [16–18]. MR mimicked CR [19], despite that animals on an MR diet consume more food than control-fed animals [16, 17]. MR reduced growth hormone signaling [18] as well as serum IGF-1. Fibroblast growth factor (FGF) was released from the liver in response to MR [20, 21].

MR in 12-month-old mice reduced body weight and adiposity, and increased physical activity, and insulin sensitivity. Mice on MR experienced increased hepatic gene expression of FGF-21, reduced insulin resistance, and reversed age-induced metabolic syndrome [21]. Mice placed on a MR diet at 6 weeks had an extended life span, and low levels of insulin, glucose, thyroid hormone T4, and IGF-I [22, 23]. MR in mice can extend life span even when initiated in mice as late as 12 months of age [24]. An MR diet also increases maximal life span in (BALB/cJ × C57BL/6 J) F1 mice with lower levels of serum IGF-I, insulin, glucose, and thyroid hormone [22]. Kidneys in MR mice were more insulin sensitive. MR may reduce the renal-function decline related to aging [24].

Oxidative stress was reduced in rats by MR. MR resulted in reduction in oxidative stress biomarkers plasma 8-hydroxydeoxyguanosine (8-OHdG) and 8-isoprostane [25]. MR decreased mitochondria reactive oxygen species (mitROS) production, oxidative damage to mitochondrial DNA, and protein oxidation [26]. Both 40 and 80% MR decreased mitochondrial ROS generation. The results show that 40% MR is sufficient to decrease ROS production and oxidative stress in rat liver [27].

An MR diet in humans had no negative side effects. Decreases in plasma levels of MET (22%) and cysteine (CYS) (15%) were observed in the MR group after 3 weeks. MR significantly decreased plasma total cholesterol, LDL, and uric acid, but had no effects on leptin, adiponectin, IGF-1, or glutathione. Restrictions in both MET and CYS may be required for maximum beneficial effects on adipokines and longevity [28].

MR diets are not practical in humans as seen in cancer studies (please *see* Chapter 9 in this volume). Recently, an orally deliverable recombinant methioninase (o-rMETase) has been developed [29] that could be used for MR-mediated life extension in place of an MR diet. MR effected by (o-rMETase) could also lower the extremely high homocysteine levels found in end-stage renal disease (ESRD).

References

1. McCay CM (1935) The effect of retarded growth upon the length of life span and upon the ultimate body size. J Nutr 10:63–79
2. Masoro EJ (1988) Food restriction in rodents, an evaluation of its role in the study of aging. J Gerontol 43:B59–B64
3. Weindruch R (1990) Caloric restriction and longevity. In: Goldstein AL (ed) Biomedical advances in aging. Plenum Press, New York, NY, pp 313–318
4. Eberly KW, Bruckner Kardoss E (1989) Immune function in aging rats, effects of germ-free status and caloric restriction. Prog Clin Biol Res 287:105–116
5. Cohen LA, Choi KW, Wang CX (1988) Influence of dietary fat, caloric restriction, and voluntary exercise on Nnitrosomethylurea-induced mammary tumorigenesis in rats. Cancer Res 48:4276–4283
6. Klurfeld DM, Welch CB, Lloyd LM, Kritchevsky D (1989) Inhibition of DMBA-induced mammary tumorigenesis by caloric restriction in rats fed high-fat diets. Int J Cancer 43:922–925
7. Semsei I, Rao G, Richardson A (1989) Changes in the ex pression of Superoxide dismutase and catalase as a function of age and dietary restriction. Biochem Biophys Res Com mun 164:620–625
8. Laganiere S, Yu BP (1989) Effect of chronic food restriction in aging rats. II. Liver cytosolic antioxidants and related enzymes. Mech Ageing Dev 48:221–230
9. Srivastava VK, Busbee DL (1992) Decreased fidelity of DNA polymerases and decreased DNA excision repair in aging mice, effects of caloric restriction. Biochem Biophys Res Commun 182:712–721
10. Orentreich N, Matias JR, DeFelice A, Zimmerman JA (1993) Low methionine ingestion by rats extends life span. J Nutr 123:269–274
11. Meehan CA, Cochran E, Mattingly M, Gorden P, Brown RJ (2015) Mild caloric restriction decreases insulin requirements in patients with type 2 diabetes and severe insulin resistance. Medicine 94:e1160
12. Weindruch R, Walford RL (1982) Dietary restriction in mice beginning at one year of age, effect on life span and spontaneous cancer incidence. Science 215:1415–1418
13. Orgeron ML, Stone KP, Wanders D, Cortez CC, Van NT, Gettys TW (2014) The impact of dietary methionine restriction on biomarkers of metabolic health. Prog Mol Biol Transl Sci 121:351–376
14. Richie JP Jr, Leutzinger Y, Parthasarathy S, Malloy V, Orentreich N, Zimmerman JA (1994) Methionine restriction increases blood glutathione and longevity in F344 rats. FASEB J 8:1302–1307
15. Malloy VL, Krajcik RA, Bailey SJ, Hristopoulos G, Plummer JD, Orentreich N (2006) Methionine restriction decreases visceral fat mass and preserves insulin action in aging male Fischer 344 rats independent of energy restriction. Aging Cell 5:305–314
16. Hasek BE, Stewart LK, Henagan TM, Boudreau A, Lenard NR, Black C, Shin J, Huypens P, Malloy VL, Plaisance EP, Krajcik RA, Orentreich N, Gettys TW (2010) Dietary methionine restriction enhances metabolic flexibility and increases uncoupled respiration in both fed and fasted states. Am J Physiol Regul Integr Comp Physiol 299:R728–R739
17. Plaisance EP, Henagan TM, Echlin H, Boudreau A, Hill KL, Lenard NR, Hasek BE, Orentreich N, Gettys TW (2010) Role of β-adrenergic receptors in the hyperphagic and hypermetabolic responses to dietary methionine restriction. Am J Physiol Regul Integr Comp Physiol 299:R740–R750
18. Ables GP, Perrone CE, Orentreich D, Orentreich N (2012) Methionine-restricted C57BL/6J mice are resistant to diet-induced obesity and insulin resistance but have low bone density. PLoS One 7:e51357
19. Masoro EJ (2005) Overview of caloric restriction and ageing. Mech Ageing Dev 126:913–922
20. Badman MK, Pissios P, Kennedy AR, Koukos G, Flier JS, Maratos-Flier E (2007) Hepatic fibroblast growth factor 21 is regulated by PPARa and is a key mediator of hepatic lipid metabolism in ketotic states. Cell Metab 5:426–437
21. Lees EK, Król E, Grant L, Shearer K, Wyse C, Moncur E, Bykowska AS, Mody N, Gettys TW, Delibegovic M (2014) Methionine restriction restores a younger metabolic phenotype in adult mice with alterations in fibroblast growth factor 21. Aging Cell 13:817–827
22. Miller RA, Buehner G, Chang Y, Harper JM, Sigler R, Smith-Wheelock M (2005) Methionine-deficient diet extends mouse lifespan, slows immune and lens aging, alters glucose, T4, IGF-I and insulin levels, and increases hepatocyte MIF levels and stress resistance. Aging Cell 4:119–125
23. Sun L, Sadighi Akha AA, Miller RA, Harper JM (2009) Life-span extension in mice by

preweaning food restriction and by methionine restriction in middle age. J Gerontol A Biol Sci Med Sci 64:711–722

24. Grant L, Lees EK, Forney LA, Mody N, Gettys T, Brown PA, Wilson HM, Delibegovic M (2016) Methionine restriction improves renal insulin signalling in aged kidneys. Mech Aging Dev 157:35–43
25. Maddineni S, Nichenametla S, Sinha R, Wilson RP, Richie JP Jr (2013) Methionine restriction affects oxidative stress and glutathione-related redox pathways in the rat. Exp Biol Med 238:392–399
26. Sanz A, Caro P, Ayala V, Portero-Otin M, Pamplona R, Barja G (2006) Methionine restriction decreases mitochondrial oxygen radical generation and leak as well as oxidative damage to mitochondrial DNA and proteins. FASEB J 20:1064–1073
27. Caro P, Gómez J, López-Torres M, Sánchez I, Naudí A, Jove M, Pamplona R, Barja G (2008) Forty percent and eighty percent methionine restriction decrease mitochondrial ROS generation and oxidative stress in rat liver. Biogerontology 9:183–196
28. Ables GP, Brown-Borg HM, Buffenstein R, Church CD, Elshorbagy AK, Gladyshev VN, Huang TH, Miller RA, Mitchell JR, Richie JP, Rogina B, Stipanuk MH, Orentreich DS, Orentreich N (2014) The first international mini-symposium on methionine restriction and lifespan. Front Genet 5:122
29. Kawaguchi K, Han Q, Li S, Tan Y, Igarashi K, Kiyuna T, Miyake K, Miyake M, Chmielowski B, Nelson SD, Russell TA, Dry SM, Li Y, Eckhardt MA, Unno M, Eilber FC, Hoffman RM (2018) Targeting methionine with oral recombinant methioninase (o-rMETase) arrests a patient-derived orthotopic xenograft (PDOX) model of BRAF-V600E mutant melanoma, implications for clinical cancer therapy and prevention. Cell Cycle 17:356–361

Chapter 20

L-[Methyl-^{11}C] Methionine-Positron-Emission Tomography (MET-PET)

Robert M. Hoffman

Abstract

Methionine (MET) dependence is a cancer-specific metabolic abnormality that is due to MET overuse for aberrant transmethylation reactions. [^{11}C]-MET is very useful for positron-emission tomography (PET) due to MET overuse in malignant tumors. Many benefits of MET-PET have been demonstrated. MET-PET can differentiate recurrent glioma and necrosis. [^{11}C]-MET-PET can also predict prognosis in gliomas better than [^{18}F]-FDG PET. [^{11}C]-MET-PET is better than MRI for predicting survival in low-grade glioma (LGG). MET-PET has greater specificity for detecting residual tumor after surgery than MRI.

Key words Cancer, Methionine dependence, Methoinine uptake, Transmethylation, Positron-emission tomography, PET imaging, MET-PET, [^{11}C]-MET, Hoffman effect

1 Overview of MET-PET

Cancer cells have an elevated requirement for methionine (MET) due to excessive and aberrant transmethylation reactions [1–5]. This phenomenon is termed the "Hoffman effect" [6–12] analogous to the "Warburg effect" [13] for excessive use of glucose by cancer cells.

MET-positron-emission tomography (PET) (MET-PET) can distinguish benign and malignant glioma better than either CT or MR imaging [14–19]. MET-PET can diagnose low-grade and malignant glial tumors in healthy cerebral cortex without disruption of the blood-brain barrier [20]. The high signal with MET-PET is due to the Hoffman effect of elevated MET uptake and use by cancer cells compared to surronding normal tissue.

MET-PET has also been used for choroidal melanoma to determine the efficacy in carbon ion beam radiotherapy (CIRT) [21]. Patients should fast for at least 6 h before MET-PET scans [21]. MET-PET can be performed 20 min after intravenous

Robert M. Hoffman (ed.), *Methionine Dependence of Cancer and Aging: Methods and Protocols*, Methods in Molecular Biology, vol. 1866, https://doi.org/10.1007/978-1-4939-8796-2_20, © Springer Science+Business Media, LLC, part of Springer Nature 2019

injection of $[^{11}C]$-MET (250–500 MBq) [20]. The $[^{11}C]$-MET uptake was more intense in choroidal melanoma than in the cerebellar cortex or occipital cortex in 87.5% of patients [21].

MET-PET provides good contrast due to the high ratio of uptake of $[^{11}C]$-MET in tumors compared to normal tissue and thus is useful for differentiating tumors from non-tumor tissue [22–24], for distinguishing tumors from treatment-induced lesions, and for correlation with histological grade in glioma [25].

MET-PET images can identify cancer cells even in a small tumor by the highly-elevated uptake of MET by the tumor. High sensitivity and accuracy of MET-PET were shown in detecting tumor recurrence with no false-negative cases [26]. MET-PET is a sensitive and accurate technique for differentiating between recurrent malignant glioma and radiation necrosis [26].

More malignant cancer cells were found in the areas of tumors with highly elevated $[^{11}C]$-MET uptake, whereas the less malignant were in tumor areas with only moderately elevated uptake [20].

$[^{18}F]$-fluorodeoxyglucose (FDG)-PET is limited by high uptake of FDG in healthy brain tissue giving poor contrast for tumor imaging, especially low-malignant tumors [20, 27, 28].

PET can demonstrate the efficacy of adjuvant therapy for remnant for astrocytoma and glioma tumor [20, 29–31].

Many studies have demonstrated the superiority of $[^{11}C]$-MET-PET over $[^{18}F]$-FDG PET [32–34]. $[^{11}]$C-MET-PET can predict prognosis in gliomas and is better than $[^{18}F]$-FDG PET and MRI in predicting survival in low-grade glioma (LGG) [35]. $[^{18}F]$-FDG has high uptake in normal brain cortex and low uptake in LGG, limiting its usefulness in tumor visualization and delineation [35–37].

$[^{11}C]$-MET uptake was greatest in the most active glioma area, and was significantly different between high-grade gliomas and LGG $[^{11}C]$-MET-PET was independent from contrast enhancement in CT or MRI. Recurrent or residual tumors had a higher $[^{11}C]$-MET uptake than primary gliomas [38].

Since postoperative changes cannot be differentiated from residual tumor by MRI, in contrast to MET-PET which has greater specificity for tumor tissue [39].

In conclusion, the use of $[^{11}C]$-MET is very effective in MET-PET imaging because the cancers use excessive MET for their aberrant excess transmethylation and therefore take up excess $[^{11}C]$-MET, compared to normal tissue [20, 21, 26, 39, 40]. In a comparison of MET-PET and fluorodeoxyglucose (FDG)-PET, MET-PET was found to be superior for glioma [35] suggesting that cancer cells may have a greater abnormal requirement for MET than the cancer cells have for glucose [2]. MET-PET is probably useful for all cancers since they are all MET dependent and use excess amounts of MET.

References

1. Hoffman RM (2015) Development of recombinant methioninase to target the general cancer-specific metabolic defect of methionine dependence: a 40-year odyssey. Expert Opin Biol Ther 15:21–31
2. Hoffman RM (2017) The wayward methyl group and the cascade to cancer. Cell Cycle 16:825–829
3. Coalson DW, Mecham JO, Stern PH, Hoffman RM (1982) Reduced availability of endogenously synthesized methionine for S-adenosylmethionine formation in methionine dependent cancer cells. Proc Natl Acad Sci U S A 79:4248–4251
4. Hoffman RM, Erbe RW (1976) High *in vivo* rates of methionine biosynthesis in transformed human and malignant rat cells auxotrophic for methionine. Proc Natl Acad Sci U S A 73:1523–1527
5. Stern PH, Hoffman RM (1984) Elevated overall rates of transmethylation in cell lines from diverse human tumors in vitro 20:663–670
6. Murakami T, Li S, Han Q, Tan Y, Kiyuna T, Igarashi K, Kawaguchi K, Hwang HK, Miyaki K, Singh AS, Nelson SD, Dry SM, Li Y, Hiroshima Y, Lwin TM, DeLong JC, Chishima T, Tanaka K, Bouvet M, Endo I, Eilber FC, Hoffman RM (2017) Recombinant methioninase effectively targets a Ewing's sarcoma in a patient-derived orthotopic xenograft (PDOX) nude-mouse model. Oncotarget 8:35630–35638
7. Kawaguchi K, Igarashi K, Li S, Han Q, Tan Y, Kiyuna T, Miyake Y, Murakami T, Chmielowski B, Nelson SD, Russell TA, Dry SM, Li Y, Unno M, Eilber FC, Hoffman RM (2017) Combination treatment with recombinant methioninase enables temozolomide to arrest a BRAF V600E melanoma growth in a patient-derived orthotopic xenograft. Oncotarget 8:85516–85525
8. Kawaguchi K, Igarashi K, Li S, Han Q, Tan Y, Miyake K, Kiyuna T, Miyake M, Murakami T, Chmielowski S, Nelson SD, Russell TA, Dry SM, Li Y, Unno M, Eilber FC, Hoffman RM (2018) Recombinant methioninase (rMETase) is an effective therapeutic for BRAF-V600E-negative as well as -positive melanoma in patient-derived orthotopic xenograft (PDOX) mouse models. Oncotarget 9:915–923
9. Igarashi K, Kawaguchi K, Li S, Han Q, Tan Y, Murakami T, Kiyuna T, Miyake K, Miyake M, Singh AS, Eckhadt MA, Nelson SD, Russell TA, Dry SM, Li Y, Yamamoto N, Hayashi K, Kimura H, Miwa S, Tsuchiya H, Singh RS, Eilber FC, Hoffman RM (2018) Recombinant methioninase in combination with DOX overcomes first-line DOX resistance in a patient-derived orthotopic xenograft nude-mouse model of undifferentiated spindle-cell sarcoma. Cancer Lett 417:168–173
10. Igarashi K, Li S, Han Q, Tan Y, Kawaguchi K, Murakami T, Kiyuna T, Miyake K, Li Y, Nelson SD, Dry SM, Singh AS, Elliott I, Russell TA, Eckhadt MA, Yamamoto N, Hayashi K, Kimura H, Miwa S, Tsuchiya H, Eilber FC, Hoffman RM (2018) Growth of a doxorubicin-resistant undifferentiated spindle-cell sarcoma PDOX is arrested by metabolic targeting with recombinant methioninase. J Cell Biochem 119:3537–3544
11. Kawaguchi K, Han Q, Li S, Tan Y, Igarashi K, Miyake K, Kiyuna T, Miyake M, Chmielowski B, Nelson SD, Russell TA, Dry SM, Li Y, Singh AS, Eckardt MA, Unno M, Eilber FC, Hoffman RM (2018) Intra-tumor L-methionine level highly correlates with tumor size in both pancreatic cancer and melanoma patient-derived orthotopic xenograft (PDOX) nude-mouse models. Oncotarget 9:11119–11125
12. Kawaguchi K, Han Q, Li S, Tan Y, Igarashi K, Kiyuna T, Miyake K, Miyake M, Chmielowski B, Nelson SD, Russell TA, Dry SM, Li Y, Eckhardt MA, Unno M, Eilber FC, Hoffman RM (2018) Targeting methionine with oral recombinant methioninase (o-rMETase) arrests a patient-derived orthotopic xenograft (PDOX) model of BRAF-V600E mutant melanoma: implications for clinical cancer therapy and prevention. Cell Cycle 17:356–361
13. Warburg O (1956) On the origin of cancer cells. Science 123:309–314
14. Derlon JM, Bourdet C, Bustany P, Chatel M, Theron J, Darcel F, Syrota A (1989) [11C]L-methionine uptake in gliomas. Neurosurgery 25:720–728
15. Mineura K, Sasajima T, Suda Y, Kowada M, Shishido F, Uemura K (1990) Amino acid study of cerebral gliomas using positron emission tomography—analysis of (11C-methyl)-L-methionine uptake index. Neurol Med Chir 30:997–1002
16. Ogawa T, Inugami A, Hatazawa J, Kanno I, Murakami M, Yasui N, Mineura K, Uemura K (1996) Clinical positron emission tomography for brain tumors: comparison of fluorodeoxyglucose F 18 and L-methyl-11C-methionine. Am J Neuroradiol 17:345–353
17. Ogawa T, Shishido F, Kanno I, Inugami A, Fujita H, Murakami M, Shimosegawa E,

Ito H, Hatazawa J, Okudera T et al (1993) Cerebral glioma: evaluation with methionine PET. Radiology 186:45–53
18. Tovi M, Lilja A, Bergstrom M, Ericsson A, Bergstrom K, Hartman M (1990) Delineation of gliomas with magnetic resonance imaging using Gd-DTPA in comparison with computed tomography and positron emission tomography. Acta Radiol 1:417–429
19. Willemsen AT, van Waarde A, Paans AM, Pruim J, Luurtsema G, Go KG, Vaalburg W (1995) In vivo protein synthesis rate determination in primary or recurrent brain tumors using L-[1-11C]-tyrosine and PET. J Nucl Med 36:411–419
20. Nariai T, Tanaka Y, Wakimoto H, Aoyagi M, Tamaki M, Ishiwata K, Senda M, Ishii K, Hirakawa K, Ohno K (2005) Usefulness of L-[methyl-^{11}C] methionine-positron emission tomography as a biological monitoring tool in the treatment of glioma. J Neurosurg 103:498–507
21. Tamura K, Yoshikawa K, Ishikawa H, Hasebe M, Tsuji H, Yanagi T, Suzuki K, Kubo A, Tsujii H (2009) Carbon-11-methionine PET imaging of choroidal melanoma and the time course after carbon ion beam radiotherapy. Anticancer Res 29:1507–1514
22. Lilja A, Lundqvist H, Olsson Y, Spannare B, Gullberg P, Langstrom B (1989) Positron emission tomography and computed tomography in differential diagnosis between recurrent or residual glioma and treatment-induced brain lesions. Acta Radiol 30:121–128
23. Ogawa T, Inugami A, Hatazawa J, Kanno I, Murakami M, Yasui N et al (1995) Clinical positron emission tomography for brain tumors: comparison of fludeoxyglucose F 18 and l-methyl-^{11}C-methionine. Am J Neuroradiol 17:345–353
24. Ogawa T, Kanno I, Shishido F, Inugami A, Higano S, Fujita H et al (1991) Clinical value of PET with^{18}F-fluorodeoxyglucose and L-methyl-^{11}C-methionine for diagnosis of recurrent brain tumor and radiation injury. Acta Radiol 32:197–202
25. De Witte O, Goldberg I, Wikler D, Rorive S, Damhaut P, Monclus M, Salmon I, Brotchi J, Goldman S (2001) Positron emission tomography with injection of methionine as a prognostic factor in glioma. J Neurosurg 95:746–750
26. Tsuyuguchi N, Takami T, Sunada I, Iwai Y, Yamanaka K, Tanaka K, Nishikawa M, Ohata K, Torii K, Morino M, Nishio A, Hara M (2004) Methionine positron emission tomography for differentiation of recurrent brain tumor and radiation necrosis after stereotactic radiosurgery—in malignant glioma. Ann Nucl Med 18:291–296
27. García-Garzon JR, Villasboas-Rosciolesi D, Baquero M, Bassa P, Soler M, Riera E (2016) A false-negative case of primary central nervous system lymphoma on 11C-methionine PET and intense 18F-FDG uptake. Clin Nucl Med 41:664–665
28. Bosnyák E, Kamson DO, Robinette NL, Barger GR, Mittal S, Juhász C (2016) Tryptophan PET predicts spatial and temporal patterns ofpost-treatment glioblastoma progression detected by contrast-enhanced MRI. J Neuro-Oncol 126:317–325
29. Jung TY, Min JJ, Bom HS, Jung S, Kim IY, Lim SH, Kim DY, Kwon SY (2017) Prognostic value of post-treatment metabolic tumor volume from ^{11}C-methionine PET/CT in recurrent malignant glioma. Neurosurg Rev 40:223–229
30. Kardan A, Satter M (2016) Advanced methionine positron-emission tomography imaging for brain tumor diagnosis, surgical planning, and treatment. In: Handbook of Neuro-oncology Neuroimaging, Academic Press, Cambridge, MA, pp 371–384
31. Kobayashi K, Hirata K, Yamaguchi S, Manabe O, Terasaka S, Kobayashi H, Shiga T, Hattori N, Tanaka S, Kuge Y, Tamaki N (2015) Prognostic value of volume-based measurements on (11)C-methionine PET in glioma patients. Eur J Nucl Med Mol Imaging 42:1071–1080
32. Chung JK, Kim YK, Kim SK, Lee YJ, Paek S, Yeo JS, Jeong JM, Lee DS, Jung HW, Lee MC (2002) Usefulness of 11C-methionine PET in the evaluation of brain lesions that are hypo- or isometabolic on 18F-FDG PET. Eur J Nucl Med Mol Imaging 29:176–182
33. Zhao C, Zhang Y, Wang J (2014) A meta-analysis on the diagnostic performance of (18) F-FDG and (11)C-methionine PET for differentiating brain tumors. Am J Neuroradiol 35:1058–1065
34. Xu W, Gao L, Shao A, Zheng J, Zhang J (2017) The performance of 11C-methionine PET in the differential diagnosis of glioma recurrence. Oncotarget 8:91030–91039
35. Singhal T, Narayanan TK, Jacobs MP, Bal C, Mantil JC (2012) 11C-methionine PET for grading and prognostication in gliomas: a comparison study with 18F-FDG PET and contrast enhancement on MRI. J Nucl Med 53:1709–1715
36. Chen W, Silverman DH (2008) Advances in evaluation of primary brain tumors. Semin Nucl Med 38:240–250

37. Singhal T, Narayanan TK, Jain V, Mukherjee J, Mantil J (2008) ^{11}C-L-methionine positron emission tomography in the clinical management of cerebral gliomas. Mol Imaging Biol 10:1–18
38. Herholz K, Hölzer T, Bauer B, Schröder R, Voges J, Ernestus RI, Mendoza G, Weber-Luxenburger G, Löttgen J, Thiel A, Wienhard K, Heiss WD (1998) 11C-methionine PET for differential diagnosis of low-grade gliomas. Neurology 50:1316–1322
39. Grosu AL, Weber WA, Riedel E, Jeremic B, Nieder C, Franz M, Gumprecht H, Jaeger R, Schwaiger M, Molls M (2005) L-(methyl-11C) methionine positron emission tomography for target delineation in resected high-grade gliomas before radiotherapy. Int J Radiat Oncol Biol Phys 63:64–74
40. Glaudemans AW, Enting RH, Heesters MA, Dierckx RA, van Rheenen RW, Walenkamp AM, Slart RH (2013) Value of 11C-methionine PET in imaging brain tumours and metastases. Eur J Nucl Med Mol Imaging 40:615–635

Chapter 21

Is the Hoffman Effect for Methionine Overuse Analogous to the Warburg Effect for Glucose Overuse in Cancer?

Robert M. Hoffman

Abstract

The general cancer-specific metabolic defect of methionine (MET) dependence is due to MET overuse for aberrant transmethylation reactions. The excess use of MET for aberrant transmethylation reactions apparently diverts methyl groups from DNA. The resulting global DNA hypomethylation is also a general phenomenon in cancer and leads to unstable genomes and aneuploid karyotypes. The excessive and aberrant use of MET in cancer is readily observed in [^{11}C]-MET-PET imaging, where high uptake of [^{11}C]-MET results in a very strong and selective tumor signal compared to normal tissue background for brain cancer and possibly other cancers. [^{11}C]-MET is superior to [^{18}C]-fluorodeoxyglucose (FDG) for PET imaging, suggesting that MET overuse in cancer ("Hoffman effect") is greater than glucose overuse in cancer ("Warburg effect").

Key words Methionine dependence, Cellular methionine, *S*-Adenosylmethionine, Transmethylation, DNA methylation, Hoffman effect

1 Introduction

1.1 Methionine Dependence in Cancer Cells

Approximately 60 years ago, Sugimura et al. [1] observed that rat tumor growth was inhibited by giving rats a diet depleted in methionine (MET). This was the first demonstration that cancer cells had an elevated requirement for MET, called MET dependence. Bertino's group subsequently showed that L5178Y mouse leukemia cells in culture required very high levels of MET in order to proliferate [2]. Subsequently, most cancer cell lines were found to be MET dependent [3, 4]. The occurrence of MET dependence among these diverse cancer types suggested that MET dependence may be a general phenomenon in cancer [5, 6].

1.2 MET-Dependent Cancer Cells Synthesize Normal Amounts of MET

MET-dependent cancer cells synthesize large amounts of MET endogenously through the reaction catalyzed by N^5-methyltetrahydropteroyl-L-glutamate: L-homocysteine *S*-methyltransferase (EC 2.1.1.13) (MET synthase) [5]. The activity of MET synthase was

Robert M. Hoffman (ed.), *Methionine Dependence of Cancer and Aging: Methods and Protocols*, Methods in Molecular Biology, vol. 1866, https://doi.org/10.1007/978-1-4939-8796-2_21,

comparable in extracts of MET-dependent malignant and normal MET-independent cells: Uptake of radioactive label from [5-^{14}C]-methyltetrahydropteroyl-L-glutamic acid (N^5-methyl-H_4PteGlu) was as great or greater in MET-dependent malignant cells as in the normal MET-independent cells. The reaction was nearly totally dependent on the addition of homocysteine, the methyl acceptor. The majority of the labeled methyl groups incorporated by MET-dependent cancer cells was recovered as MET. Thus MET dependence in cancer cells is not due to inability to synthesize and incorporate MET from homocysteine and N^5-methyl-H_4PteGlu [6, 7].

1.3 Low Levels of Endogenous MET and S-Adenosylmethionine in Cancer Cells Under MET Restriction

Despite the normal or greater-than-normal MET synthesis in MET-dependent cancer cells, the level of free MET and *S*-adenosylmethionine (AdoMET), the universal methyl donor, was very low in MET-dependent cancer cells under MET restriction (MR). The low AdoMET/AdoHCY ratio occurring in MET-dependent cancer cells under MR probably limits the growth of MET-dependent cells in MR conditions [8].

1.4 Enhanced Rates of Transmethylation in Cancer Cells

Cancer cells have enhanced overall rates of transmethylation compared to normal cells which may be the basis of the MET dependence and may be responsible for low free MET levels and the low AdoMET and low AdoMET/AdoHCY ratio in cancer cells, under MR [9]. The elevated MET use in cancer cells has been termed the "Hoffman effect" [10, 11] (*see* **Notes 1** and **2**).

1.5 MET-Dependent Cancer Cells Arrest in S/G_2 Phase of the Cell Cycle Under MET Restriction

MET-dependent cancer cells arrest in the S/G_2 phases of the cell cycle under conditions of MR [12, 13].

1.6 MET-Independent Revertants

Rare cells from MET-dependent cancer cell lines regained the ability to grow normally under MR and were thereby termed MET-independent revertants [14]. An increase in MET synthase activity was not necessary for reversion to MET independence [12, 14]. The revertants also had much lower transmethylation rates than parental MET-dependent cell lines further indicating that excessive transmethylation is the basis of MET dependence [6, 15].

MET-independent revertant cells also revert for other properties of malignancy and become more normal-like indicating further a relationship between altered MET metabolism and oncogenic transformation [16].

1.7 Discovery and Description of DNA Hypomethylation in Cancer Cells

Genome-wide DNA hypomethylation of human cancer cells was first described by our laboratory in the early 1980s [17], and has been found in almost all types of cancers [18–21]. Other groups subsequently confirmed our discovery [22–24]. Perucho et al. [25] used a biochemical quantitative assay to determine genome-wide hypomethylation in the gastric mucosa of gastric cancer patients and non-cancer patients with *H. pylori* infection, as well as global DNA hypomethylation in gastric tumors suggesting an epigenetic field defect of DNA hypomethylation in gastric cancer [26]. The degree of DNA hypomethylation in primary tumors was significantly associated with tumor progression [25]. Consistent with the Perucho et al. results, Liteplo and Kerbel [27] found that high-metastatic variants of a melanoma had more extensive DNA hypomethylation than the low metastatic parental cells [25].

1.8 Diversion of Methyl Groups in MET-Dependent Cancer Cells

A MET-dependent cancer cell line was cultured under conditions of MR and found to have increased methylation of both an endogenous substrate and *Escherichia coli* RNA but decreased DNA methylation [28]. These results indicated that methyl groups were being diverted from their normal sites, including DNA, in MET-dependent cancer cells [6].

1.9 From Perturbed Methionine Metabolism to DNA Hypomethylation to a Destabilized Genome to Aneuploidy to Cancer (Fig. 1)

We previously suggested that the premalignant DNA hypomethylation, such as that observed by Perucho et al. [25], results from the unbalanced excess transmethylation which diverts methyl groups to where they are not available for normal DNA methylation. The excess transmethylation rate explains the MET dependence or "MET addition" of cancer cells and overuse of MET. Hypomethylation of DNA then results in the initiation of aneuploidy and subsequent speciation to autonomous cancer [29].

2 Conclusion

MET overuse and concomitant MET dependence are possibly universal in cancer and seem to be more intensive and extensive than aerobic glycolysis observed in cancer. Altered MET metabolism [30] may be the basis of cancer.

3 Notes

1. [^{11}C]-MET is very effective in positron-emission tomography (PET) imaging (MET-PET), since the cancers use excessive MET for their aberrant excess transmethylation and therefore take up excess [^{11}C]-MET [31–35]. In a comparison of MET-PET and fluorodeoxyglucose (FDG)-PET, MET-PET was found to be superior for glioma [36] suggesting that

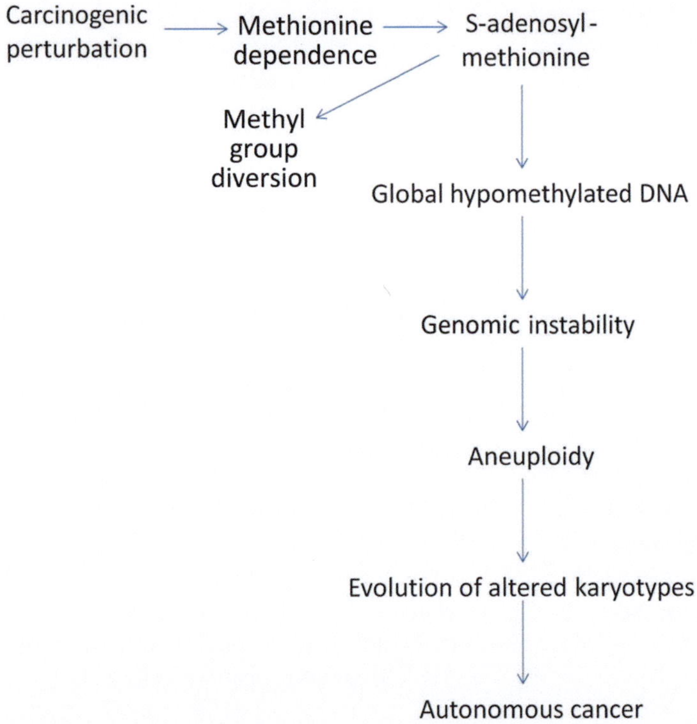

Fig. 1 The wayward methyl group and the cascade to cancer [6]

cancers may have a greater abnormal requirement for MET than glucose when compared to normal tissue [6].

2. The elevated use of glucose by cancer cells, even under aerobic conditions, has been termed the "Warburg effect" [37, 38]. The elevated use of MET by cancer cells has been termed the "Hoffman effect." The PET results described above suggest that the Hoffman effect may be more significant than the Warburg effect. Thompson has stated that metabolic reprogramming is a cancer "hallmark" [39], the "uitimate designation" in cancer. Six metabolic "hallmarks" observed in cancer, are listed by Thompson, but he states "few tumors display all 'hallmarks'" [39]. Perhaps a 7th "hallmark" is altered methionine metabolism, which may be found in all cancers.

References

1. Sugimura T, Birnbaum SM, Winitz M, Greenstein JP (1959) Quantitative nutritional studies with water-soluble, chemically defined diets. VIII. The forced feeding of diets each lacking in one essential amino acid. Arch Biochem Biophys 81:448–455
2. Chello PL, Bertino JR (1973) Dependence of 5-methyltetrahydrofolate utilization by L5178Y murine leukemia cells in vitro on the presence of hydroxycobalamin and transcobalamin II. Cancer Res 33:1898–1904
3. Mecham JO, Rowitch D, Wallace CD, Stern PH, Hoffman RM (1983) The metabolic defect of methionine dependence occurs frequently in human tumor cell lines. Biochem Biophys Res Commun 117:429–434

4. Tan Y, Xu M, Hoffman RM (2010) Broad selective efficacy of recombinant methioninase and polyethylene glycol-modified recombinant methioninase on cancer cells *in vitro*. Anticancer Res 30:1041–1046
5. Hoffman RM (2015) Development of recombinant methioninase to target the general cancer-specific metabolic defect of methionine dependence: a 40-year odyssey. Expert Opin Biol Ther 15:21–31
6. Hoffman RM (2017) The wayward methyl group and the cascade to cancer. Cell Cycle 16:825–829
7. Hoffman RM, Erbe RW (1976) High in vivo rates of methionine biosynthesis in transformed human and malignant rat cells auxotrophic for methionine. Proc Natl Acad Sci U S A 73:1523–1527
8. Coalson DW, Mecham JO, Stern PH, Hoffman RM (1982) Reduced availability of endogenously synthesized methionine for S-adenosylmethionine formation in methionine dependent cancer cells. Proc Natl Acad Sci U S A 79:4248–4251
9. Stern PH, Hoffman RM (1984) Elevated overall rates of transmethylation in cell lines from diverse human tumors in vitro 20:663–670
10. Murakami T, Li S, Han Q, Tan Y, Kiyuna T, Igarashi K, Kawaguchi K, Hwang HK, Miyaki K, Singh AS, Hiroshima Y, Lwin TM, DeLong JC et al (2017) Recombinant methioninase effectively targets a Ewing's sarcoma in a patient-derived orthotopic xenograft (PDOX) nude-mouse model. Oncotarget 8:35630–35638
11. Kawaguchi K, Igarashi K, Li S, Han Q, Tan Y, Kiyuna T, Miyake Y, Murakami T, Chmielowski B, Nelson SD, Russell TA, Dry SM, Li Y et al (2017) Combination treatment with recombinant methioninase enables temozolomide to arrest a BRAF V600E melanoma growth in a patient-derived orthotopic xenograft. Oncotarget 8:85516–85525
12. Hoffman RM, Jacobsen SJ (1980) Reversible growth arrest in simian virus 40-transformed human fibroblasts. Proc Natl Acad Sci U S A 77:7306–7310
13. Yano S, Li S, Han Q, Tan Y, Bouvet M, Fujiwara T, Hoffman RM (2014) Selective methioninase-induced trap of cancer cells in S/G_2 phase visualized by FUCCI imaging confers chemosensitivity. Oncotarget 5:8729–8736
14. Hoffman RM, Jacobsen SJ, Erbe RW (1978) Reversion to methionine independence by malignant rat and SV40-transformed human fibroblasts. Biochem Biophys Res Commun 82:228–234
15. Judde JG, Ellis M, Frost P (1989) Biochemical analysis of the role of transmethylation in the methionine dependence of tumor cells. Cancer Res 49:4859–4865
16. Hoffman RM, Jacobsen SJ, Erbe RW (1979) Reversion to methionine independence in simian virus 40-transformed human and malignant rat fibroblasts is associated with altered ploidy and altered properties of transformation. Proc Natl Acad Sci U S A 76:1313–1317
17. Diala ES, Hoffman RM (1982) Hypomethylation of HeLa cell DNA and the absence of 5-methylcytosine in SV40 and adenovirus (type 2) DNA: analysis by HPLC. Biochem Biophys Res Commun 107:19–26
18. Diala ES, Cheah MSC, Rowitch D, Hoffman RM (1983) Extent of DNA methylation in human tumor cells. J Natl Cancer Inst 71:755–764
19. Feinberg AP, Tycko B (2004) The history of cancer epigenetics. Nat Rev Cancer 4:143–153
20. Park JH, Park J, Choi JK et al (2011) Identification of DNA methylation changes associated with human gastric cancer. BMC Med Genet 4.82
21. Yoshida T, Yamashita S, Takamura-Enya T et al (2011) Alu and Satalpha hypomethylation in Helicobacter pylori-infected gastric mucosae. Int J Cancer 128:33–39
22. Feinberg AP, Vogelstein B (1983) Hypomethylation distinguishes genes of some human cancers from their normal counterparts. Nature 301:89–92
23. Feinberg AP, Vogelstein B (1983) Hypomethylation of ras oncogenes in primary human cancers. Biochem Biophys Res Commun 111:47–54
24. Khan R, Zhang XY, Supakar PC, Ehrlich KC, Ehrlich M (1988) Human methylated DNA-binding protein. Determinants of a pBR322 recognition site. J Biol Chem 263:14374–14383
25. Leodolter A, Alonso S, González B, Ebert MP, Vieth M, Röcken C, Wex T, Peitz U, Malfertheiner P, Perucho M (2015) Somatic DNA hypomethylation in *H. pylori*-associated high-risk gastritis and gastric cancer: enhanced somatic hypomethylation associates with advanced stage cancer. Clin Transl Gastroenterol 6:e85
26. Ushijima T, Hattori N (2012) Molecular pathways: involvement of Helicobacter pylori-triggered inflammation in the formation of an epigenetic field defect, and its usefulness as

cancer risk and exposure markers. Clin Cancer Res 18:923–929

27. Liteplo RG, Kerbel RS (1987) Reduced levels of DNA 5-methylcytosine in metastatic variants of the human melanoma cell line MeWo. Cancer Res 47:2264–2267
28. Tisdale MJ (1980) Effect of methionine deprivation on methylation and synthesis of macromolecules. Br J Cancer 42:121–128
29. Bloomfield M, McCormack A, Mandrioli D, Fiala C, Aldaz CM, Duesberg P (2014) Karyotypic evolutions of cancer species in rats during the long latent periods after injection of nitrosourea. Mol Cytogenet 7:71
30. Borrego SL, Fahrmann J, Datta R, Stringari C, Grapov D, Zeller M, Chen Y, Wang P, Baldi P, Gratton E, Fiehn O, Kaiser P (2016) Metabolic changes associated with methionine stress sensitivity in MDA-MB-468 breast cancer cells. Cancer Metab 4:9
31. Grosu AL, Weber WA, Riedel E, Jeremic B, Nieder C, Franz M, Gumprecht H, Jaeger R, Schwaiger M, Molls M (2005) L-(methyl-11C) methionine positron emission tomography for target delineation in resected high-grade gliomas before radiotherapy. Int J Radiat Oncol Biol Phys 63:64–74
32. Glaudemans AW, Enting RH, Heesters MA, Dierckx RA, van Rheenen RW, Walenkamp AM, Slart RH (2013) Value of 11C-methionine PET in imaging brain tumours and metastases. Eur J Nucl Med Mol Imaging 40:615–635
33. Tsuyuguchi N, Takami T, Sunada I, Iwai Y, Yamanaka K, Tanaka K, Nishikawa M, Ohata K, Torii K, Morino M, Nishio A, Hara M (2004) Methionine positron emission tomography for differentiation of recurrent brain tumor and radiation necrosis after stereotactic radiosurgery--in malignant glioma. Ann Nucl Med 18:291–296
34. Nariai T, Tanaka Y, Wakimoto H, Aoyagi M, Tamaki M, Ishiwata K, Senda M, Ishii K, Hirakawa K, Ohno K (2005) Usefulness of L-[methyl-11C] methionine-positron emission tomography as a biological monitoring tool in the treatment of glioma. J Neurosurg 103:498–507
35. Tamura K, Yoshikawa K, Ishikawa H, Hasebe M, Tsuji H, Yanagi T, Suzuki K, Kubo A, Tsujii H (2009) Carbon-11-methionine PET imaging of choroidal melanoma and the time course after carbon ion beam radiotherapy. Anticancer Res 29:1507–1514
36. Singhal T, Narayanan TK, Jacobs MP, Bal C, Mantil JC (2012) 11C-methionine PET for grading and prognostication in gliomas: a comparison study with 18F-FDG PET and contrast enhancement on MRI. J Nucl Med 53:1709–1715
37. Warburg O (1956) On the origin of cancer cells. Science 123:309–314
38. Weinhouse S, Warburg O, Burk D, Schade AL (1956) On respiratory impairment in cancer cells. Science 124:267–272
39. Pavlova NN, Thompson CB (2016) The emerging hallmarks of cancer metabolism. Cell metabolism 23:27–47

Chapter 22

Recombinant Methioninase as a DNA Demethylation Agent

Robert M. Hoffman and David Machover

Abstract

This chapter reviews the effect of methionine (MET) restriction, via treatment with recombinant methioninase (rMETase), on DNA methylation of cancer cells. CCRF-CEM human cancer cells were treated with rMETase under subcytotoxic conditions. The rMETase-treated cells contained significantly lower levels of genomic methylated DNA than did untreated control cells. DNA methylation was measured by incorporation of the methyl group of [^{3}H]methyl-*S*-adenosylmethionine into DNA and by methylation-sensitive arbitrarily-primed PCR. DNA hypomethylation effected by rMETase was of similar extent to that effected by treatment of the cells with the DNA methyltransferase inhibitor 5-azacytidine.

Key words Recombinant methioninase, Cancer cells, DNA hypomethylation, Malignancy

1 Introduction

1.1 DNA Hypomethylation in Cancer

Global DNA hypomethylation is a general characteristic of human cancer, as originally discovered by our laboratory [1, 2]. DNA hypomethylation is an early event in the formation of cancer as it appears in premalignant tissue [3]. The progression of DNA hypomethylation may be driven by "oncogenes" [4].

Perucho et al. [5] observed that *H. pylori* appears to cause a field defect of DNA hypomethylation in a region of the gastric mucosa prior to cancer development that is not reversed by *H. pylori* eradication. Perucho et al. [5] also observed that enhanced DNA hypomethylation was associated with a more invasive and advanced-stage type of gastric cancer.

Consistent with the above observation, the more metastatic melanoma sublines were, the more extensively they were hypomethylated in their DNA [6]. Also, global DNA hypomethylation increases as cervical dysplasia progresses to cervical carcinoma [7]. Compared to benign tumors, atypical and malignant meningiomas were observed to have increased global DNA hypomethylation [8] (*see* **Notes 1** and **2**).

Robert M. Hoffman (ed.), *Methionine Dependence of Cancer and Aging: Methods and Protocols*, Methods in Molecular Biology, vol. 1866, https://doi.org/10.1007/978-1-4939-8796-2_22, © Springer Science+Business Media, LLC, part of Springer Nature 2019

1.2 DNA Hypomethylation Leads to Aneuploidy

Jaenish et al. generated mice with a mutant DNA methyltransferase 1 (DNMT1) allele which reduced DNMT1 expression to 10% of normal levels and resulted in genome-wide hypomethylation. The mutant mice developed T-cell lymphomas which had a high frequency of chromosome 15 trisomy. Also, DNMT-deficient HCT-116 colon cancer cells had a high degree of genome instability leading to aneuploidy, including many novel chromosomal translocations [9]. DNA hypomethylation therefore seems to cause chromosomal instability, aneuploidy, and subsequent cancer [10].

1.3 Relationship of the Elevated Methionine (MET) Requirements of Cancer Cells and DNA Hypomethylation

The elevated methionine (MET) use in cancer cells has been termed the "Hoffman effect" [11], analogous to the "Warburg effect" for enhanced glucose utilization in cancer [12]. Cancer cells are abnormally dependent on MET due to abnormally elevated transmethylation reactions that are poorly understood [13]. The consequent depletion of AdoMET by these transmethylation reactions [14] appears to result in hypomethylation of DNA in cancer cells, since the MET methyl group may be diverted to a methyl sink in the cancer cells, and thereby not sufficiently available for normal DNA methylation. Rare cells from MET-dependent cancer cell lines regained the normal ability to grow in MET-restricted medium. These cell lines were termed MET-independent revertants [15, 16]. MET-independent revertants also had much lower basal transmethylation rates than parental MET-dependent cell lines [17].

We then demonstrated that MET-independent revertants of cancer cells concomitantly reverted for characteristics associated with cancer. Thus, the MET-independent revertants become more normal-like [16]. These results indicate that aberrant elevated transmethylation is crucial in cancer (*see* **Notes 1–3**).

2 Materials [18]

1. CCRF-CEM or other cancer cells.
2. RPMI 1640 (Life Technologies, Inc., Gaithersburg, MD) supplemented with 10% fetal bovine serum (Life Technologies, Inc.) and antibiotics (50 μg/mL streptomycin and 50 units/mL penicillin) at 37 °C in an atmosphere containing 5% CO_2.
3. [^{3}H]methyl-*S*-adenosylmethionine (78 Ci/mmol; New England Nuclear Life Science Products, Inc., Boston, MA).
4. rMETase from *E. coli* expressing the *Pseudomonas putida* methioninase gene (AntiCancer Inc., San Diego, CA).
5. 5-Azacytidine (Sigma Chemical Co., St. Louis, MO).
6. Proteinase K (Roche Diagnostics, Meylan, France).

7. Recombinant *SssI* CpG methylase (New England Biolabs, Beverly, MA).
8. 50 mM NaCl, 10 mM MgCl, and 1 mM DTT.
9. Dithiothreitol (DTT).
10. Ion-exchange filter (Whatman DE81).
11. Ethanol.
12. Pico-Fluor 40 (Packard Instruments, Groningen, The Netherlands) scintillation mixture or equivalent.
13. Scintillation counter (LKB Wallac, Turku, Finland), or equivalent.

3 Methods [18]

1. Test the effect of recombinant methioninase (rMETase) as a single agent for cytotoxicity on cancer cells over a concentration range of 0.02–0.225 unit/mL.
2. Measure cell viability after exposure to rMETase for 3, 6, and 72 h with the 3-(4,5-dimethylthiazol-2-yl)-2,5-diphenyltetrazolium bromide (MTT) colorimetric assay, as described previously [19, 20].
3. Measure incorporation of the methyl group of [^{3}H]methyl-*S*-adenosylmethionine in DNA, which positively correlates with the extent of DNA hypomethylation, after treatment of cancer cells with rMETase at 0.2 unit/mL for 6 h and at 0.02 units/mL for 72 h in order to effect DNA hypomethylation.
4. Treat cancer cells for 48 h with 0.3 μM 5-azacytidine in order to effect DNA hypomethylation [21–24] and measure as described above.
5. Treat genomic DNA from 10^7 cancer cells with proteinase K and then extract as described previously [25].
6. Make a reaction mixture with 0.5 μg DNA, 1 μCi [^{3}H]methyl-*S*-adenosylmethionine (78 Ci/mmol), 3 units of recombinant *SssI* CpG methylase and buffer [10 mM Tris–HCL (pH 7.9), 50 mM NaCl, 10 mM MgCl, and 1 mM DTT.
7. After incubation at 30 °C for 1 h to enable DNA (5-cytosine) methylation, isolate DNA on an ion-exchange filter (Whatman DE81) wash in PBS, and then wash in ethanol.
8. Assay the dried filter for radioactivity with Pico-Fluor 40 scintillation mixture in a scintillation counter.
9. Express methylation in dpm/0.5 μg DNA. Do statistical analysis with the Wilcoxon's test.

4 Results

4.1 rMETase Decreases Genomic DNA Methylation Levels in CCRF-CEM Cells

Total genomic DNA methylation was measured by incorporation of the [^{3}H]methyl group from [^{3}H]methyl-*S*-adenosylmethionine (SAM) in DNA through the action of *Sss*I CpG methylase (Fig. 1). DNA methylation rates of the above reaction were increased over the untreated control by 1.54 and 1.45 by treatment of CCRF-CEM cells with rMETase at 0.2 units/mL for 6 h and 0.02 units/mL for 72 h, respectively. These results indicate that rMETase was causing DNA hypomethylation in CCRF-CEM cells [18].

4.2 5-Azacytidine Decreases Genome DNA Methylation Levels in CCRF-CEM Cells

DNA methylation rates were also increased by 5-azacytidine (5-AzaCr) (0.3 μM) for 48 h by 1.52 sold over control.

Statistically-significant differences in DNA methylation rates compared to the control were found both in rMETase-treated cells ($P = 0.005$) and in 5-azacytidine-treated cells ($P = 0.02$). The demethylating effect of rMETase was similar to that of 5-AzaCr ($P = 0.9$) [18] (*see* **Note 4**).

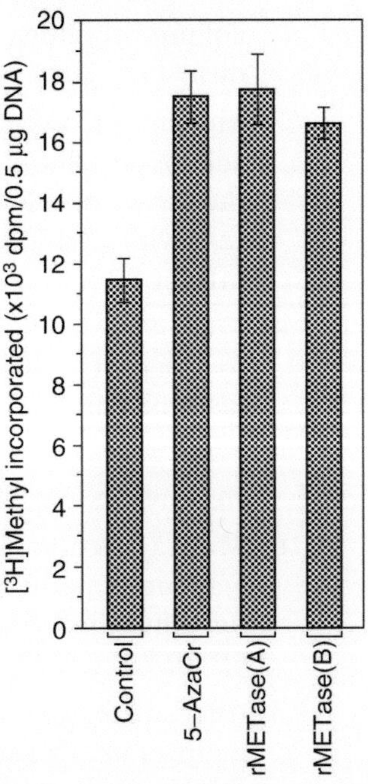

Fig. 1 Effect of rMETase on DNA methylation of CCRF-CEM cells. DNA methylation was measured by incorporation of the methyl radical from L-[*methyl*-^{3}H]SAM in genomic DNA. Histograms represent DNA methylation by *Sss*I CpG methylase in untreated control cells, in cells exposed to 0.3 μM 5-AzaCr for 48 h, and in cells exposed to rMETase at 0.2 unit/mL for 6 h [*rMETase(A)*] and 0.02 unit/mL for 72 h [*rMETase(B)*]. *Columns* represent the mean of two to six determinations, each done in duplicate. *Bars,* SE [18]

5 Notes

1. We previously suggested that the premalignant DNA hypomethylation, such as that observed by Perucho et al. [5], results from the unbalanced excess transmethylation which diverts methyl groups where they are not available for normal methylation processes such as DNA methylation [27]. The excess transmethylation rate explains the "MET dependence" of cancer cells. Hypomethylated DNA then results in the initiation of aneuploidy and subsequent speciation to autonomous cancer [25, 28].
2. We proposed that carcinogenesis is initiated by perturbation of MET metabolism and transmethylation ("metabolic reprogramming") resulting in DNA hypomethylation, thereby destabilizing the karyotype, which sets off a chain reaction of aneuploidizations as Duesberg [26] proposes, which generates evermore abnormal karyotypes and eventually cancer-specific combinations [27, 28].
3. Every hypothesis should be testable and be able to be negated. The present hypothesis for example predicts that sublethal reduction of DNA methylation, as observed with rMETase, may make cancer cells more malignant [18].
4. The methyl(5-cytosine) levels of DNA are determined by the radioactivity incorporated in DNA [^{3}H]methyl from [^{3}H] methyl-*S*-adenosylmethionine, the methyl donor for CpG methylase. DNA-bound radioactivity increases with increasing levels of unmethylated DNA [18].

References

1. Diala ES, Hoffman RM (1982) Hypomethylation of HeLa cell DNA and the absence of 5-methylcytosine in SV40 and adenovirus (type 2) DNA: analysis by HPLC. Biochem Biophys Res Commun 107:19–26
2. Diala ES, Cheah MSC, Rowitch D, Hoffman RM (1983) Extent of DNA methylation in human tumor cells. J Natl Cancer Inst 71:755–764
3. Goelz SE, Vogelstein B, Hamilton SR, Feinberg AP (1985) Hypomethylation of DNA from benign and malignant human colon neoplasms. Science 228:187–190
4. Mudbhary R, Hoshida Y, Chernyavskaya Y, Jacob V, Villanueva A, Fiel MI, Chen X, Kojima K, Thung S, Bronson RT, Lachenmayer A, Revill K, Alsinet C, Sachidanandam R, Desai A, Senbanerjee S, Ukomadu C, Llovet JM, Sadler KC (2014) UHRF1 overexpression drives DNA hypomethylation and hepatocellular carcinoma. Cancer Cell 25:196–209
5. Leodolter A, Alonso S, González B, Ebert MP, Vieth M, Röcken C, Wex T, Peitz U, Malfertheiner P, Perucho M (2015) Somatic DNA hypomethylation in H. pylori-associated high-risk gastritis and gastric cancer: enhanced somatic hypomethylation associates with advanced stage cancer. Clin Transl Gastroenterol 6:e85
6. Liteplo RG, Kerbel RS (1987) Reduced levels of DNA 5-methylcytosine in metastatic variants of the human melanoma cell line MeWo. Cancer Res 47:2264–2267
7. Kim YI, Giuliano A, Hatch KD, Schneider A, Nour MA, Dallal GE, Selhub J, Mason JB (1994) Global DNA hypomethylation

increases progressively in cervical dysplasia and carcinoma. Cancer 74:893–899
8. Gao F, Shi L, Russin J, Zeng L, Chang X, He S, Chen TC, Giannotta SL, Weisenberger DJ, Zada G, Mack WJ, Wang K (2013) DNA methylation in the malignant transformation of meningiomas. PLoS One 8:e54114
9. Karpf AR, Matsui S (2005) Genetic disruption of cytosine DNA methyltransferase enzymes induces chromosomal instability in human cancer cells. Cancer Res 65:8635–8639
10. Gaudet F, Hodgson JG, Eden A, Jackson-Grusby L, Dausman J, Gray JW, Leonhardt H, Jaenisch R (2003) Induction of tumors in mice by genomic hypomethylation. Science 300:489–492
11. Murakami T, Li S, Han Q, Tan Y, Kiyuna T, Igarashi K, Kawaguchi K, Hwang HK, Miyaki K, Singh AS, Nelson SD, Dry SM, Li Y, Hiroshima Y, Lwin TM, DeLong JC, Chishima T, Tanaka K, Bouvet M, Endo I, Eilber FC, Hoffman RM (2017) Recombinant methioninase effectively targets a Ewing's sarcoma in a patient-derived orthotopic xenograft (PDOX) nude mouse model. Oncotarget 8:35630–35638
12. Warburg O (1956) On the origin of cancer cells. Science 123:309–314
13. Stern PH, Hoffman RM (1984) Elevated overall rates of transmethylation in cell lines from diverse human tumors. In Vitro 20:663–670
14. Coalson DW, Mecham JO, Stern PH, Hoffman RM (1982) Reduced availability of endogenously synthesized methionine for S-adenosylmethionine formation in methionine dependent cancer cells. Proc Natl Acad Sci U S A 79:4248–4251
15. Hoffman RM, Jacobsen SJ, Erbe RW (1978) Reversion to methionine independence by malignant rat and SV40-transformed human fibroblasts. Biochem Biophys Res Commun 82:228–234
16. Hoffman RM, Jacobsen SJ, Erbe RW (1979) Reversion to methionine independence in simian virus 40-transformed human and malignant rat fibroblasts is associated with altered ploidy and altered properties of transformation. Proc Natl Acad Sci U S A 76:1313–1317
17. Judde JG, Ellis M, Frost P (1989) Biochemical analysis of the role of transmethylation in the methionine dependence of tumor cells. Cancer Res 49:4859–4865
18. Machover D, Zittoun J, Saffroy R, Broët P, Giraudier S, Magnaldo T, Goldschmidt E, Debuire B, Orrico M, Tan Y, Mishal Z, Chevallier O, Tonetti C, Jouault H, Ulusakarya A, Tanguy ML, Metzger G, Hoffman RM (2002) Treatment of cancer cells with methioninase produces DNA hypomethylation and increases DNA synthesis. Cancer Res 62:4685–4689
19. Machover D, Zittoun J, Broe¨t P, Metzger G, Orrico M, Goldschmidt E, Schilf A, Tonetti C, Tan Y, Delmas-Marsalet B, Luccioni C, Falissard B, Hoffman RM (2001) Cytotoxic synergism of methioninase in combination with 5-fluorouracil and folinic acid. Biochem Pharmacol 61:867–876
20. Carmichael J, Degraff WG, Gazdar AF, Minna JD, Mitchell JB (1987) Evaluation of a tetrazolium-based semiautomated colorimetric assay: assessment of chemosensitivity testing. Cancer Res 47:936–942
21. Robertson KD, Jones PA (2000) DNA methylation: past, present and future directions. Carcinogenesis 21:461–467
22. Widschwendter M, Jones PA (2002) The potential prognostic, predictive, and therapeutic values of DNA methylation in cancer. Clin Cancer Res 8:17–21
23. Jutterman R, Li E, Jaenisch R (1994) Toxicity of 5-aza-2-deoxycytidine to mammalian cells is mediated primarily by covalent trapping of DNA methyltransferase rather than DNA demethylation. Proc Natl Acad Sci U S A 91:11797–11801
24. Karpf AR, Moore BC, Ririe TO, Jones DA (2001) Activation of the p53 DNA damage response pathway after inhibition of DNA methyltransferase by 5-aza-2-deoxycytidine. Mol Pharmacol 59:751–757
25. Sambrook J, Russell DW (2000) Isolation of high-molecular-weight DNA from mammalian cells using proteinase K and phenol. In: Molecular cloning: a laboratory manual, vol 1, 3rd edn. Cold Spring Harbor Laboratory Press, Cold Spring Harbor, NY, pp 6.4–6.12
26. Duesberg P, Li R (2003) Multistep carcinogenesis: a chain reaction of aneuploidizations. Cell Cycle 2:202–210
27. Hoffman RM (2017) The wayward methyl group and the cascade to cancer. Cell Cycle 16:825–829
28. Hoffman RM (2017) Is DNA methylation the new guardian of the genome? Molecular Cytogenetics 10:11

Chapter 23

Homocysteine, Thioretinaco Ozonide, and Oxidative Phosphorylation in Cancer and Aging: A Proposed Clinical Trial Protocol

Kilmer S. McCully

Abstract

The objective of the proposed clinical interventional trial is to demonstrate the efficacy of a novel therapeutic strategy in subjects with cancer and hyperhomocysteinemia. Following discovery of abnormal homocysteine thiolactone metabolism in cultured malignant cells, thioretinamide, the amide synthesized from retinoic acid and homocysteine thiolactone, and thioretinaco, the complex formed from cobalamin and thioretinamide, were demonstrated to have antineoplastic, anticarcinogenic, and anti-atherogenic properties in animal models. Retinol, ascorbate, and homocysteine thiolactone are necessary for biosynthesis of thioretinamide and thioretinaco by cystathionine synthase and for formation of thioretinaco ozonide from thioretinamide, cobalamin, and ozone. Thioretinaco ozonide is required for prevention of abnormal oxidative metabolism, aerobic glycolysis, suppressed immunity, and hyperhomocysteinemia in cancer.

The pancreatic enzyme therapy of cancer promotes catabolism of proteins, nucleic acids, and glycosaminoglycans with excess homocysteinylated amino groups resulting from abnormal accumulation of homocysteine thiolactone in malignant cells. Dietary deficiencies of pyridoxal, folate, cobalamin, and nitriloside contribute to hyperhomocysteinemia in cancer, and in protein energy malnutrition. A deficiency of dietary sulfur amino acids downregulates cystathionine synthase, causing hyperhomocysteinemia.

The organic sulfur compound diallyl trisulfide increases hydrogen sulfide production from homocysteine in animal models, inhibits Stat3 signaling in cancer stem cells, and produces apoptosis of malignant cells. The furanonaphthoquinone compound napabucasin inhibits Stat3 signaling and causes mitochondrial dysfunction, decreased oxidative phosphorylation, and apoptosis of malignant cells. The protocol of the proposed clinical trial in subjects with myelodysplasia consists of thioretinamide and cobalamin as precursors of thioretinaco ozonide, combined with pancreatic enzyme extracts, diallyl trisulfide, napabucasin, nutritional modification to minimize processed foods, vitamin supplements, essential amino acids, and beneficial dietary fats and proteins.

Key words Adenosyl methionine, Apoptosis, Cystathionine synthase, Diallyl trisulfide, Homocysteine thiolactone, Hyperhomocysteinemia, Myelodysplasia, Napabucasin, Oxidative phosphorylation, Pancreatic enzymes, Thioretinamide, Thioretinaco ozonide, Clinical trial

Robert M. Hoffman (ed.), *Methionine Dependence of Cancer and Aging: Methods and Protocols*, Methods in Molecular Biology, vol. 1866, https://doi.org/10.1007/978-1-4939-8796-2_23, © Springer Science+Business Media, LLC, part of Springer Nature 2019

1 Introduction

Since publication of the monograph on the chemical pathology of homocysteine [1–5], new discoveries and interpretations concerning the structure and function of cystathionine synthase have increased our understanding of this problem in such diverse fields as protein energy malnutrition, pancreatic enzyme function in therapy of malignant disease, aerobic glycolysis by malignant cells, function of ascorbate in oxidation of the sulfur atom of homocysteine, and metabolic blockade of sulfur oxidation in malignant cells [6]. In degenerative diseases of aging, including cancer, atherosclerosis, and neurodegenerative and autoimmune diseases, abnormal homocysteine metabolism is demonstrated by observation of elevated levels of homocysteine that is bound to plasma proteins by disulfide bonds [7].

Abnormal homocysteine metabolism was first implicated in the etiology of degenerative diseases by observation of accelerated arteriosclerosis in children with hyperhomocysteinemia caused by two different enzymatic disorders resulting from inherited deficiency of cystathionine synthase or methionine synthase [8]. Accelerated arteriosclerosis was subsequently demonstrated in a child with deficiency of methylene tetrahydrofolate reductase, a third inherited enzymatic disorder causing hyperhomocysteinemia [9]. In all three of these enzymatic disorders, elevation of blood levels of homocysteine is implicated in the pathogenesis of arteriosclerosis by a direct effect of homocysteine on the metabolic activity of arterial cells and tissues.

Abnormal homocysteine thiolactone metabolism was demonstrated in cultures of cells from malignant tissues [10]. The results of this study show that cultured malignant cells contain a metabolic blockade of the oxidation of the sulfur atom of homocysteine thiolactone to sulfate, leading to accumulation of homocysteine thiolactone within malignant cells. Homocysteine thiolactone reacts with the free amino groups of macromolecules, forming peptide bonds that cause homocysteinylation of the amino groups of proteins, nucleic acids, and glycosaminoglycans. This metabolic blockade within malignant cells is ascribed to deficiency of a derivative of homocysteine thiolactone that normally occurs within nonmalignant cells.

The formation of homocysteine thiolactone from methionine in malignant cells is catalyzed by methionyl t-RNA synthase by an error editing reaction [11]. Abnormal homocysteine thiolactone metabolism in malignant cells is hypothesized to result from a deficiency of or a failure to synthesize an *N*-substituted derivative of homocysteine thiolactone [10]. According to this hypothesis, normal cells contain a derivative of homocysteine thiolactone that facilitates sulfate formation from homocysteine thiolactone. The concentration of this hypothetical derivative is believed to be diminished during the carcinogenic transformation of normal to malignant cells through the action of carcinogenic chemicals, radiation, microbes, or chronic inflammation. The function of this hypothetical derivative in normal cells is to prevent accumulation of homocysteine thiolactone by catalyzing its conversion to phosphoadenosine phosphosulfate; sulfate esters of glycosaminoglycans, steroids, and other compounds; and sulfate ions. Decreased concentration of this hypothetical derivative in malignant cells leads to the characteristic metabolic abnormalities of malignancy, which are attributable to excessive accumulation of homocysteine thiolactone. According to this concept, the increased growth rate, aggregation of nucleoproteins, altered expression of developmentally suppressed genes, degradation of cellular membranes, and abnormalities of oxidative metabolism, such as aerobic glycolysis, are attributable to increased intracellular accumulation of homocysteine thiolactone within malignant cells. Treatment of animals with transplanted malignant neoplasms with homocysteine thiolactone perchlorate causes necrosis within malignant neoplasms, because of increased accumulation of homocysteine thiolactone within malignant tissues [12].

1.1 Discovery of Thioretinamide, Thioretinaco, and Thioretinaco Ozonide

The identity of the hypothetical derivative of homocysteine thiolactone that prevents growth of malignant tumors in animals was elucidated by organic synthesis of antineoplastic compounds containing homocysteine thiolactone. Arachidonoyl homocysteine thiolactone amide and pyridoxal homocysteine thiolactone enamine decrease the growth of transplanted murine mammary adenocarcinoma [13]. *N*-maleyl homocysteine thiolactone amide, *N*-maleimide homocysteine thiolactone amide, and rhodium trichloride oxalyl homocysteine thiolactone amide suppress the growth of transplanted neoplasms in animals [14, 15]. Encapsulation of *N*-maleimide homocysteine thiolactone amide within liposomes greatly enhances its antineoplastic activity [16]. Structural analysis of these biologically active derivatives of homocysteine thiolactone shows that the hypothetical chemopreventive derivative of homocysteine thiolactone in normal cells is active in a lipid-soluble form, contains a conjugated double-bond system with a carbonyl group adjacent to the nitrogen atom of homocysteine thiolactone, and forms a complex with a transition metal atom that enhances antineoplastic activity.

Homocysteine thiolactone reacts by organic synthesis with retinoic acid to form *N*-homocysteine thiolactonyl retinamide (NHTR), known as thioretinamide [17]. Thioretinamide reacts with cobalamin to form the complex, *N*-homocysteine thiolactonyl retinamido cobalamin ($(NHTR)_2Co$), known as thioretinaco [18]. Both thioretinamide and thioretinaco have anticarcinogenic and antineoplastic activities in mice treated with a carcinogen and in mice with transplanted neoplasms. The method of synthesis of thioretinamide was significantly improved by use of *N*-ethyl-*N′*-(3-dimethylaminopropyl) carbodiimide in the reaction mixture [19]. This method replaces the conjugation agent, dicyclohexylcarbodiimide, in the reaction mixture of the original method and produces pure thioretinamide in 72% of theoretical yield. This pure thioretinamide and its complex with cobalamin, thioretinaco, have anti-atherogenic activity in rats treated with parenteral homocysteine thiolactone [19]. The anticarcinogenic, antineoplastic, antiviral, and antiaging activities of thioretinaco ozonide are enhanced by use of membranergic compositions, specifically the polypeptide cytokines, alpha-interferon, beta-interferon, and gamma-interferon [20]. A therapeutically active composition of thioretinaco ozonide for providing anticarcinogenic, antineoplastic, antiviral, anti-atherogenic, and antiaging benefits is formed by thioretinaco ozonide, complexed with adenosine triphosphate and oxygen within an ozone-resistant liposomal carrier [21].

1.2 Ascorbate, Homocysteine Thiolactone Oxidation, and Growth Hormone

Studies of homocysteine thiolactone metabolism in the liver of scorbutic guinea pigs that are deprived of dietary ascorbate disclosed a failure of oxidation of homocysteine thiolactone to homocysteine and sulfate, as well as a pathway for synthesis of phosphoadenosine phosphosulfate from the sulfur atom of homocysteine thiolactone [22]. Homocysteic acid, the oxidized sulfonic acid derivative of homocysteine, promotes growth in normal animals and promotes growth and release of insulin-like growth factor, IGF-1, in hypophysectomized animals that are treated with thyroxine [23]. Young animals and hypophysectomized animals convert more homocysteine thiolactone to homocysteic acid and other oxidized homocysteine derivatives than older or normal animals [24].

Cultured cells that are deficient in cystathionine synthase and unable to convert homocysteine to cystathionine are able to oxidize the sulfur atom of homocysteine thiolactone to sulfate, demonstrating a pathway for sulfate synthesis that is independent of conversion of homocysteine to cystathionine, cysteine, and sulfate [25]. The pathway for synthesis of sulfate from homocysteine thiolactone involves synthesis of thioretinamide from homocysteine thiolactone and retinoic acid and subsequent oxidation of thioretinamide to sulfite, alpha-keto-butyrate, and retinoic acid by superoxide [2].

In the 1930s ascorbic acid was found to influence the growth of cancer in animals, mainly acting to extend their life span [26]. Moreover, the amount of ascorbic acid in the tissues of animals with cancer is decreased, further suggesting the possibility of a therapeutic action in human patients with cancer. Otto Warburg discovered the role of cytochrome enzymes in cellular respiration [27]. Later he demonstrated that cancer cells and embryonic cells have a characteristic mode of cellular respiration known as aerobic glycolysis in which glucose is converted to lactic acid instead of conversion to carbon dioxide, the mode of cellular respiration of normal cells [28]. Ascorbic acid inhibits cellular respiration and glycolysis of cancer cells [29]. Controversial studies showed that massive doses of ascorbic acid cause regression of some advanced human cancers and extended the life span of patients with terminal malignancy, compared with historical controls [30]. Later in the 1980s controlled studies showed that massive doses of ascorbic acid have minor beneficial effects on side effects of chemotherapy and radiation therapy and produce a slight increase in survival times of human cancer patients [31].

1.3 Biosynthesis of Thioretinamide and Thioretinaco by Cystathionine Synthase

Nutritional studies demonstrated that the hyperhomocysteinemia of protein energy malnutrition is associated with reduction in levels of plasma transthyretin, the plasma protein that transports retinol-binding protein and thyroxine [32]. The metabolic disorder caused by protein energy malnutrition consists of decreased synthesis and downregulation of the activity of cystathionine synthase, leading to hyperhomocysteinemia and decreased synthesis of cystathionine and cysteine [33]. Transthyretin contains abundant tryptophan, and the plasma level of transthyretin declines in protein energy malnutrition because of dietary deficiency of tryptophan and other essential amino acids, leading to decreased endogenous synthesis of transthyretin. Plasma transthyretin is a sensitive indicator of protein energy malnutrition [34]. Decreased plasma transthyretin in protein energy malnutrition is accompanied by elevation of plasma homocysteine [35].

The heme-oxygenase function of cystathionine synthase catalyzes the generation of superoxide radical from dioxygen [36]. Retinoic acid enhances the stimulation by thyroid hormone of heme oxygenase activity in the liver of thyroidectomized rats, demonstrating interaction between retinoic acid and the heme group of heme oxygenase [37]. *N*-(4-hydroxyphenyl)-retinamide, known as fenretinide, induces apoptosis in retinal cells through increased generation of reactive oxygen species and through increased expression of heme oxygenase [38]. Investigation of the properties of fenretinide demonstrates anti-neoplastic potential, based on animal and clinical studies, because of the ability of this synthetic retinamide to induce apoptosis in malignant cells [39].

Taken together, these observations [31–38] indicate that retinol is delivered to cells by the retinol-binding protein component of transthyretin, and the heme oxygenase function of cystathionine synthase is responsible for the oxidation of retinol to retinoic acid and the simultaneous reaction of retinoic acid with homocysteine thiolactone to produce thioretinamide [5]. This process is catalyzed by binding of dehydroascorbate to the heme group of cystathionine synthase and production of superoxide radical from dioxygen. In catalyzing this reaction of retinol with superoxide radical, dehydroascorbate is simultaneously reduced to semidehydroascorbate, and thioretinamide is formed by the reaction of homocysteine thiolactone with enzyme-bound retinoic acid. Thioretinamide is subsequently further metabolized to alpha-ketobutyrate, hydrogen sulfide, and retinoic acid, and this pathway is facilitated by oxidation of hydrogen sulfide to sulfite and sulfate by superoxide [2].

This formulation of the synthesis of thioretinamide from retinol and homocysteine thiolactone by the heme-oxygenase function of cystathionine synthase explains the failure of sulfate synthesis from homocysteine thiolactone in experimental scurvy and the function of dehydroascorbate in sulfate synthesis [22]. Thioretinamide is a precursor of thioretinaco by reaction with cobalamin [18]. Presumably the biosynthesis of thioretinaco is facilitated by interaction of the corrin group of cobalamin with the heme group of cystathionine synthase. Thioretinaco ozonide catalyzes the process of oxygen utilization in oxidative phosphorylation by forming a complex with adenosine triphosphate (ATP) [2]. The synthesis of thioretinaco from thioretinamide is facilitated by thyroxine that is transported by plasma transthyretin, explaining how oxidative metabolism is stimulated by thyroxine [37]. Only higher eukaryotes contain cystathionine synthase with a heme functional group, and the cystathionine synthase of yeast and flagellates contains no heme functional group [40]. Since embryonic and malignant cells are deficient in the activity of cystathionine synthase [41], these observations explain why malignant cells are deficient in oxidation of homocysteine thiolactone to sulfate by the heme oxygenase function of cystathionine synthase.

Retinoids, including all-trans-retinoic acid, have been evaluated for prevention of carcinogenesis in bronchial and oral tissues [42]. Retinoic acid causes remissions in cases of acute promyelocytic leukemia [43, 44]. Synthetic retinoids, such as fenretinide, are antiproliferative and induce apoptosis in breast cancer cells [38, 45]. Fenretinide is bound to retinol-binding protein, a component of transthyretin, and is eliminated from plasma by loss of retinol-binding protein through glomerular filtration [46]. It is likely that thioretinamide can also be bound to retinol-binding protein for transport to tissues by plasma transthyretin, but no evidence has been reported to support this suggestion.

In a recent study [47], the active site of oxidative phosphorylation and ATP synthesis in mitochondria is proposed to consist of two molecules of thioretinamide bound to cobalamin, forming thioretinaco, complexed with ozone, oxygen, nicotinamide adenine dinucleotide, and inorganic phosphate, $TR_2CoO_3O_2NAD^+H_2PO_4^-$. Reduction of the pyridinium nitrogen of the nicotinamide group by an electron from electron transport complexes initiates polymerization of phosphate with adenosine diphosphate, yielding nicotinamide riboside and ATP bound to thioretinaco ozonide oxygen. A second electron reduces oxygen to hydroperoxyl radical, releasing

ATP from the active site. A proton gradient is created within F1F0 ATPase complexes of mitochondria by reaction of protons with reduced nicotinamide riboside and with hydroperoxide radical, yielding reduced nicotinamide riboside and hydroperoxide and creating the mitochondrial membrane potential. The hyperhomocysteinemia of aging and dementia is attributed to decreased biosynthesis of adenosyl methionine by thioretinaco ozonide and ATP, causing decreased allosteric activation of cystathionine synthase and decreased allosteric activation of methylenetetrahydrofolate reductase, resulting in dysregulation of methionine metabolism.

1.4 The Trophoblastic Origin of Malignant Cells

The embryologist John Beard discovered that trophoblastic cells of the embryo, which invade the uterine endometrium and myometrium during implantation of the fertilized embryo, are related to the asexual cycle of cellular organisms and are converted to placental cytotrophoblastic and syncytiotrophoblastic cells by the action of enzymes produced by the pancreas of the developing fetus [48]. Based on the concept that trophoblastic cells, which are distributed within developing tissues of the fetus, are similar in their cellular behavior to malignant cells, Beard introduced the pancreatic enzyme treatment of cancer in 1902. This treatment consists of injecting enzymes and proenzymes extracted from porcine pancreas into patients with various forms of primary or metastatic cancer. The trophoblastic theory of the origin of cancer is based on the assumption that malignant stem cells originate from the trophoblastic cells which migrate from the yolk sac of the developing embryo into somatic tissues, as described by Beard.

Human fetal and malignant cells produce small quantities of chorionic gonadotrophin [49]. This hormone is produced in large quantities by the highly-malignant tumor of placenta, choriocarcinoma. These observations provide evidence for the trophoblastic origin of malignant cells. Although the origin of adult stem cells in normal human tissues is incompletely understood, the sensitivity of trophoblastic cells to oncolysis by pancreatic enzymes and proenzymes forms the theoretical basis for this therapeutic approach [50, 51]. This sensitivity is related to the accumulation of homocysteinylated enzymes, plasma proteins, and cellular proteins, ribonucleic acid, deoxyribonucleic acid, and glycosaminoglycans that occurs by reaction of excess homocysteine thiolactone, which accumulates during aging, atherogenesis, carcinogenesis, and autoimmune diseases, with the free amino groups of these macromolecules [2, 52]. Pancreatic extracts contain active trypsin, chymotrypsin, elastase, amylase, lipase, ribonuclease, and deoxyribonuclease, as well as proenzyme precursors of these digestive enzymes. These enzymes are capable of hydrolyzing the homocysteinylated proteins, nucleic acids, and glycosaminoglycans that accumulate in malignant tissues and in the tissues of aging persons.

The enzyme cystathionase (cystathionine γ-lyase) is absent from the liver of human fetus and premature infants, and the activities of the enzymes, cystathionine synthase and adenosyl methionine synthase, are at a level of about 15–25% of adult human liver [53]. This discovery shows that the transsulfuration pathway for conversion of homocysteine to cystathionine, cysteine, and sulfate is inactive in fetal tissues. Therefore, the pathway for synthesis of sulfate from homocysteine thiolactone, involving synthesis of thioretinamide from retinol and homocysteine thiolactone and subsequent oxidation of thioretinamide to sulfite and sulfate by superoxide, is the source of sulfate groups of glycosaminoglycans utilized in the growth of fetal cells and tissues. The fetal cystathionine synthase assayed in human tissues contains the heme-oxygenase function of the enzyme, since sulfate groups of glycosaminoglycans and other molecules are synthesized from the sulfur atom of methionine and homocysteine in embryonic tissues. A recent study proposes participation of thioretinaco ozonide and the active site of oxidative phosphorylation in the biosynthesis of phosphoadenosine phosphosulfate, the coenzymatic precursor of sulfate esters, from NAD^+ and hydrosulfate [54].

1.5 Glycolysis, Nitrilosides, and Hydrogen Sulfide in Malignant Cells

In the early twentieth century Warburg discovered that embryonic tissues and malignant cells are unable to utilize oxygen for cellular metabolism but instead metabolize glucose to lactate as a source of cellular energy [28]. In other studies, Warburg showed that carcinogenic chemicals decrease normal cellular respiration by irreversible inhibition of oxygenases and by irreversible inhibition of transport of electrons by cytochrome enzyme systems. These findings are supported by the demonstration of deficient succinic dehydrogenase and cytochrome-oxidase activities within malignant tissues [55].

Taken together these early observations [28, 55] can be interpreted as examples of the clonal selection of malignant cells from trophoblastic stem cells that are deficient in the heme oxygenase activity of cystathionine synthase. The resulting failure of oxidation of retinol to retinoic acid and failure of reaction of retinoic acid with homocysteine thiolactone to produce thioretinamide by these malignant cells will lead to deficient formation of thioretinaco and failure of oxidative phosphorylation, catalyzed by thioretinaco ozonide [2]. The failure of oxidative phosphorylation by malignant cell clones that are deficient in the heme-oxygenase function of cystathionine synthase, resulting from decreased production of thioretinaco ozonide from cobalamin and thioretinamide, will lead to an embryonic form of metabolism in which ATP synthesis is dependent upon production of lactate from glucose, otherwise known as aerobic glycolysis.

Nitrilosides are substances containing nitrile groups produced by plants. The most important plant nitriloside is amygdalin (mandelonitrile β-diglucoside), other nitrilosides are dhurrin (hydroxymandelonitrile β-glucoside), lotaustralin (methylethylketone-cyanohydrin β-glucoside), and linamarin (acetone-cyanohydrin β-glucoside) [56]. Malignant cells contain glucosidase, the enzyme that metabolizes amygdalin and other nitrilosides to cyanide. Normal cells contain rhodanese, a sulfotransferase enzyme that catalyzes thiocyanate synthesis from cyanide and hydrogen sulfide. Malignant cells contain insufficient rhodanese to prevent accumulation of cyanide. Therefore, the prevention and control of growth of malignant cells and tissues by dietary nitrilosides are attributable to the consequent accumulation of cyanide within malignant cells. The reaction of cyanide with the cobalt atom of thioretinaco inactivates thioretinaco ozonide, thereby preventing oxidative phosphorylation [4]. Indeed hydrogen cyanide causes regression of transplanted sarcoma in rats [56]. This system of chemical surveillance against the growth of trophoblastic malignant cell clones is promoted by dietary or supplemental consumption of amygdalin and other plant nitrilosides.

Hydrogen sulfide is generated from homocysteine by cystathionine synthase and cystathionase, and low levels of hydrogen sulfide decrease oxidative stress and ameliorate pathological conditions such as ischemia-reperfusion injury, hypertension, and renal failure [57]. Hydrogen sulfide is a key gasotransmitter in sensing oxygen availability in tissues [58]. The reducing properties of hydrogen sulfide are responsible for scavenging the reactive oxygen species production induced by increased blood levels of homocysteine, inhibiting myocardial injury [59]. Increased production of hydrogen sulfide from homocysteine, metabolized from homocysteinylated proteins, nucleic acids, and glycosaminoglycans of apoptotic cells by pancreatic enzymes, will promote catabolism of homocysteine and conversion of the sulfur atom of homocysteine to thiocyanate by reaction of hydrogen sulfide with the cyanide generated from dietary nitrilosides.

1.6 Hydrogen Sulfide, Diallyl Trisulfide, and Apoptosis of Malignant Cells

The enzymes cystathionine synthase, cystathionase (cystathionine γ-lyase), and 3-mercaptopyruvate sulfotransferase produce hydrogen sulfide from cysteine [60]. In an experimental mouse model hydrogen sulfide attenuates neurodegeneration and neurovascular dysfunction induced by intracerebral administration of homocysteine. Hydrogen sulfide was found to attenuate myocardial ischemia-reperfusion injury by preservation of oxygen consumption by mitochondria [61]. The beneficial vascular effects of the allyl-sulfide constituents of garlic, diallyl trisulfide, and diallyl disulfide are mediated by hydrogen sulfide [62].

The allyl sulfides, diallyl trisulfide and diallyl disulfide, are responsible for the homocysteine-lowering effects of aged garlic extract observed in folate-deficient rats, by increasing adenosyl methionine in liver, which impairs the remethylation of homocysteine to methionine and enhances conversion of homocysteine to cystathionine by cystathionine synthase [63]. In an animal model diallyl trisulfide protects against ethanol-induced oxidative stress and apoptosis by stimulating cystathionine synthase and cystathionase activities, thereby increasing production of hydrogen sulfide by cystathionine γ-lyase [64]. In diabetic rats diallyl trisulfide protects against the oxidative stress and apoptosis induced by hyperglycemia by stimulating production of hydrogen sulfide derived from cystathionine gamma-lyase [65, 66]. These studies support the function of hydrogen sulfide in mediating the beneficial effects of diallyl trisulfide, diallyl disulfide, and other allyl sulfides on platelet aggregation, hypertension, elevated homocysteine, elevated cholesterol, oxidative stress, and apoptosis occurring in cardiovascular disease. Diallyl trisulfide is the most potent diallyl sulfide compound in providing beneficial effects, compared with diallyl disulfide and diallyl sulfide, which are less potent. The unsaturated allyl groups of these polysulfide compounds facilitate their entry through plasma membranes into cells, since the corresponding saturated propyl derivatives have no beneficial cardiovascular effects.

The allyl sulfides diallyl trisulfide and diallyl disulfide have not only beneficial cardioprotective effects, but also potent antineoplastic and anticarcinogenic effects as documented by many studies on these compounds. Treatment of cultured human glioblastoma cells with allyl sulfides causes production of reactive oxygen species and induction of apoptosis by activation of the JNK-1 pathway [67]. In this study increases in intracellular free calcium [Ca^{2+}], expression of calreticulin, and activation of caspase-4 indicate involvement of endoplasmic reticulum stress and decreased mitochondrial membrane potential in induction of apoptosis, resulting in reduced cell viability. The potential efficacy of diallyl trisulfide in treatment of human glioblastoma is attributed to the ability of this compound to penetrate the blood–brain barrier, increasing its concentration within glioblastoma cells.

Diallyl trisulfide induces apoptosis in cultured human breast cancer cells through activation of c-jun N-terminal kinase (JNK) and activator protein-1 (AP-1) [68]. Diallyl trisulfide causes apoptosis and reduced cell viability in cultured human breast cancer cells and transgenic mouse breast cancer cells, whereas cultured normal breast-ductal cells were resistant to growth inhibition and induction of apoptosis by diallyl trisulfide [69]. Human breast cancer cells in culture which are exposed to diallyl trisulfide exhibit suppression of matrix metalloproteinase 2/9 (MMP-2/9) by blocking the nuclear factor kappa B (NFκB) and ERK/MAPK signaling pathways, potentially inhibiting migration and invasion of metastatic breast cancer [70]. Another study demonstrates targeting and growth inhibition of breast cancer stem cells by diallyl trisulfide through inhibition of forkhead box Q1 (FoxQ1) [71].

In studies of human skin cancer diallyl trisulfide was demonstrated to inhibit growth of human melanoma cells and basal-cell carcinoma cells in culture by increasing the levels of intracellular reactive oxygen species, leading to DNA damage, and by inducing G_2/M mitotic arrest, endoplasmic-reticulum stress, and mitochondria-mediated apoptosis, including the caspase-dependent and caspase-independent pathways [72].

In a study of cultured human pancreatic cancer cells, diallyl trisulfide was demonstrated to produce apoptosis and suppression of growth, but non-tumorigenic pancreatic ductal epithelial cells were significantly more resistant to suppression of growth and induction of apoptosis by diallyl trisulfide, compared with pancreatic cancer cells [73]. Pancreatic cancer evolves from dysplastic epithelial precursor cells, termed pancreatic intraepithelial neoplasia (PanIN). Different degrees of dysplasia are classified as PanIN-1, PanIN-2, and PanIN-3, regarding progression of the dysplastic changes to malignant and invasive pancreatic adenocarcinoma cells. Diallyl sulfides, including diallyl trisulfide, are potentially effective in preventing progression of PanIN cells to the malignant phenotype, delaying the onset of invasive pancreatic cancer.

In a study of human promyelocytic leukemia cells in culture, garlic oil and onion oil were demonstrated to inhibit cellular proliferation and induce differentiation, an effect that was similar to the effect of retinoic acid on differentiation [74]. There was no cellular toxicity of garlic oil, as assayed by release of lactate dehydrogenase from cells, and the analysis of garlic oil by gas chromatography-mass spectroscopy revealed diallyl disulfide 56.6%, methyl allyl disulfide 12.0%, diallyl trisulfide 11.8%, diallyl sulfide 1.94%, and dimethyl trisulfide 1.4%. The toxic effects of retinoic acid therapy are obviated by the use of thioretinamide, which is unassociated with toxicity.

1.7 Furanonaphthoquinones, Napabucasin, Diallyl Trisulfide, and Inhibition of Stat3 Signaling

In screening for synthetic furanonaphthoquinone compounds with cytotoxic activity toward various leukemia cells and multiple myeloma cells, it was demonstrated that 2-methyl-naphtho[2,3-*b*]furan-4,9 dione (FNQ3) decreases the growth and increases apoptosis within cultured human leukemia and myeloma cell lines [75]. Normal control cell lines are resistant to the cytotoxic effects of FHQ3, requiring a tenfold increase in concentration to produce apoptosis and growth inhibition. The cytotoxic effect of FNQ3 is mediated by mitochondrial collapse, as measured by depolarization of the mitochondrial membrane, resulting in appearance of a sub-G1 (apoptotic) population of cultured cells. Moreover, FNQ3 markedly enhances granulocytic differentiation of human myeloid leukemia cells in the presence of low concentrations of retinoic acid or dihydroxy vitamin D3. The mitochondrial dysfunction induced by FNQ3 can be interpreted as competitive inhibition of electron transfer from respiratory complexes to the active site of oxidative phosphorylation, as mediated by coenzyme Q-10, resulting in a decreased proton flow to F1F0 complexes and the resulting decreased membrane potential [3].

Multiple naphthoquinones isolated from the bark and roots of an African shrub, *Newbouldia laevis*, used in traditional medicine were demonstrated to have prominent antifungal and antibacterial properties [76]. Additional furanonaphthoquinones, atraric acid, and a benzofuran were also isolated from the stem barks of *Newbouldia laevis* [77]. In a similar study of the roots of the "roble real" tree of Puerto Rico and the Dominican Republic, *Ekmanianthe longiflora*, multiple furanonaphthoquinones with anticancer and antimicrobial activity were found to have cytotoxic effects in cultured human breast and lung cancer cell lines [78]. Studies of naphthoquinones and analogs from *Avicennia* (mangrove) trees disclosed inhibitory effects against mouse-skin tumor formation in carcinogenesis testing [79]. Synthetic derivatives of furanonaphthoquinones isolated from plants were demonstrated to have cytotoxic activity against human tumor cells incubated against KB cells [80]. The basis for toxicity was considered by the authors to be related to "intercalation within DNA and free radicals." Two newly discovered cytotoxic naphthoquinones were isolated from roots and stems of the Madagascar plant, *Mendoncia cowanii* (vahimpianaomby), and found to be cytotoxic for human ovarian cancer cell lines [81]. All of these furanonaphthoquinones with cytotoxic activity potentially affect mitochondrial function through inhibition of electron transfer, as mediated by coenzyme Q-10, from respiratory complexes to the active site of oxidative phosphorylation. Malignant cells are more susceptible to the cytotoxic effects of these furanonaphthoquinones because of the lower concentration of thioretinaco ozonide within the mitochondrial membranes of malignant cells, compared with normal cells.

The signal transducer and activator of transcription 3 (Stat3) is frequently detected in breast cancer cell lines but not in normal breast epithelial cells. A virtual database screening protocol disclosed a natural product molecule, deoxytetrangomycin, an angucycline antibiotic (National Cancer Institute 628869) with potent inhibitory activity against Stat3 activity in human breast cancer cell lines [82]. A systematic study of naphthoquinone derivatives with inhibitory activity against Stat3 signaling in cancer stem cells disclosed a novel class of furanonaphthoquinone molecules with inhibitory activity against cancer stem-cell proliferation [83]. The most active of these compounds is napabucasin, 2-carboxymethyl-naphtho[2,3-*b*]furan-4,9-dione, which inhibits gene transcription dependent upon Stat3, thereby suppressing gene expression of cancer stemness, blocking spherogenesis of cultured cancer cells, and causing apoptosis of a wide variety of cancer-cell types [84]. In a study of human prostate cancer-cell cultures, napabucasin was demonstrated to increase apoptosis, and inhibit cell proliferation, cell motility, cell survival, and colony-formation ability of prostate cancer stem cells [85]. Moreover, an in vivo study demonstrated that napabucasin inhibits growth of prostate-cancer xenografts established from these cancer cell cultures in athymic mice.

Diallyl trisulfide, the cancer-chemopreventive constituent of garlic, inhibits phosphorylation of Stat3 in prostate cancer cells in culture and in vivo [86]. In this study diallyl trisulfide inhibited nuclear translocation of Stat3 and dimerization of Stat3 in prostate cancer cell lines. In addition, diallyl trisulfide inhibited prostate-cancer development in a transgenic-mouse model, correlating with a decrease in phosphorylated Stat3. Diallyl trisulfide also inhibited migration of prostate cancer cells, an indicator of metastatic potential, in an in vitro membrane-migration assay. In a study of mouse colitis induced by dextran sulfate, diallyl trisulfide suppressed Stat3 and NF-κB expression, resulting in decreased inflammation of the colon [87].

1.8 A Proposed Clinical Trial Protocol

Based on the preceding rationale, a proposed clinical trial is recommended to demonstrate the efficacy of the thioretinamide protocol in human subjects with myelodysplasia syndrome (MDS). The thioretinamide protocol will be implemented in a prospective nutritional-metabolic clinical multicenter interventional trial. This trial will include groups of subjects with myelodysplastic syndrome that are randomized into treatment groups in comparison with groups receiving conventional therapy. The expected results of the trial will demonstrate the efficacy of the thioretinamide protocol for control of malignant disease as exemplified by myelodysplastic syndrome, in direct comparison with current therapeutic strategy. The technologies addressed in the proposed trial relate to new understanding of the abnormal homocysteine metabolism underlying cancer. The critical aspects of these new technologies include catabolism of homocysteinylated macromolecules; biosynthesis of thioretinaco and thioretinaco ozonide from retinol, thioretinamide, cobalamin, and ozone; apoptosis of cancer stem cells by allyl sulfides and furanonaphthoquinones; catabolism of homocysteine by cystathionine synthase; formation of transthyretin from essential amino acids; and control of homocysteine metabolism by beneficial dietary fats and proteins.

The protocol of the proposed trial consists of thioretinamide and cobalamin as precursors of thioretinaco ozonide, combined with pancreatic enzyme extracts, diallyl trisulfide, napabucasin, nutritional modification to minimize processed foods, vitamin supplements, essential amino acids, beneficial dietary fats, and proteins. In Phase I of the proposed trial a small group of 20 normal healthy volunteers will be given escalating doses of thioretinamide with the full protocol. Homocysteine levels in plasma, chemistry and hematology parameters, and clinical observation will be monitored to assess safety of the protocol. In Phase II of the proposed trial

100 subjects with myelodysplastic syndrome will be given a therapeutic dose of thioretinamide with the full protocol. The subjects will be observed for prevention of leukemia, hemorrhages, infections, vascular adverse events, and autoimmune disease. The proposed trial is designed to demonstrate the efficacy of the thioretinamide protocol in prevention and therapy of myelodysplastic syndrome and its complications. The advantage of this novel approach is the lack of toxicity of the protocol and its potential for inducing complete remission of MDS. The design of the trial permits comparison of outcomes of Phase II of the thioretinamide protocol with the outcomes of conventional azacytidine therapy for myelodysplastic syndrome. Successful completion of the proposed trial will for the first time provide clinical evidence for implementation of the thioretinamide protocol for prevention and treatment of leukemia, anemia, hyperhomocysteinemia, autoimmune complications, and adverse vascular events in myelodysplastic syndrome.

1.9 Hyperhomocysteinemia, Vascular Disease, Autoimmunity, and Myelodysplastic Syndrome

Patients with myelodysplastic syndrome have an increased risk of development of leukemia, vascular disease, and autoimmune disease. Hyperhomocysteinemia, oxidative cell damage, and adverse cardiovascular events were observed in a study of 33 cases of myelodysplastic syndrome [88]. Hyperhomocysteinemia was observed in 42% of myelodysplasia cases, 4 of 5 cases with cardiovascular events, and 9 of 15 cases with associated autoimmune disease, including rheumatoid arthritis, Behcet's disease, antiplatelet antibodies, and anti-mitochondrial antibodies. Elevation of malondialdehyde, an indicator of oxidative stress, was observed in all myelodysplasia cases. Autoimmune manifestations, such as systemic vasculitis, dermal vasculitis, arthritis, glomerulonephritis, and relapsing polychondritis, occur in approximately 10% of cases of MDS [89]. Moreover, laboratory evidence of autoimmune phenomena, including hyperglobulinemia, hypoglobulinemia, antinuclear antibodies, anti-DNA antibodies, rheumatoid factor positivity, and anti-erythrocyte antibodies occur in approximately two-thirds of MDS cases.

Oxygen metabolites and total antioxidant activity were found to be elevated in 44% of myelodysplasia cases in a subsequent study of 50 cases [90]. The karyotypes of these cases were normal in 31 cases, complex in 6, and in the remaining cases single-chromosome abnormalities were present in chromosomes 5, 7, 8, 20, or Y. In a study of 61 cases of myelodysplasia, the plasma levels of cysteine, homocysteine, and cysteinyl glycine were elevated in all cases, compared with healthy controls [91]. The plasma levels of total and oxidized glutathione and nitrite were significantly depressed in all myelodysplasia cases, compared with healthy controls, demonstrating increased oxidative stress. There was no correlation with serum iron or ferritin levels in myelodysplasia cases, excluding iron overload as a factor in the increased oxidative stress associated with myelodysplasia. The antioxidant, *N*-acetyl cysteine, and the differentiating agent, all-*trans*-retinoic acid, were demonstrated to restore effective hematopoiesis in cultured bone marrow cells from myelodysplasia cases [92]. This finding supports the presumed role of retinoic acid as a precursor of thioretinamide and thioretinaco in restoring hematopoiesis in myelodysplasia.

1.10 Azacytidine Therapy of Myelodysplastic Syndrome

Myelodysplastic syndrome encompasses a heterogeneous group of clonal hematological stem cell disorders characterized by cytopenias and a hypercellular, dysplastic bone marrow [93]. The hypercellular bone marrow includes megaloblastic maturation, dysplastic megakaryocytes, erythroid hyperplasia, impaired maturation of the myeloid series, increased blasts, and ringed sideroblasts in some cases. In peripheral blood smears monocytosis, macrocytosis, immature myeloid and erythroid forms, and pseudo Pelger-Huet cells are identified. The International Prognostic Scoring System (IPSS) classifies patients as low risk, intermediate-1 risk, intermediate-2 risk, and high risk, depending upon the number of cytopenias, cytogenetic profile, and percentage of blasts in the bone marrow. Low-risk patients have a median survival of 5.7 years, intermediate-1 patients 3.5 years, intermediate-2 patients 1.2 years, and high-risk patients 0.4 years. The scoring system for the IPSS classification depends upon the percentage of marrow blasts; presence of normal, intermediate, or complex karyotypes; and number of cytopenias.

The choice of standard management of MDS must be tailored to each patient because of the diversity of clinical presentations [93]. Life-threatening anemia, neutropenia, or thrombocytopenia is treated with red blood cell transfusions, platelet transfusions, or antibiotics as supportive therapy. However, dependence upon transfusions and supportive therapy does not lead to complete remission or cure of MDS. Beyond supportive therapy, the available options for treatment of MDS are (1) hematopoietic growth factors such as erythropoietin, darbepoietin, or granulocyte colony-stimulating factor (G-CSF); (2) immunomodulatory agents such as lenalidomide, antithymocyte globulin (ATG), cyclosporine A (CsA), or thalidomide; (3) low-dose chemotherapy with cytarabine; (4) intensive chemotherapy with cytarabine plus an anthracycline; (5) allogeneic blood or bone marrow stem cell transplantation; or (6) hypomethylating agents, 5-azacytidine or decitabine. With the exception of blood or bone marrow stem cell transplantation, none of these therapeutic protocols is curative, and most MDS patients are not candidates for transplantation therapy because of age and comorbidities. The remaining protocols can induce partial remissions and survival benefit but are not curative in most MDS patients. Fewer than half of MDS cases show any hematological improvement from available therapeutic modalities, and the majority of MDS patients experience little benefit from current therapeutics.

The hypomethylating agents 5-azacytidine and 5-*aza*-2′-deoxycytidine are phosphorylated and covalently incorporated into DNA as 5-*aza*-dCTP during the S phase of cell division. The bound azacytidine residues inhibit DNA transmethylases, causing hypomethylation of CpG promoter regions, leading to progressive loss of methylation of DNA. Hypomethylating agents also promote myeloid differentiation in vitro at doses much lower than required for cytotoxicity [93]. The use of 5-azacytidine for treatment of MDS was approved in 2004, and a recent review and meta-analysis document the prolonged survival and increased time to leukemic transformation by this therapeutic modality [94]. Histone-deacetylase inhibitors have been combined with 5-azacytidine, but this therapeutic option is not currently approved for therapy of MDS. The limited efficacy of these drugs in treatment of MDS, the many cycles of therapy required for inducing partial responses, and the lack of understanding of the processes by which these drugs benefit MDS are limitations in the effective management of MDS. Mouse models of MDS have been analyzed to understand the molecular basis for the preleukemic nature of MDS. However, the molecular basis for increased apoptosis observed in these mouse models is not understood, and reactive-oxygen species generation, dysfunction of mitochondrial membranes, and effects on apoptosis by Bcl2-signaling proteins have been suggested to play a role [94].

A range of side effects of azacytidine include anemia, neutropenia, and thromobocytopenia, effects that are characteristic of MDS, and careful monitoring of patients under treatment with this drug is required to adjust dosage and to prevent complications of these adverse effects [95]. Azacytidine is also hepatotoxic, and its use is contraindicated in the therapy of hepatocellular carcinoma because of causing hepatic coma and early mortality. Azacytidine is nephrotoxic, and elevated creatinine, kidney failure, and uremia have been reported in patients treated with intravenous azacytidine and other chemotherapeutic agents. Azacytidine can cause severe fetal damage, and its use is contraindicated in pregnancy. Azacytidine can cause nausea, vomiting, fever, diarrhea, constipation, bruising, petechiae, rigors, weakness, hypokalemia, and many other side effects, some of which can be severe or fatal [95].

1.11 Autoimmunity and Stat3 Signaling in MDS

A fraction of MDS patients (18/349) and patients with aplastic anemia (AA) (16/140) have been found to contain mutations in Stat3 signaling, which are attributed to somatic mutations in cytotoxic T-cell lymphocytes [96]. In addition, patients with T-cell large granular lymphocytic leukemia (LGL) associated with MDS or AA also have mutations in Stat3 signaling. According to the authors, "Stat3-mutated LGL clones may facilitate a persistently dysregulated autoimmune activation, responsible for the primary induction of bone marrow failure in a subset of AA and MDS patients." These findings support the "immune hypothesis" by which an immune-mediated myelosuppression in MDS leads to a preleukemic phenotype [97]. A study of patients with high-risk MDS revealed a correlation between Stat3/Stat5 signaling and responsiveness to azacytidine therapy, predicting event-free survival [98]. These findings suggest that inhibition of Stat3/Stat5 signaling may provide a therapeutic strategy for overcoming resistance to azacytidine therapy.

In patients with germline loss-of-function mutations of Stat3, immunodeficiency syndromes are observed, and germline gain-of-function mutations of Stat3 are associated with MDS, T-cell large-granular lymphocytic leukemia, and aplastic anemia [99]. These gain-of-function *STAT3* mutations confer increased Stat3 transcription, impaired cytokine signaling, and diminished T-regulatory cell function. The authors suggest a rationale for use of inhibitors of Stat3 for therapeutic benefit in patients with gain-of-function *STAT3* mutations. In support of this concept, autoimmunity, hypogammaglobulinemia, lymphoproliferation, and mycobacterial disease were demonstrated in patients with activating mutations in *STAT3* [100].

In knockout mice with $STAT3^{-}/^{-}$ mutations crossed with $CD4^{+}$ mice, T-helper 17 lymphocytes were found to be absent from intestinal lamina propria [101]. Experimental autoimmune encephalomyelitis (EAE) requires Stat3 activation, and the $STAT3^{-}/^{-}$ $CD4^{+}$ mice were found to be resistant to EAE. Mitigation of disease was also demonstrated in $STAT3^{-}/^{-}$ $CD4^{+}$ mice with induced autoimmune pneumonitis. These findings were interpreted to indicate that pathogenic $T_{H}17$ cells are dependent upon Stat3 signaling and that inhibition of this signaling pathway results in mitigation of autoimmune disease progression. The authors suggest that Stat3 inhibition may provide a therapeutic target for autoimmune diseases. In a study of knockout mice with $p53^{-}/^{-}$ mutations crossed with CD45.1 mice, spontaneous autoimmunity was ameliorated by inhibition of the Stat3 signaling pathway and suppression of $T_{H}17$ effectors [102]. This study identifies a critical function of the tumor-suppressor oncogene p53 in suppressing autoimmunity through the Stat3 pathway and $T_{H}17$ differentiation.

A study of experimental MDS in adult mice treated with ethyl nitrosourea (ENU) demonstrated that the dysplastic bone-marrow cells were accompanied by a decrease in CD45 (common leukocyte antigen) and an increase in CD71 (transferrin receptor) [103]. Upregulation of the JAK/STAT signaling pathway was demonstrated, suggesting that aberrant signaling may lead to the affected hematopoietic lineages in MDS. In an experimental model of lupus nephritis, which is observed in MDS, metformin was found to suppress autoimmunity in *Roquin sanroque* mutant mice ($Rc3h1^{san}/^{san}$) through attenuation of mTOR/STAT3 signaling [104].

1.12 Rationale of the Thioretinamide Protocol for Therapy of MDS

Since MDS is a premalignant abnormality of bone marrow stem cells, the benefit of the thioretinamide protocol in the proposed clinical trial is expected to result from increased endogenous biosynthesis of thioretinaco ozonide from thioretinamide in dysplastic cells and regenerative cells of bone marrow, conversion of aerobic glycolysis of dysplastic cells to oxidative phosphorylation, and inhibition of premalignant bone marrow stem cells through down-regulation of Stat3 signaling by diallyl trisulfide and napabucasin. The thioretinamide protocol is a patented method for treatment and prevention of degenerative diseases of aging [105]. Addition of allyl sulfides, naphthoquinones, and pancreatic enzymes to the thioretinamide protocol provides a patented thioretinamide composition to promote apoptosis of malignant cells while preventing apoptosis of normal cells [106].

The thioretinamide protocol combines administration of thioretinamide, allyl sulfides especially dially trisulfide, and naphthoquinones, especially napabucasin, with pancreatic enzymes for enzymatic degradation of homocysteinylated proteins, nucleic acids, and glycosaminoglycans, together with vitamins, amino acids, and nitrilosides to enhance metabolic conversion of homocysteine thiolactone and retinol to thioretinamide by cystathionine synthase, to promote apoptosis of malignant cells and inhibit apoptosis of normal cells, and to promote biosynthesis of thioretinaco from thioretinamide and cobalamin in regenerative cells, thereby enhancing immune function and preventing the development and progression of MDS, and related immune-system impairment.

The outcome of the Phase I and Phase II trials of the thioretinamide protocol will demonstrate safety of this nontoxic strategy for effective treatment of myelodysplastic syndrome. In addition, successful outcome of the trial will demonstrate prevention of progression of myelodysplastic syndrome; reduction of transfusion requirements; prevention of cytopenias, hemorrhage, and infections; prevention of progression to leukemia; prevention of autoimmune manifestations of MDS; prevention of hyperhomocysteinemia, acute coronary syndrome, stroke, amputation, and renal failure; and prevention of mortality, in comparison with current supportive measures and conventional therapeutics.

2 Materials and Supplies

Synthetic thioretinamide: Custom synthesis by cGMP pharmaceutical manufacturing facility for 6 kg of product with accompanying master drug file to document analysis, stability characteristics, residual solvent, forced degradation (if required), and encapsulation for oral administration, 75 mg/capsule (*see* **Note 1**).

Glandular pancreas (pork): Allergy Research Group, distributed by Nutricology, 425 mg/capsule, 20 capsules/day in 5 doses, total 8.5 g/day (*see* **Note 2**).

Garlic oil: 300 mg/capsule from Vitacost.

Napabucasin: MedChem Express, 300 mg/capsule.

S-adenosyl methionine (SAMe): Stabilized, enteric coated, from Vitacost, 200 mg/tablet.

Pyridoxal-5-phosphate: Vitacost, 50 mg/tablet.

Methyl-cobalamin, sublingual from Vitacost, Quickdots, 1000 μg.

Coenzyme Q10: Vitacost, 200 mg/capsule.

Methyl-folate: From Jarrow, distributed by Vitacost, 400 μg/capsule.

Vitamin C complex, buffered with bioflavonoids from Vitacost, 1000 mg/capsule.

Nicotinamide riboside (Niagen): LiveCellResearch.com, 250 mg/capsule.

Apricot kernels (Sunfood), 8 kernels, 30 mg vitamin B17.

Mixed essential amino acids: Solgar, distributed by Vitacost, containing 75 mg each of 8 amino acids per capsule.

Cod liver oil: Lemon flavored, Norwegian, distributed by Vitacost.

3 Methods

3.1 Phase 1 Trial

1. Give 20 healthy volunteers, aged 25–70, single ascending doses of 75, 150, and 300 mg/day of thioretinamide sequentially for a period of 4 weeks together with the full protocol of pancreatic enzymes 1.7 g five times per day (8.5 g/day), garlic oil capsules 1.2 g/day, napabucasin 300 mg/day, adenosyl methionine 200 mg/day, pyridoxal phosphate 50 mg/day, methyl cobala min 1000 μg sublingual/day, methyl folate 400 μg/day, nicotinamide riboside 250 mg/day, ascorbate with mixed bioflavonoids 1 g/day, apricot kernels 500 mg/day, coenzyme Q10 200 mg/day, cod liver oil 15 mL/day, and mixed essential amino acids 75 mg each/day.
2. Adjust diet during the trial period to eliminate all processed foods containing sugar, white flour, powdered milk, protein hydrolyzates, natural flavoring extracts, and alcohol.
3. Increase dietary consumption of berries, nuts, beans, molasses, fruits, raw vegetables, steamed vegetables, fish, and fresh meats to provide approximately 2000 kCal per day.

4. Monitor fasting plasma homocysteine, basic metabolic panel, and complete blood count before and following each ascending dose of thioretinamide.
5. Monitor mucosal surfaces, epidermal surface of skin, gastrointestinal function, evidence of hair loss, papilledema, hepatosplenomegaly, bone swelling, and bleeding, and measure blood pressure, height, and body weight before and after each ascending dose of thioretinamide for determination of safety of each dose.
6. During the Phase l trial, enter a small number of subjects (3–5) into the trial at the lowest dose of thioretinamide (75 mg/day).
7. If no adverse effects are observed after 4 weeks, enter a second group of subjects (3–5) into the trial at the intermediate dose (150 mg/day).
8. If adverse effects are observed in any of the subjects after 4 weeks, treat an additional small number of subjects (3–5) with the same dose for 4 weeks.
9. If no adverse effects are observed at the intermediate dose, treat a small number of subjects (3–5) with the highest dose of thioretinamide (300 mg/day) for 4 weeks.
10. Determine the maximum tolerated dose of thioretinamide when one of the subjects in the particular dose level experiences toxic effects of thioretinamide.
11. Determine the optimal dose of thioretinamide by the minimum dose required to lower plasma homocysteine levels to 8–10 μM.

3.2 Phase 2 Trial

1. Give a group of 28 of 100 subjects with newly-diagnosed myelodysplastic syndrome the optimal dose of thioretinamide for lowering plasma homocysteine, as determined from the results of the Phase 1 trial of the thioretinamide protocol.
2. Give thioretinamide together with the full protocol of pancreatic enzymes 1.7 g five times per day (8.5 g/day), garlic oil capsules 1.2 g/day, napabucasin 300 mg/day, adenosyl methionine 200 mg/day, pyridoxal phosphate 50 mg/day, methyl cobalamin 1000 μg sublingual/day, methyl folate 400 μg/day, nicotinamide riboside 250 mg/day, ascorbate with mixed bioflavonoids 1 g/day, apricot kernels 500 mg/day, coenzyme Q10 200 mg/day, cod liver oil 15 ml/day, and mixed essential amino acids 75 mg each/day.
3. Adjust the diet during the trial period to eliminate all processed foods containing sugar, white flour, powdered milk, protein hydrolyzates, natural flavoring extracts, and alcohol.

4. Increase dietary consumption of berries, nuts, beans, molasses, fruits, raw vegetables, steamed vegetables, fish, and fresh meats to provide approximately 2000 kCal per day.
5. Monitor fasting plasma homocysteine, basic metabolic panel, and complete blood count, and bone marrow biopsy and smear, before and after each 6 months on the thioretinamide protocol.
6. Monitor requirements for red cell or platelet transfusions, iron infusions, erythropoietin therapy, and determination of anemia, leukocytopenia, and thrombocytopenia, before and after each 6 months on the thioretinamide protocol.
7. Monitor marrow cellularity, erythropoiesis, granulopoiesis, thrombopoieses, and fibrosis for evidence of ineffective hemopoiesis and dyshemopoiesis, hypoplastic hemopoiesis, and oligoblastic leukemias.
8. Determine cytogenetic analysis for occurrence of chromosomal abnormalities, 5q-syndrome, and monosomy 7.
9. Continue the accrual period for 12 months, and the period of observation will last 12 months for each subject.
10. Monitor subjects for progression of myelodysplasia from preleukemic states, including acquired refractory anemia with or without ringed sideroblasts, cytopenia with hyperplastic marrow, or chronic monocytosis, aplastic anemia, and hypoplastic neutropenia to oligoblastic leukemias, including smoldering myelogenous leukemia; determine the interval from entry into the Phase 2 trial to progression to preleukemic and oligoblastic leukemic states.
11. Determine the therapeutic efficacy of the thioretinamide protocol by decreased transfusion requirements, reversal of anemia or cytopenia, and a delayed interval of progression to preleukemic and oligoblastic leukemic states.
12. Observe biological activity of the thioretinamide protocol in greater than 20% of 28 subjects with myelodysplasia. Recruit 72 additional subjects to determine the response rate in the entire group of 100 subjects.
13. Determine the effectiveness of the thioretinamide protocol by comparison with treatment of myelodysplastic subjects as they would be treated in accepted clinical practice.
14. Observation of biological activity of the thioretinamide protocol is greater than 20% of subjects to recommend a subsequent randomized Phase 3 trial.

3.3 Investigational New Drug License

The US Food and Drug Administration (FDA) regulations require application for an Investigational New Drug (IND) License for all clinical trials conducted by investigators in the

USA. According to the USA Code of Federal Regulations 21 § CFR 312, "An investigational new drug for which an IND is in effect in accordance with this part is exempt from the premarketing approval requirements that are otherwise applicable and may be shipped lawfully for the purpose of conducting clinical investigation of that drug." The purpose of the IND is to assure the safety and rights of human subjects in Phase 1 studies and to assure that the quality of the scientific evaluation of drugs is adequate to permit an evaluation of the drug's effectiveness and safety in Phase 2 and Phase 3 trials. A detailed description of the research plan, the qualifications of the investigators, approval by Institutional Review Boards of participating sites, and a description of the composition, manufacture, stability, and control of the drug are required by the IND application process. Approval of the application for the IND license by the FDA is required before Phase 1; Phase 2 of the proposed trial can commence. An annual report of the progress of the clinical trial is required by the FDA, and any adverse events require timely reporting to the FDA. The results of the clinical trial are reported to the FDA upon conclusion of each phase of the trial.

4 Notes

1. The custom synthesis of thioretinamide is by the method of Kazimir and Wilson [19]. This patented method [107] is in the public domain, and no royalties are due.
2. Glandular pancreatic extract is prepared by lyophilization of fresh pancreas from New Zealand pigs, according to the method of Gonzalez [51]. Porcine pancreas extract is more potent than sheep or cow pancreas extract. Porcine pancreas extract contains proenzymes that are stabilized by the lyophilization process.

References

1. McCully KS (1993) Chemical pathology of homocysteine. I. Atherogenesis. Ann Clin Lab Sci 23:477–493
2. McCully KS (1994) Chemical pathology of homocysteine. II. Carcinogenesis and homocysteine thiolactone metabolism. Ann Clin Lab Sci 24:27–59
3. McCully KS (1994) Chemical pathology of homocysteine. III. Cellular function and aging. Ann Clin Lab Sci 24:134–152
4. McCully KS (2009) Chemical pathology of homocysteine. IV. Excitotoxicity, oxidative stress, endothelial dysfunction, and inflammation. Ann Clin Lab Sci 39:219–232
5. McCully KS (2011) Chemical pathology of homocysteine. V. Thioretinamide, thioretinaco, and cystathionine synthase function in degenerative diseases. Ann Clin Lab Sci 41:300–313
6. McCully KS (2016) Homocysteine metabolism, atherosclerosis, and diseases of aging. Compr Physiol 6:401–475
7. Blom H (2001) Diseases and drugs associated with hyperhomocysteinemia. In: Carmel R,

Jacobsen DW (eds) Homocysteine in health and disease. Cambridge University Press, Cambridge, pp 331–340

8. McCully KS (1969) Vascular pathology of homocysteinemia: implications for the pathogenesis of arteriosclerosis. Am J Pathol 56:111–128
9. Kanwar YS, Manaligod JR, Wong WK (1976) Morphologic studies in a patient with homocystinuria due to 5,10-methylenetetrahydrofolate reductase deficiency. Pediatr Res 10:598–609
10. McCully KS (1976) Homocysteine thiolactone metabolism in malignant cells. Cancer Res 36:3198–3202
11. Jakubowski H, Goldman E (1993) Synthesis of homocysteine thiolactone by methionyl-tRNA synthetase in cultured malignant cells. FEBS Lett 317:237–240
12. McCully KS (1981) Homocysteine thiolactone as a tumor promoter. US Patent 4,255,443, 10 Mar 1981
13. McCully KS, Clopath P (1977) Homocysteine compounds which influence the growth of a malignant neoplasm. Chemotherapy 23:44–49
14. McCully KS (1983) Homocysteine thiolactone salts and use thereof as antineoplastic agents. US Patent 4,383,994, 17 May 1983
15. McCully KS, Vezeridis MP (1987) Antineoplastic activity of a rhodium trichloride complex of oxalyl homocysteine thiolactone. Cancer Investig 5:25–30
16. McCully KS, Vezeridis MP (1985) Antineoplastic activity of *N*-maleamide homocysteine thiolactone amide encapsulated within liposomes. Proc Soc Exp Biol Med 180:57–61
17. McCully KS, Vezeridis MP (1987) Chemopreventive and antineoplastic activity of *N*-homocysteine thiolactonyl retinamide. Carcinogenesis 8:1559–1562
18. McCully KS, Vezeridis MP (1989) Chemopreventive effect of *N*-homocysteine thiolactonyl retinamido cobalamin on carcinogenesis by ethyl carbamate in mice. Proc Soc Exp Biol Med 191:346–351
19. Kazimir M, Wilson FR (2002) Prevention of homocysteine thiolactone induced atherosclerosis in rats. Res Commun Molec Pharmacol 5(6):179–198
20. McCully KS (1996) Thioretinaco ozonide and enhanced biological activity of thioretinaco ozonide in combination with interferon. US Patent 5,565,558, 15 Oct 1996
21. McCully KS (2004) Enhanced liposomal thioretinaco ozonide compositions and liposomal carrier. US Patent 6,696,082, 24 Feb 2004
22. McCully KS (1971) Homocysteine metabolism in scurvy, growth and arteriosclerosis. Nature 231:391–392
23. Clopath P, Smith VC, McCully KS (1976) Growth promotion by homocysteic acid. Science 192:372–374
24. McCully KS (1975) Growth disorders and homocysteine metabolism. Ann Clin Lab Sci 5:147–152
25. McCully KS (1972) Macromolecular basis for homocysteine-induced changes in proteoglycan structure in growth and arteriosclerosis. Am J Pathol 66:83–95
26. Hanck A (1986) Ascorbic acid and cancer. In: Myeskens FL Jr, Prasad KN Eds, Vitamins and cancer, Humana Press, Clifton, NJ, pp 365–397
27. Warburg O (1931) The oxygen-transferring ferment of respiration. Nobel Lecture, 10 Dec 1931
28. Warburg O (1956) On the origin of cancer cells. Science 123:309–314
29. Schon R, Menke KH, Negelein E (1961) The influence of heavy metal ions on the Ehrlich ascites tumor cells of mice and the effect of cysteine. Z Physiol Chem 323:155–163
30. Cameron E, Campbell A (1974) The orthomolecular treatment of cancer. II. Clinical trial of high-dose ascorbic acid supplements in advanced human cancer. Chem Biol Interact 9:285–315
31. Cameron E, Pauling L (1978) Supplemental ascorbate in the supportive treatment of cancer: reevaluation of survival times in terminal human cancer. Proc Natl Acad Sci U S A 75:4538–4542
32. Ingenbleek Y, Hardillier E, Jung L (2002) Subclinical malnutrition is a determinant of hyperhomocysteinemia. Nutrition 18:40–46
33. Ingenbleek Y, McCully KS (2012) Vegetarianism produces subclinical malnutrition, hyperhomocysteinemia and atherogenesis. Nutrition 28:148–152
34. Ingenbleek Y, De Visscher M, De Nayer P et al (1972) Measurement of prealbumin as index of protein-calorie malnutrition. Lancet 2(7768):106–109
35. Ingenbleek Y (2009) Hyperhomocysteinemia is a biomarker for sulfur-deficiency in human morbidities. Open Clin Chem J 2:49–60
36. Carballal S, Madzelan P, Zinola CF et al (2008) Dioxygen reactivity and heme redox potential of truncated human cystathionine β-synthase. Biochemistry 47:3194–3202

37. Smith TJ, Drummond GS (1991) Retinoic acid can enhance the stimulation by thyroid hormone of heme oxygenase activity in the liver of thyroidectomized rats. Biochim Biophys Acta 1075:119–122
38. Samuel W, Kutty RK, Nagineni S et al (2006) N-(4-hydroxyphenyl) retinamide induces apoptosis in human retinal pigment epithelial cells: retinoic acid receptors regulate apoptosis, reactive oxygen species generation, and the expression of heme oxygenase-1 and Gadd153. J Cell Physiol 209:854–865
39. Hail N Jr, Kim HJ, Lotan R (2006) Mechanisms of fenretinide-induced apoptosis. Apoptosis 11:1677–1694
40. Miles EW, Kraus JP (2004) Cystathionine β-synthase: structure, function, regulation, and location of homocystinuria-causing mutations. J Biol Chem 279:29871–29874
41. Kim J, Hong SJ, Park JH et al (2009) Expression of cystathionine β-synthase is downregulated in hepatocellular carcinoma and associated with poor prognosis. Oncol Rep 21:1449–1454
42. Hong WK, Sporn MB (1997) Recent advances in chemoprevention of cancer. Science 278:1073–1077
43. Huang ME, Ye YI, Chen SR (1988) Use of all-*trans*-retinoic acid in the treatment of acute promyelocytic leukemia. Blood 72:567–572
44. Chomienne C, Ballerini P, Balitrand N et al (1989) Retinoic acid therapy for promyelocytic leukaemia. Lancet 334(8665):746–747
45. Simeone AM, Tari AM (2004) How retinoids regulate breast cancer cell proliferation and apoptosis. Cell Mol Life Sci 61:1475–1484
46. Moise AR, Noy N, Palczewski K, Blaner WS (2007) Delivery of retinoid-based therapies to target tissues. Biochemistry 46:4449–4458
47. McCully KS (2015) The active site of oxidative phosphorylation and the origin of hyperhomocysteinemia in aging and dementia. Ann Clin Lab Sci 45:222–225
48. Beard J (1911) The enzymatic treatment of cancer and its scientific basis. Chatto & Windus, London, 1911, republished by New Spring Press, New York, 2010 with a foreword by Nicholas Gonzalez
49. Acevedo HF, Tong JY, Hartsock RJ (1995) Human chorionic gonadotropin-beta subunit gene expression in cultured human fetal and cancer cells of different types and origins. Cancer 76:1467–1475
50. Novak JF, Trynka F (2005) Proenzyme therapy of cancer. Anticancer Res 25:1157–1178
51. Gonzalez N, Isaacs L (2009) The trophoblast and the origins of cancer. New Spring Press, New York
52. Perla-Kajan J, Twardowski T, Jakubowski H (2007) Mechanisms of homocysteine toxicity in humans. Amino Acids 32:561–572
53. Gaull G, Sturman JA, Raiha NCR (1972) Development of mammalian sulfur metabolism: absence of cystathionase in fetal tissues. Pediatr Res 6:538–547
54. McCully KS (2016) Homocysteine, thioretinaco ozonide, oxidative phosphorylation, biosynthesis of phosphoadenosine phosphosulfate and the pathogenesis of atherosclerosis. Ann Clin Lab Sci 46:701–704
55. Schneider WC, Potter VR (1943) Biocatalysts in cancer tissue. III. Succinic dehydrogenase and cytochrome oxidase. Cancer Res 3:353–357
56. Krebs ET Jr (1962) The nitrilosides in the prevention and control of cancer. McNaughton Foundation, Los Angeles, pp 1–21
57. Sen U, Basu P, Abe OA et al (2009) Hydrogen sulfide ameliorates hyperhomocysteinemia-associated chronic renal failure. Am J Physiol Renal Physiol 297:F410–F419
58. Olson KR, Whitfield NL (2010) Hydrogen sulfide and oxygen sensing in the cardiovascular system. Antioxid Redox Signal 12:1219–1234
59. Chang L, Geng B, Yu F et al (2008) Hydrogen sulfide inhibits myocardial injury induced by homocysteine in rats. Amino Acids 34:573–585
60. Polhemus DJ, Lefer DJ (2014) Emergence of hydrogen sulfide as an endogenous gaseous signaling molecule in cardiovascular disease. Circ Res 114:730–737
61. Elrod JW, Calvert JW, Morrison J et al (2007) Hydrogen sulfide attenuates myocardial ischemia-reperfusion injury by preservation of mitochondrial function. Proc Natl Acad Sci U S A 104:15560–15565
62. Benavides GA, Squadrito GL, Mills RW et al (2007) Hydrogen sulfide mediates the vasoactivity of garlic. Proc Natl Acad Sci U S A 104:17977–17982
63. Yeh YY, Yeh SM (2006) Homocysteine-lowering action is another potential cardiovascular protective factor of aged garlic extract. J Nutr 136:745S–749S
64. Chen LY, Chen Q, Zhu XJ et al (2016) Diallyl trisulfide protects against ethanol-induced oxidative stress and apoptosis via a hydrogen sulfide-mediated mechanism. Int Immunopharmacol 36:23–30

65. Tsai CY, Wang CC, Lai TY et al (2013) Antioxidant effects of diallyl trisulfide on high glucose-induced apoptosis are mediated by the PI3K/Akt-dependent activation of Nrf2 in cardiomyocytes. Int J Cardiol 168:1286–1297
66. Tsai CY, Wen SY, Shibu MA et al (2015) Diallyl trisulfide protects against high glucose-induced cardiac apoptosis by stimulating the production of cystathionine gamma-lyase-derived hydrogen sulfide. Int J Cardiol 195:300–310
67. Das A, Banik NL, Ray SK (2007) Garlic compounds generate reactive oxygen species leading to activation of stress kinases and cysteine proteases for apoptosis in human glioblastoma T98G and U87MG cells. Cancer 110:1083–1094
68. Na HK, Kim EH, Choi MA et al (2012) Diallyl trisulfide induces apoptosis in human breast cancer cells through ROS-mediated activation of JNK and AP-1. Biochem Pharmacol 84:1241–1250
69. Chandra-Kuntal K, Lee J, Singh SV (2013) Critical role for reactive oxygen species in apoptosis induction and cell migration inhibition by diallyl trisulfide, a cancer chemopreventive component of garlic. Breast Cancer Res Treat 138:69–79
70. Liu Y, Zhu P, Wang Y et al (2015) Antimetastatic therapies of the polysulfide diallyl trisulfide against triple-negative breast cancer (TNBC) via suppression MMP2/9 by blocking NF-κB and ERK/MAPK signaling pathways. PLoS One 10:e1023781
71. Kim SH, Kaschula CH, Priedigkeit N et al (2016) Forkhead box Q1 is a novel target of breast cancer stem cell inhibition by diallyl trisulfide. J Biol Chem 291:13495–13508
72. Wang HC, Pao J, Lin SY et al (2012) Molecular mechanisms of garlic-derived allyl sulfides in the inhibition of skin cancer progression. Ann N Y Acad Sci 1271:44–52
73. Ma HB, Huang S, Yin XR et al (2014) Apoptotic pathway induced by diallyl trisulfide in pancreatic cancer cells. World J Gastroenterol 20:193–203
74. Seki T, Tsuji K, Hayato Y et al (2000) Garlic and onion oils inhibit proliferation and induce differentiation of HL-60 cells [human promyelocytic leukemia cells]. Cancer Lett 160:29–35
75. Desmond JC, Kawabata H, Mueller-Tidow C et al (2005) The synthetic furanonapthoquinone induces growth arrest, apoptosis and differentiation in a variety of leukaemias and multiple myeloma cells. Brit J Haematol 131:520–529
76. Gafner S, Wolfender JL, Nianga M et al (1996) Antifungal and antibacterial napthoquinones from *Newbouldia laevis* roots. Phytochemistry 42:1315–1320
77. Gormann R, Kaloga M, Li XC et al (2003) Furanonaphthoquinones, atraric acid and a benzofuran from stem barks of *Newbouldia laevis*. Phytochemistry 64:583–587
78. Peraza-Sanchez SR, Chavez D, Chai HB et al (2000) Cytotoxic constituents of the roots of *Ekmanianthe longiflora*. J Nat Prod 63:492–495
79. Itoigawa M, Ito C, Tan HTW et al (2001) Cancer chemopreventive activity of naphthoquinones and their analogs from *Avicennia* plants. Cancer Lett 174:135–139
80. Ogawa M, Koyanagi J, Sugaya A et al (2006) Cytotoxic activity toward KB cells of 2-substituted naphtho[2,3-*b*]furan-4,9-diones and their related compounds. Biosci Biotechnol Biochem 70:1009–1012
81. Williams RB, Norris A, Miller JS et al (2006) Two new cytotoxic naphthoquinones from *Mendoncia cowanii* from the rainforest of Madagascar. Planta Med 72:564–566
82. Song H, Wang R, Wang S, Lin J (2005) A low-molecular weight compound discovered through virtual database screening inhibits Stat3 function in breast cancer cells. Proc Natl Acad Sci U S A 102:4700–4705
83. Jiang Z, Chiang JL, Leggett D (2014) STAT3 pathway inhibitors and cancer stem cell inhibitors. US Patent 8,877,803, 4 Nov 2014
84. Li Y, Rogoff HA, Keates S et al (2015) Suppression of cancer relapse and metastasis by inhibiting cancer stemness. Proc Natl Acad Sci U S A 112:1839–1844
85. Zhang Y, Jin Z, Zhou H et al (2016) Suppression of prostate cancer progression by cancer cell stemness inhibitor napabucasin. Cancer Med 5:1251–1258
86. Chandra-Kuntal K, Singh SV (2010) Diallyl trisulfide inhibits activation of Signal Transducer and Activator of Transcription 3 in prostate cancer cells in culture and in vivo. Cancer Prev Res (Phila) 3:1473–1483
87. Lee HJ, Lee HG, Choi KS et al (2013) Diallyl trisulfide suppresses dextran sodium sulfate-induced mouse colitis: NFκB and STAT3 as potential targets. Biochem Biophys Res Commun 437:267–273
88. Cortelezzi A, Fracchiolla NS, Bamonti-Catena F et al (2001) Hyperhomocysteinemia in myelodysplastic syndromes: specific

association with autoimmunity and cardiovascular disease. Leuk Lymphoma 41:147–150

89. Giannouli S, Kanellopoulou T, Voulegarelis M (2012) Myelodysplasia and autoimmunity. Curr Opin Rheumatol 24:97–102

90. Fracchiolla NS, Catena FB, Novembrino C et al (2003) Possible association between reactive oxygen metabolites and karyotypic abnormalities in myelodysplastic syndromes. Haematologica 88:594–597

91. Pimkova K, Chrastinova L, Suttnar J et al (2014) Plasma levels of aminothiols, nitrite, nitrate, and malondialdehyde in myelodysplastic syndromes in the context of clinical outcomes and as a consequence of iron overload. Oxidative Med Cell Longev 2014:416028

92. Cortelezzi A, Cattaneo C, Sarina B et al (1999) Efficacy of N-acetylcysteine and all-*trans*-retinoic acid in restoring in vitro effective hemopoiesis in myelodysplastic syndromes. Leuk Res 24:129–137

93. Nimer SD (2008) Myelodysplastic syndromes. Blood 111:4841–4851

94. Gurion R, Vidal L, Gafter-Gvilli A et al (2010) 5-azacytidine prolongs overall survival in patients with myelodysplastic syndrome—a systematic review and meta-analysis. Haematologica 95:303–310

95. "Prescribing information—Azacytidine for Infection" (2016) fda.gov United States Food and Drug Administration

96. Jerez A, Clemente MJ, Makishima H et al (2013) STAT3 mutations indicate the presence of subclinical T-cell clones in a subset of aplastic anemia and myelodysplasia syndrome patients. Blood 122:2453–2459

97. Schultz KR (2013) STAT3 mutations and persistence of autoimmunity. Blood 122:2295–2296

98. Mitiades P, Lamprianidou E, Vassilakopoulos TP et al (2016) The Stat 3/5 signaling biosignature in hematopoietic stem/progenitor cells predicts response and outcome in myelodysplastic syndrome patients treated with azacytidine. Clin Cancer Res 22:1958–1968

99. Milner JD, Vogel TP, Forbes L et al (2015) Early-onset lymphoproliferation and autoimmunity caused by germline *STAT3* gain-of-function mutations. Blood 125:591–599

100. Haapaniemi EM, Kaustio M, Rajala HLM et al (2015) Autoimmunity, hypogammaglobulinemia, lymphoproliferation, and mycobacterial disease in patients with activating mutations in *STAT3*. Blood 125:639–648

101. Harris TJ, Grosso JF, Yen HR et al (2007) An in vivo requirement for STAT3 signaling in TH17 development and TH17-dependent autoimmunity. J Immunol 179:4313–4317

102. Zhang S, Zheng M, Kibe R et al (2011) Trp53 negatively regulates autoimmunity via the STAT3-Th17 axis. FASEB J 25:2387–2398

103. Daw S, Chatterjee R, Law A et al (2016) Analysis of hematopathology and alteration of JAK1/STAT3/STAT5 signaling axis in experimental myelodysplastic syndrome. Chem Biol Interact 260:176–185

104. Lee SY, Moon SJ, Kim EK et al (2017) Metformin suppresses systemic autoimmunity in *Roquin*$^{san/san}$ mice through inhibiting B cell differentiation into plasma cells via regulation of AMPK/mTOR/STAT3. J Immunol 198:2661–2670

105. McCully KS (2015) Compositions and method for utilization of thioretinamide in therapy of diseases of aging. US Patent No. 9,216,209. 22 Dec 2015

106. McCully KS (2017) Thioretinamide compositions for the apoptosis of malignant cells while preventing the apoptosis of normal cells and related methods. US Continuing Patent Application S.N. 15/475,103, 30 Mar 2017

107. Kazimir M, Wilson R (2000) Method for synthesis of N-homocysteine thiolactonyl retinamide. US Patent 6,054,595, 25 Apr 2000

Chapter 24

Afterword: Oral Methioninase—Answer to Cancer and Fountain of Youth?

Robert M. Hoffman, Qinghong Han, Kei Kawaguchi, Shukuan Li, and Yuying Tan

Abstract

The elevated methionine (MET) requirement of cancer cells is termed MET dependence and is possibly the only known general metabolic defect in cancer. Targeting MET by recombinant methioninase (rMETase) can arrest the growth of cancer cells in vitro and in vivo due to their elevated requirement for MET. rMETase can also potentiate chemotherapy drugs active in S phase due to the selective arrest of cancer cells in S/G_2 phase during MET restriction (MR). We previously reported that rMETase, administrated by intraperitoneal injection (ip-rMETase), could inhibit tumor growth in mouse models of cancer including patient-derived orthotopic xenograft (PDOX) mouse models. We subsequently compared ip rMETase and oral rMETase (o-rMETase) on a melanoma PDOX mouse model. o-rMETase was significantly more effective than ip-rMETase to inhibit tumor growth without overt toxicity. The combination of o-rMETase + ip rMETase was significantly more effective than either monotherapy and completely arrested tumor growth. Thus, o-rMETase is effective as an anticancer agent with the potential of clinical development for chronic cancer therapy as well as for cancer prevention. o-rMETase may also have potential as an antiaging agent for healthy people, since MR has been shown to extend the life span of a variety of different organisms.

Key words Recombinant methioninase, Methionine dependence, Oral administration, Pyridoxal-L-phosphate, Melanoma, PDOX, Nude mice, Orthotopic

1 Introduction

An excessive requirement for methionine (MET), termed MET dependence, appears to be a general metabolic defect in cancer (*see* **Note 1**) [1–9]. We have previously shown that cancer cell growth can be selectively arrested by MET restriction (MR) in vitro and in vivo, such as with recombinant methioninase (rMETase) [10–13] (*see* **Notes 2–4**). rMETase can arrest tumors in patient-derived orthotopic xenograft (PDOX) models

Robert M. Hoffman (ed.), *Methionine Dependence of Cancer and Aging: Methods and Protocols*, Methods in Molecular Biology, vol. 1866, https://doi.org/10.1007/978-1-4939-8796-2_24, © Springer Science+Business Media, LLC, part of Springer Nature 2019

[14–22]. rMETase can also potentiate chemotherapy active in S phase due to the selective arrest of cancer cells in S phase during MR [23–27].

In previous studies, we established a PDOX nude mouse model of a BRAF V600E-mutant melanoma (*see* **Notes 5–7**) [15, 28–30]. rMETase administered intraperitoneally (i.p.) in combination with a first-line melanoma drug, temozolomide (TEM), regressed the PDOX melanoma. The combination of TEM, first-line therapy, and i.p. rMETase was significantly more efficacious than either monotherapy [15].

We review in this chapter that oral rMETase (o-rMETase) is highly effective in the BRAF V600E-mutant melanoma PDOX and discuss implications of this result for cancer therapy as well as anti-aging.

2 Materials

1. Athymic *nu/nu* nude mice, 4–6 weeks old (AntiCancer Inc., San Diego, CA).
2. 6-0 Nylon suture (Ethilon, Ethicon, Inc., NJ, USA).
3. pAC-1 rMETase high-expression clone (AntiCancer Inc.).
4. Recombinant L-methionine α-deamino-γ-mercaptomethane lyase (methioninase, METase) [EC 4.4.1.11] (AntiCancer Inc.): rMETase is a homotetrameric PLP enzyme of 172 kDa molecular mass [31] (AntiCancer Inc., San Diego, CA).
5. Pyridoxal-L-phosphate (PLP) (Sigma Aldrich, St. Louis, MO).
6. Stainless steel gavage needles (Fine Science Tools, Foster City, CA).
7. Phosphate-buffered saline (PBS).
8. Ketamine mixture: 20 mg/kg ketamine, 15.2 mg/kg xylazine, and 0.48 mg/kg acepromazine maleate (Henry Scheim, New York, NY).
9. DEAE Sepharose FF.
10. Sephacryl S-200HR.
11. ActiClean Etox.

2.1 Patient-Derived Tumor

1. A 75-year-old female patient was previously diagnosed with a BRAF V600E melanoma of the right chest wall. The tumor was previously resected in the Department of Surgery, University of California, Los Angeles (UCLA). Written informed consent was provided by the patient, and the Institutional Review Board (IRB) of UCLA approved this experiment [15, 28–30].

3 Methods

3.1 Mice

1. Use athymic *nu/nu* nude mice.
2. Maintain mice in a barrier facility in a high-efficacy particulate arrestance (HEPA)-filtered rack under standard conditions of 12-h light/dark cycles.
3. Feed the mice an autoclaved laboratory rodent diet.
4. Conduct all animal studies in accordance with the principles and procedures outlined in the National Institutes of Health Guide for the Care and Use of Animals under Assurance Number A3873-1.
5. Perform all mouse surgical procedures and imaging with the animals anesthetized by subcutaneous injection of a ketamine mixture.
6. Monitor the response of the mice during surgery to ensure adequate depth of anesthesia.
7. Observe the mice on a daily basis and sacrifice by CO_2 inhalation if they meet the following humane endpoint criteria: severe tumor burden (more than 20 mm in diameter), prostration, significant body weight loss, difficulty breathing, rotational motion, and body-temperature drop [14–22].

3.2 Establishment of PDOX Models of Melanoma by Surgical Orthotopic Implantation (SOI)

1. Harvest subcutaneously-grown patient-derived BRAF V600E mutant melanoma from nude mice and cut into small fragments (3 mm^3).
2. After additional nude mice are anesthetized with the ketamine solution described above, make a 5 mm skin incision on the right chest into the chest wall and split to make space for the melanoma tissue fragment.
3. Implant a single tumor fragment orthotopically into the space to establish the PDOX model.
4. Close the wound with a 6-0 nylon suture (*see* **Note 8**) [15, 28–30].

3.3 Recombinant Methioninase (rMETase)

1. Use recombinant L-methionine α-deamino-γ-mercaptomethane lyase (recombinant methioninase [rMETase]) [EC 4.4.1.11] from *Pseudomonas putida* cloned and produced in *Escherichia coli*. rMETase is a homotetrameric PLP enzyme of 172 kDa molecular mass [31].

3.4 rMETase Production

1. Use the pAC-1 rMETase high-expression clone expressed in *E. coli* for rMETase production.
2. Use the fermentation procedure for host *E. coli* cells and the purification protocol for rMETase as previously described:

Purify rMETase by three different steps using columns of DEAE Sepharose FF and Sephacryl S-200HR, and ActiClean Etox, which is designed for eliminating endotoxin [31] (*see* **Note 4**).

3.5 Formulation of o-rMETase and Pyridoxal-L-Phosphate (PLP) Supplementation

1. Add PLP (1.0 mL of 20 mmol/L) to 200 mL drinking water and make fresh daily.
2. Administer rMETase daily by gavage using a stainless feeding needle (100 units [2.0 mg] in phosphate-buffered saline [PBS]).

3.6 Treatment Study Design in the PDOX Model of Melanoma

1. Randomize BRAF V600E-mutant melanoma PDOX nude mice into four groups of five mice each: untreated control; ip-rMETase (100 units intraperitoneally [i.p.], 14 consecutive days); o-rMETase (100 units, orally by gavage [p.o.], 14 consecutive days); and o-rMETase+ip-rMETase (100 units, p.o. + 100 units, i.p., 14 consecutive days).

3.7 Determination of Plasma MET

1. Measure the plasma MET concentration using a pre-column derivatization, followed by high-performance liquid chromatography (HPLC) separation based on a previously described method [32].
2. Use a 10 μL plasma sample or MET standard.
3. Identify the plasma MET by retention time of standard MET.
4. The limit of detection is 0.5 μM MET. The upper limit of detection for MET assay is 100 μM.

3.8 Statistical Analysis

1. Use JMP version 11.0 for statistical analyses.
2. Determine significant differences for continuous variables using the Mann-Whitney *U*-test.
3. Express line graph average values and show error bar SD. A probability value of $P \leq 0.05$ is considered statistically significant.

4 Results

o-rMETase ($p = 0.0086$) and ip-rMETase ($p = 0.005$) significantly inhibited the BRAF V600E melanoma PDOX model. The combination of o-rMETase+ip-rMETase was significantly more effective than either alone (Figs. 1 and 2) (*see* **Note 9**).

Posttreatment plasma MET levels were significantly decreased by ip-rMETase or o-rMETase compared to untreated control (Fig. 3).

Body weight loss was not observed in any treatment group (Fig. 4). There were no animal deaths in any group. These results showed the safety of o-rMETase and its potential for chronic cancer treatment in the clinic (*see* **Note 10**).

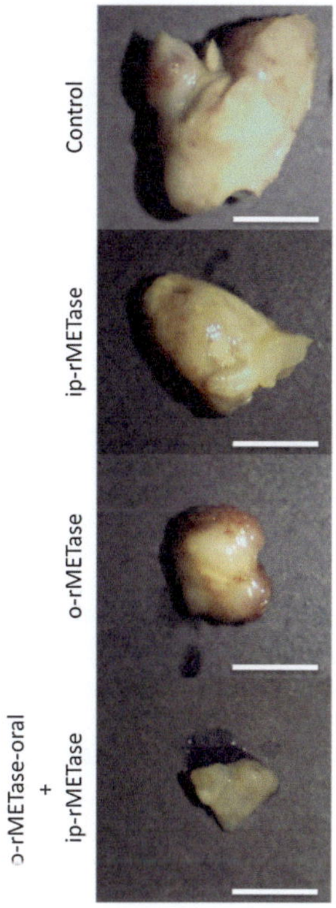

Fig. 1 Photographs of representative tumors from the untreated control and treatment groups of the BRAF V600E-mutant melanoma PDOX. Tumors were resected on day 15 of treatment. Scale bar: 5 mm [19]

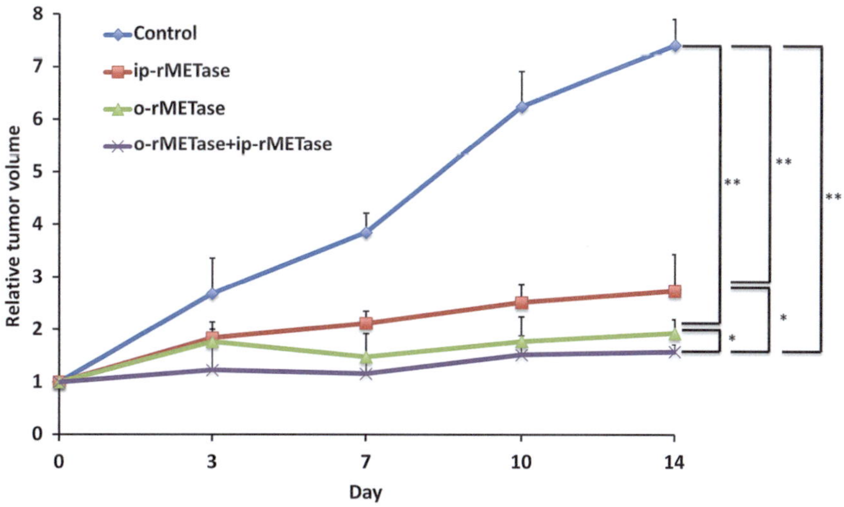

Fig. 2 Quantitative efficacy of ip-rMETase, o-rMETase, and combination of ip-rMETase and o-rMETase on the BRAF V600E-mutant melanoma PDOX. Line graph shows relative tumor volume at each point relative to the initial tumor volume. $^{**}p < 0.01$, $^{*}p < 0.05$. Error bars: ±SD [19]

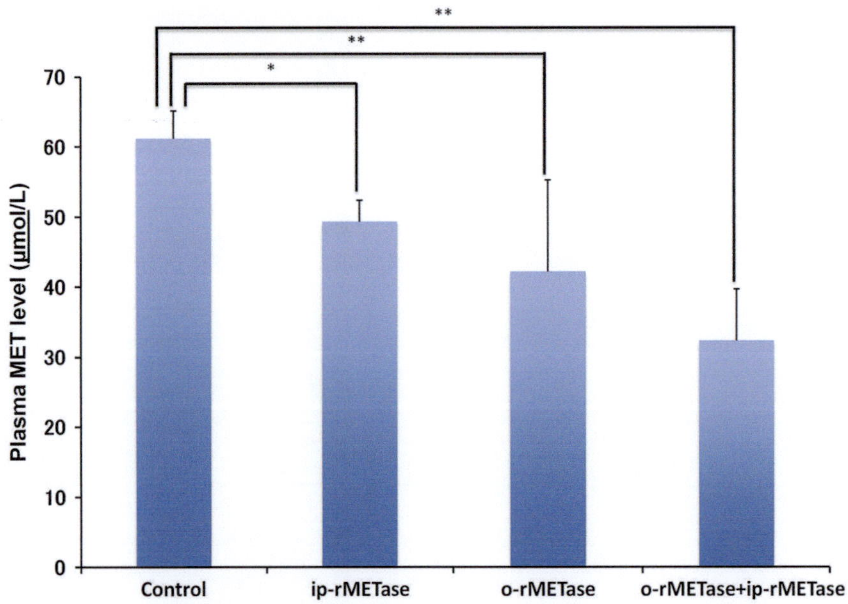

Fig. 3 Effect of ip-rMETase and o-rMETase on plasma rMETase levels. Bar graphs show plasma MET levels in each group at posttreatment. $^{**}p < 0.01$, $^{*}p < 0.05$. Error bars: $\pm$SD [19]

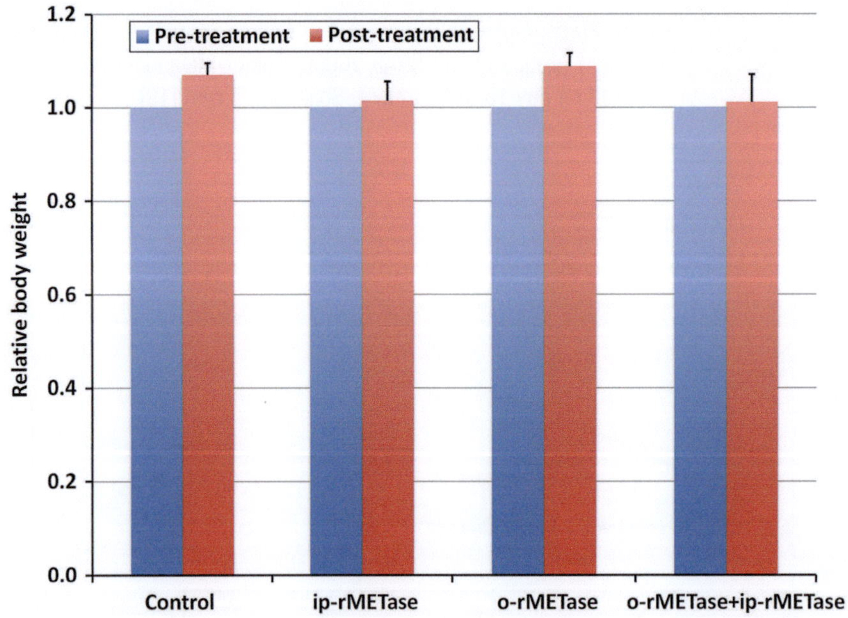

Fig. 4 Effect of ip-rMETase, o-rMETase, and combination of ip-rMETase and o-rMETase on the BRAF V600E-mutant melanoma PDOX mouse body weight. Bar graph shows mouse body weight in each treatment group at pre- and posttreatment. There were no significant differences between any treatment group and untreated control [19]

5 Discussion

o-rMETase can easily be self-administered orally; o-rMETase could be used for chronic cancer treatment or cancer prevention. A lower dose of o-rMETase could be used throughout life as an anti-aging drug (please *see* Chapter 19 of this volume).

6 Notes

1. MET dependence is a general metabolic defect in cancer. MET dependence is due to excessive use of MET for aberrant transmethylation reactions, termed the "Hoffman effect," analogous to the Warburg effect for elevated glucose use in cancer [1–9, 14, 33–38].
2. The excessive and aberrant use of MET in cancer is observed in [^{11}C]-MET-PET imaging, where high uptake of [^{11}C]-MET results in a very strong and selective tumor signal compared with normal tissue background. [^{11}C]-MET is superior to [^{18}C] fluorodeoxyglucose (FDG)-PET indicating MET dependence is more cancer-specific than glucose dependence [8, 9].
3. MET is sourced mainly from food. However, MR through diets with low protein content does not allow the maintenance of good nutritional status (please *see* Chapter 9 of this volume). In addition, MR by dietary intervention is limited since MET is also sourced from protein breakdown with tumors and other tissues [1]. Further reduction of plasma MET and thereby tumor MET has been achieved with the use of rMETase [10, 14, 15, 36, 39].
4. Our laboratory cloned *Pseudomonas putida* rMETase into *E. coli* for large-scale production [31].
5. It has been demonstrated that MR induces a selective S/G_2-phase cell-cycle arrest of cancer cells in vitro and in vivo [23–25, 33, 34].
6. This chapter reviews the power of the PDOX model to identify effective therapy for recalcitrant cancer. Toward this goal of precision personalized oncology, our laboratory pioneered the patient-derived orthotopic xenograft (PDOX) nude mouse model with the technique of surgical orthotopic implantation (SOI), including pancreatic [17, 21, 37, 38, 40, 41], breast [42], ovarian [43], lung [44], cervical [45], colon [46–48], stomach [49], sarcoma [14, 16, 18, 20, 50–63], and melanoma [15, 17, 19, 28–30, 64].
7. We reported recently on the efficacy of ip-rMETase against Ewing's sarcoma in a PDOX model. ip-rMETase effectively

reduced tumor growth compared to untreated control. Serum and tumor MET levels were lower in the ip-rMETase group [14].

8. The melanoma PDOX was transplanted on the chest wall of nude mice to match the site in which it grew in the patient.
9. In a previous study, the BRAF V600E-mutant melanoma PDOX was sensitive to ip-rMETase and increased TEM efficacy in combination [15].
10. It was a surprising result that o-rMETase was effective against the BRAF V600E-mutant melanoma PDOX and is more effective than ip-rMETase. The use of o-rMETase opens many possibilities for nontoxic chronic cancer treatment and for cancer prevention as well as for general life-span extension, since MET is also a target of aging [Chapter 19 of the present volume].

References

1. Hoffman RM (2015) Development of recombinant methioninase to target the general cancer-specific metabolic defect of methionine dependence: a 40-year odyssey. Expert Opin Biol Ther 15:21–31
2. Hoffman RM, Erbe RW (1976) High *in vivo* rates of methionine biosynthesis in transformed human and malignant rat cells auxotrophic for methionine. Proc Natl Acad Sci U S A 73:1523–1527
3. Stern PH, Mecham JO, Wallace CD, Hoffman RM (1983) Reduced free-methionine in methionine-dependent SV40-transformed human fibroblasts synthesizing apparently normal amounts of methionine. J Cell Physiol 117:9–14
4. Stern PH, Wallace CD, Hoffman RM (1984) Altered methionine metabolism occurs in all members of a set of diverse human tumor cell lines. J Cell Physiol 119:29–34
5. Stern PH, Hoffman RM (1984) Elevated overall rates of transmethylation in cell lines from diverse human tumors. In Vitro 20:663–670
6. Hoffman RM (1984) Altered methionine metabolism, DNA methylation and oncogene expression in carcinogenesis: a review and synthesis. Biochim Biophys Acta 738:49–87
7. Coalson DW, Mecham JO, Stern PH, Hoffman RM (1982) Reduced availability of endogenously synthesized methionine for S-adenosylmethionine formation in methionine dependent cancer cells. Proc Natl Acad Sci U S A 79:4248–4251
8. Hoffman RM (2017) Is DNA methylation the new guardian of genome? Mol Cytogenetics 10:11
9. Hoffman RM (2017) The wayward methyl group and the cascade to cancer. Cell Cycle 16:825–829
10. Tan Y, Sun X, Xu M, Tan X-Z, Sasson A, Rashidi B, Han Q, Tan X-Y, Wang X, An Z, Sun F-X, Hoffman RM (1999) Efficacy of recombinant methioninase in combination with cisplatin on human colon tumors in nude mice. Clin Cancer Res 5:2157–2163
11. Kokkinakis DM, Hoffman RM, Frenkel EP, Wick JB, Han Q, Xu M, Tan Y, Schold SC (2001) Synergy between methionine stress and chemotherapy in the treatment of brain tumor xenografts in athymic mice. Cancer Res 61:4017–4023
12. Mecham JO, Rowitch D, Wallace CD, Stern PH, Hoffman RM (1983) The metabolic defect of methionine dependence occurs frequently in human tumor cell lines. Biochem Biophys Res Commun 117:429–434
13. Yoshioka T, Wada T, Uchida N, Maki H, Yoshida H, Ide N, Kasai H, Hojo K, Shono K, Maekawa R, Yagi S, Hoffman RM, Sugita K (1998) Anticancer efficacy *in vivo* and *in vitro*, synergy with 5-fluorouracil, and safety of recombinant methioninase. Cancer Res 58:2583–2587
14. Murakami T, Li S, Han Q, Tan Y, Kiyuna T, Igarashi K, Kawaguchi K, Hwang HK, Miyaki K, Singh AS, Hiroshima Y, Lwin TM,

DeLong JC, Chishima T, Tanaka K, Bouvet M, Endo I, Eilber FC, Hoffman RM (2017) Recombinant methioninase effectively targets a Ewing's sarcoma in a patient-derived orthotopic xenograft (PDOX) nude-mouse model. Oncotarget 8:35630–35638

15. Kawaguchi K, Igarashi K, Li S, Han Q, Tan Y, Kiyuna T, Miyake Y, Murakami T, Chmielowski B, Nelson SD, Russell TA, Dry SM, Li Y, Unno M, Eilber FC, Hoffman RM (2017) Combination treatment with recombinant methioninase enables temozolomide to arrest a BRAF V600E melanoma growth in a patient-derived orthotopic xenograft. Oncotarget 8:85516–85525
16. Igarashi K, Kawaguchi K, Li S, Han Q, Tan Y, Murakami T, Kiyuna T, Miyake K, Miyake M, Singh AS, Eckhadt MA, Nelson SD, Russell TA, Dry SM, Li Y, Yamamoto N, Hayashi K, Kimura H, Miwa S, Tsuchiya H, Singh RS, Eilber FC, Hoffman RM (2018) Recombinant methioninase in combination with DOX overcomes first-line DOX resistance in a patient-derived orthotopic xenograft nude-mouse model of undifferentiated spindle-cell sarcoma. Cancer Lett 417:168–173
17. Kawaguchi K, Han Q, Li S, Tan Y, Igarashi K, Miyake K, Kiyuna T, Miyake M, Chmielowski B, Nelson SD, Russell TA, Dry SM, Li Y, Singh AS, Eckardt MA, Unno M, Eilber FC, Hoffman RM (2018) Intra-tumor L-methionine level highly correlates with tumor size in both pancreatic cancer and melanoma patient-derived orthotopic xenograft (PDOX) nude-mouse models. Oncotarget 9:11119–11125
18. Igarashi K, Li S, Han Q, Tan Y, Kawaguchi K, Murakami T, Kiyuna T, Miyake K, Li Y, Nelson SD, Dry SM, Singh AS, Elliott I, Russell TA, Eckhadt MA, Yamamoto N, Hayashi K, Kimura H, Miwa S, Tsuchiya H, Eilber FC, Hoffman RM (2018) Growth of a doxorubicin-resistant undifferentiated spindle-cell sarcoma PDOX is arrested by metabolic targeting with recombinant methioninase. J Cell Biochem 119:3537–3544
19. Kawaguchi K, Han Q, Li S, Tan Y, Igarashi K, Kiyuna T, Miyake K, Miyake M, Chmielowski B, Nelson SD, Russell TA, Dry SM, Li Y, Eckhardt MA, Unno M, Eilber FC, Hoffman RM (2018) Targeting methionine with oral recombinant methioninase (o-rMETase) arrests a patient-derived orthotopic xenograft (PDOX) model of BRAF-V600E mutant melanoma: implications for clinical cancer therapy and prevention. Cell Cycle 17:356–361
20. Igarashi K, Kawaguchi K, Kiyuna T, Miyake K, Miyake M, Li S, Han Q, Tan Y, Zhao M, Li Y, Nelson SD, Dry SM, Singh AS, Elliott I, Russell TA, Eckardt MA, Yamamoto N, Hayashi K, Kimura H, Miwa S, Tsuchiya H, Eilber FC, Hoffman RM (2018) Tumor-targeting *Salmonella typhimurium* A1-R combined with recombinant methioninase and cisplatinum eradicates an osteosarcoma cisplatinum-resistant lung metastasis in a patient-derived orthotopic xenograft (PDOX) mouse model: decoy, trap and kill chemotherapy moves toward the clinic. Cell Cycle 17:801–809
21. Kawaguchi K, Miyake K, Han Q, Li S, Tan Y, Igarashi K, Lwin TM, Higuchi T, Kiyuna T, Miyake M, Oshiro H, Bouvet M, Unno M, Hoffman RM (2018) Targeting altered cancer methionine metabolism with recombinant methioninase (rMETase) overcomes partial gemcitabine-resistance and regresses a patient-derived orthotopic xenograft (PDOX) nude mouse model of pancreatic cancer. Cell Cycle 21:1–6
22. Igarashi K, Kawaguchi K, Li S, Han Q, Tan Y, Gainor E, Kiyuna T, Miyake K, Miyake M, Singh AS, Eckhadt MA, Nelson SD, Russell TA, Dry SM, Li Y, Higuchi T, Oshiro H, Yamamoto N, Hayashi K, Kimura H, Miwa S, Tsuchiya H, Eilber FC, Hoffman RM (2018) Recombinant methioninase combined with doxorubicin (DOX) regresses a DOX-resistant synovial sarcoma in a patient-derived orthotopic xenograft (PDOX) mouse model. Oncotarget 9:19263–19272
23. Hoffman RM, Jacobsen SJ (1980) Reversible growth arrest in simian virus 40-transformed human fibroblasts. Proc Natl Acad Sci U S A 77:7306–7310
24. Stern PH, Hoffman RM (1986) Enhanced *in vitro* selective toxicity of chemotherapeutic agents for human cancer cells based on a metabolic defect. J Natl Cancer Inst 76:629–639
25. Guo H, Lishko VK, Herrera H, Groce A, Kubota T, Hoffman RM (1993) Therapeutic tumor-specific cell cycle block induced by methionine starvation *in vivo*. Cancer Res 53:5676–5679
26. Yano S, Li S, Han Q, Tan Y, Bouvet M, Fujiwara T, Hoffman RM (2014) Selective methioninase-induced trap of cancer cells in S/G_2 phase visualized by FUCCI imaging confers chemosensitivity. Oncotarget 5:8729–8736
27. Yano S, Takehara K, Zhao M, Tan Y, Han Q, Li S, Bouvet M, Fujiwara T, Hoffman RM (2016) Tumor-specific cell-cycle decoy by

Salmonella typhimurium A1-R combined with tumor-selective cell-cycle trap by methioninase overcome tumor intrinsic chemoresistance as visualized by FUCCI imaging. Cell Cycle 15:1715–1723

28. Kawaguchi K, Murakami T, Chmielowski B, Igarashi K, Kiyuna T, Unno M, Nelson SD, Russell TA, Dry SM, Li Y, Eilber FC, Hoffman RM (2016) Vemurafenib-resistant BRAF-V600E mutated melanoma is regressed by MEK targeting drug trametinib, but not cobimetinib in a patient-derived orthotopic xenograft (PDOX) mouse model. Oncotarget 7:71737–71743
29. Kawaguchi K, Igarashi K, Murakami T, Chmiewloski B, Kiyuna T, Zhao M, Zhang Y, Singh A, Unno M, Nelson SD, Russell T, Dry SM, Li Y, Eilber FC, Hoffman RM (2016) Tumor-targeting *Salmonella typhimurium* A1-R combined with temozolomide regresses malignant melanoma with a BRAF-V600 mutation in a patient-derived orthotopic xenograft (PDOX) model. Oncotarget 7:85929–85936
30. Kawaguchi K, Igarashi K, Murakami T, Zhao M, Zhang Y, Chmielowski B, Kiyuna T, Nelson SD, Russell TA, Dry SM, Li Y, Unno M, Eilber FC, Hoffman RM (2017) Tumor-targeting *Salmonella typhimurium* A1-R sensitizes melanoma with a BRAF-V600E mutation to vemurafenib in a patient-derived orthotopic xenograft (PDOX) nude mouse model. J Cell Biochem 118:2314–2319
31. Tan Y, Xu M, Tan X, Tan X, Wang X, Saikawa Y, Nagahama T, Sun X, Lenz M, Hoffman RM (1997) Overexpression and large-scale production of recombinant L-methionine-alpha- deamino-gamma-mercaptomethane-lyase for novel anticancer therapy. Protein Expr Purif 9:233–245
32. Jones BN, Gilligan JP (1983) o-Phthaldialdehyde precolumn derivatization and reversed-phase high-performance liquid chromatography of polypeptide hydrolysates and physiological fluids. J Chromatogr 266:471–482
33. Kokkinakis DM, von Wronski MA, Vuong TH, Brent TP, Schold SC Jr (1997) Regulation of O6-methylguanine-DNA methyltransferase by methionine in human tumour cells. Br J Cancer 75:779–788
34. Kokkinakis DM, Schold SC Jr, Hori H, Nobori T (1997) Effect of long-term depletion of plasma methionine on the growth and survival of human brain tumor xenografts in athymic mice. Nutr Cancer 29:195–204
35. Lishko VK, Lishko OV, Hoffman RM (1993) The preparation of endotoxin-free L-methionine-alpha-deamino-gamma-mercaptomethane-lyase (L-methioninase) from Pseudomonas putida. Protein Expr Purif 4:529–533
36. Tan Y, Zavala J Sr, Xu M, Zavala J Jr, Hoffman RM (1996) Serum methionine depletion without side effects by methioninase in metastatic breast cancer patients. Anticancer Res 16:3937–3942
37. Hiroshima Y, Zhang Y, Murakami T, Maawy A, Miwa S, Yamamoto M, Yano S, Sato S, Momiyama M, Mori R, Matsuyama R, Chishima T, Tanaka K, chikawa Y, Bouvet M, Endo I, Zhao M, Hoffman RM (2014) Efficacy of tumor-targeting *Salmonella typhimurium* A1-R in combination with anti-angiogenesis therapy on a pancreatic cancer patient-derived orthotopic xenograph (PDOX) and cell line mouse models. Oncotarget 5:12346–12357
38. Fu X, Guadagni F, Hoffman RM (1992) A metastatic nude-mouse model of human pancreatic cancer constructed orthotopically with histologically intact patient specimens. Proc Natl Acad Sci U S A 89:5645–5649
39. Tan Y, Zavala J Sr, Han Q, Xu M, Sun X, Tan X, Tan X, Magana R, Geller J, Hoffman RM (1997) Recombinant methioninase infusion reduces the biochemical endpoint of serum methionine with minimal toxicity in high-stage cancer patients. Anticancer Res 17:3857–3860
40. Hiroshima Y, Maawy A, Zhang Y, Murakami T, Momiyama M, Mori R, Matsuyama R, Katz MH, Fleming JB, Chishima T, Tanaka K, Ichikawa Y, Endo I, Hoffman RM, Bouvet M (2014) Metastatic recurrence in a pancreatic cancer patient derived orthotopic xenograft (PDOX) nude mouse model is inhibited by neoadjuvant chemotherapy in combination with fluorescence-guided surgery with an anti-CA 19–9-conjugated fluorophore. PLoS One 9:e114310
41. Hiroshima Y, Maawy AA, Katz MH, Fleming JB, Bouvet M, Endo I, Hoffman RM (2015) Selective efficacy of zoledronic acid on metastasis in a patient-derived orthotopic xenograph (PDOX) nude-mouse model of human pancreatic cancer. J Surg Oncol 111:311–315
42. Fu X, Le P, Hoffman RM (1993) A metastatic-orthotopic transplant nude-mouse model of human patient breast cancer. Anticancer Res 13:901–904
43. Fu X, Hoffman RM (1993) Human ovarian carcinoma metastatic models constructed in nude mice by orthotopic transplantation of histologically-intact patient specimens. Anticancer Res 13:283–286

44. Wang X, Fu X, Hoffman RM (1992) A new patient-like metastatic model of human lung cancer constructed orthotopically with intact tissue via thoracotomy in immunodeficient mice. Int J Cancer 51:992–995
45. Hiroshima Y, Zhang Y, Zhang N, Maawy A, Mii S, Yamamoto M, Uehara F, Miwa S, Yano S, Murakami T, Momiyama M, Chishima T, Tanaka K, Ichikawa Y, Bouvet M, Murata T, Endo I, Hoffman RM (2015) Establishment of a patient-derived orthotopic xenograph (PDOX) model of HER-2-positive cervical cancer expressing the clinical metastatic pattern. PLoS One 10:e0117417
46. Fu X, Besterman JM, Monosov A, Hoffman RM (1991) Models of human metastatic colon cancer in nude mice orthotopically constructed by using histologically intact patient specimens. Proc Natl Acad Sci U S A 88:9345–9349
47. Metildi CA, Kaushal S, Luiken GA, Talamini MA, Hoffman RM, Bouvet M (2014) Fluorescently-labeled chimeric anti-CEA antibody improves detection and resection of human colon cancer in a patient-derived orthotopic xenograft (PDOX) nude mouse model. J Surg Oncol 109:451–458
48. Hiroshima Y, Maawy A, Metildi CA, Zhang Y, Uehara F, Miwa S, Yano S, Sato S, Murakami T, Momiyama M, Chishima T, Tanaka K, Bouvet M, Endo I, Hoffman RM (2014) Successful fluorescence-guided surgery on human colon cancer patient-derived orthotopic xenograft mouse models using a fluorophore-conjugated anti-CEA antibody and a portable imaging system. J Laparoendosc Adv Surg Tech A 24:241–247
49. Furukawa T, Kubota T, Watanabe M, Kitajima M, Hoffman RM (1993) Orthotopic transplantation of histologically intact clinical specimens of stomach cancer to nude mice: correlation of metastatic sites in mouse and individual patient donors. Int J Cancer 53:608–612
50. Kawaguchi K, Igarashi K, Kiyuna T, Miyake K, Miyake M, Murakami T, Chmielowski B, Nelson SD, Russell TA, Dry SM, Li Y, Singh AS, Unno M, Eilber FC, Hoffman RM (2018) Individualized doxorubicin sensitivity testing of undifferentiated soft tissue sarcoma (USTS) in a patient-derived orthotopic xenograft (PDOX) model demonstrates large differences between patients. Cell Cycle 17:627–633
51. Murakami T, DeLong J, Eilber FC, Zhao M, Zhang Y, Zhang N, Singh A, Russell T, Deng S, Reynoso J, Quan C, Hiroshima Y, Matsuyama R, Chishima T, Tanaka K, Bouvet M, Chawla S, Endo I, Hoffman RM (2016) Tumor-targeting *Salmonella typhimurium* A1-R in combination with doxorubicin eradicate soft tissue sarcoma in a patient-derived orthotopic xenograft PDOX model. Oncotarget 7:12783–12790
52. Hiroshima Y, Zhao M, Zhang Y, Zhang N, Maawy A, Murakami T, Mii S, Uehara F, Yamamoto M, Miwa S, Yano S, Momiyama M, Mori R, Matsuyama R, Chishima T, Tanaka K, Ichikawa Y, Bouvet M, Endo I, Hoffman RM (2015) Tumor-targeting *Salmonella typhimurium* A1-R arrests a chemo-resistant patient soft-tissue sarcoma in nude mice. PLoS One 10:e0134324
53. Kiyuna T, Murakami T, Tome Y, Kawaguchi K, Igarashi K, Zhang Y, Zhao M, Li Y, Bouvet M, Kanaya F, Singh A, Dry S, Eilber FC, Hoffman RM (2016) High efficacy of tumor-targeting *Salmonella typhimurium* A1-R on a doxorubicin- and dactolisib-resistant follicular dendritic-cell sarcoma in a patient-derived orthotopic xenograft PDOX nude mouse model. Oncotarget 7:33046–33054
54. Murakami T, Singh AS, Kiyuna T, Dry SM, Li Y, James AW, Igarashi K, Kawaguchi K, DeLong JC, Zhang Y, Hiroshima Y, Russell T, Eckardt MA, Yanagawa J, Federman N, Matsuyama R, Chishima T, Tanaka K, Bouvet M, Endo I, Eilber FC, Hoffman RM (2016) Effective molecular targeting of CDK4/6 and IGF-1R in a rare FUS-ERG fusion CDKN2A-deletion doxorubicin-resistant Ewing's sarcoma in a patient-derived orthotopic xenograft (PDOX) nude-mouse model. Oncotarget 7:47556–47564
55. Hiroshima Y, Zhang Y, Zhang N, Uehara F, Maawy A, Murakami T, Mii S, Yamamoto M, Miwa S, Yano S, Momiyama M, Mori R, Matsuyama R, Chishima T, Tanaka K, Ichikawa Y, Bouvet M, Endo I, Hoffman RM (2015) Patient-derived orthotopic xenograft (PDOX) nude mouse model of soft-tissue sarcoma more closely mimics the patient behavior in contrast to the subcutaneous ectopic model. Anticancer Res 35:697–701
56. Igarashi K, Murakami T, Kawaguchi K, Kiyuna T, Miyake K, Zhang Y, Nelson SD, Dry SM, Li Y, Yanagawa J, Russell TA, Singh AS, Tsuchiya H, Elliott I, Eilber FC, Hoffman RM (2017) A patient-derived orthotopic xenograft (PDOX) mouse model of an cisplatinum-resistant osteosarcoma lung metastasis that was sensitive to temozolomide and trabectedin: implications for precision oncology. Oncotarget 8:62111–62119
57. Igarashi K, Kawaguchi K, Kiyuna T, Murakami T, Miwa S, Nelson SD, Dry SM, Li Y, Singh A, Kimura H, Hayashi K,

Yamamoto N, Tsuchiya H, Eilber FC, Hoffman RM (2017) Temozolomide combined with irinotecan caused regression in an adult pleomorphic rhabdomyosarcoma patient-derived orthotopic xenograft (PDOX) nude-mouse model. Oncotarget 8:75874–75880

58. Igarashi K, Kawaguchi K, Murakami T, Kiyuna T, Miyake K, Nelson SD, Dry SM, Li Y, Yanagawa J, Russell TA, Singh AS, Yamamoto N, Hayashi K, Kimura H, Miwa S, Tsuchiya H, Eilber FC, Hoffman RM (2017) Intra-arterial administration of tumor-targeting *Salmonella typhimurium* A1-R regresses a cisplatin-resistant relapsed osteosarcoma in a patient-derived orthotopic xenograft (PDOX) mouse model. Cell Cycle 16:1164–1170

59. Murakami T, Kiyuna T, Kawaguchi K, Igarashi K, Singh AS, Hiroshima Y, Zhang Y, Zhao M, Miyake K, Nelson SD, Dry SM, Li Y, DeLong JC, Lwin TM, Chishima T, Tanaka K, Bouvet M, Endo I, Eilber FC, Hoffman RM (2017) The irony of highly-effective bacterial therapy of a patient-derived orthotopic xenograft (PDOX) model of Ewing's sarcoma, which was blocked by Ewing himself 80 years ago. Cell Cycle 16:1046–1052

60. Igarashi K, Kawaguchi K, Murakami T, Kiyuna T, Miyake K, Singh A, Nelson SD, Dry SM, Li Y, Yamamoto N, Hayashi K, Kimura H, Miwa S, Tsuchiya H, Eilber FC, Hoffman RM (2017) High efficacy of pazopanib on an undifferentiated spindle-cell sarcoma resistant to first-line therapy is identified with a patient-derived orthotopic xenograft (PDOX) nude mouse model. J Cell Biochem 118:2739–3743

61. Kiyuna T, Murakami T, Tome Y, Kawaguchi K, Igarashi K, Miyake K, Kanaya F, Singh A, Eilber FC, Hoffman RM (2017) Analysis of stroma labeling during multiple passage of a sarcoma imageable patient-derived orthotopic xenograft (iPDOX) in red fluorescent protein transgenic nude mice. J Cell Biochem 118:3367–3371

62. Igarashi K, Kawaguchi K, Murakami T, Kiyuna T, Miyake K, Yamamoto N, Hayashi K, Kimura H, Nelson SD, Dry SM, Li Y, Singh AS, Miwa S, Odani A, Eilber FC, Tsuchiya H, Hoffman RM (2017) A novel anionic-phosphate-platinum complex effectively targets an undifferentiated pleomorphic sarcoma better than cisplatinum and doxorubicin in a patient-derived orthotopic xenograft (PDOX). Oncotarget 8:63353–63359

63. Miyake K, Murakami T, Kiyuna T, Igarashi K, Kawaguchi K, Miyake M, Li Y, Nelson SD, Dry SM, Bouvet M, Elliott IA, Russell TA, Singh AS, Eckardt MA, Hiroshima Y, Momiyama M, Matsuyama R, Chishima T, Endo I, Eilber FC, Hoffman RM (2017) The combination of temozolomide-irinotecan regresses a doxorubicin-resistant patient-derived orthotopic xenograft (PDOX) nude-mouse model of recurrent Ewing's sarcoma with a *FUS-ERG* fusion and CDKN2A deletion: direction for third-line patient therapy. Oncotarget 8:103129–103136

64. Yamamoto M, Zhao M, Hiroshima Y, Zhang Y, Shurell E, Eilber FC, Bouvet M, Noda M, Hoffman RM (2016) Efficacy of tumor-targeting *Salmonella typhimurium* A1-R on a melanoma patient-derived orthotopic xenograft (PDOX) nude-mouse model. PLoS One 11:e0160882

Epilogue: Why Do We Keep Mis-targeting Cancer Chemotherapy When the Methionine Target Has Been Obvious for More than a Half-Century?

Robert M. Hoffman

Key words Methionine dependence, Recombinant methioninase, Oral administration, Pyridoxal-L-phosphate, Targeted therapy

"Targeted therapy" has been a paradigm for cancer treatment for at least 20 years. At approximately the end of the twentieth century, angiogenesis was a major target for cancer therapy. Folkman's great discovery that growing tumors need new blood vessels for growth [1] became the dominant paradigm. Many candidate angiogenesis inhibitors were developed. The primary example is a monoclonal antibody to vascular endothelial growth factor (VEGF) ("bevacizumab," which was commercialized by Genentech-Roche as "Avastin"). However, Avastin has had only moderate efficacy [2] due to lack of sufficient antitumor activity and dose-limiting toxicity since normal tissues also require angiogenesis. Thus, bevacizumab lacks anticancer selectivity. In 1998, Jim Watson, who co-discovered the structure of DNA, stated in the NY times of Dr. Folkman that he "will cure cancer in 2 years with angiogenesis therapy" [3].

Another recent target for cancer therapy has been "tyrosine kinase inhibitors." This paradigm got its start with the drug imatinib commercialized as "Gleevec" [4]. Gleevec showed good activity against chronic myelogenous leukemia (CML) due to a chromosome translocation affecting the tyrosine kinase enzyme. Gleevec also showed efficacy against a rare sarcoma called gastrointensive stromal tumor (GIST) [5]. However, Gleevec has not shown high efficacy against other cancer types. Following Gleevec, a whole series of tyrosine kinase inhibitors was used for CML, GIST, and melanoma [6], as well as other tumor types with modest success.

In the past few years, there has been a rebirth of "immuno oncology" that has had many cycles since the time of William

Robert M. Hoffman (ed.), *Methionine Dependence of Cancer and Aging: Methods and Protocols*, Methods in Molecular Biology, vol. 1866, https://doi.org/10.1007/978-1-4939-8796-2,

B. Coley and Coley's toxins at the turn of the twentieth century [7]. The 1980s saw a highly-publicized surge of immuno-oncology led by Steve Rosenberg of the NCI, who developed lymphokine-activated killer (LAK) cells to treat kidney and other cancers [8]. Although there was much publicity, LAK cell therapy, where a cancer patient's T cells were removed and amplified in the presence of interleukin-2, had only limited efficacy. In the past few years, "immuno-oncology" has re-emerged under a slightly different guise targeting "immune checkpoint inhibitors" with antibodies against the "immune checkpoints" PD-1 and PD-L1 [9] that are claimed to overcome immune inhibition against tumors. In this new incarnation of immuno-oncology the T cells of cancer patients are also modified genetically ex vivo with "CAR-T therapy" (chimeric antigen receptor). In either iteration, LAK or CAR-T therapy, the activated T cells must penetrate tumors which appears to be a severe limitation [10, 11].

Cytotoxic chemotherapy was originally developed in the 1940s, 1950s, and 1960s for childhood and adult leukemia and lymphoma, with great success. However, when cytotoxic chemotherapy was applied to solid tumors, the success was very limited, since cytotoxic chemotherapy targets dividing cells (the reason for chemotherapy-induced hair loss) and in solid tumors dividing cells are a minor population, with the quiescent cells resisting chemotherapy [12]. So, here we are late in the second decade of the twenty-first century and patients with metastatic solid cancer have about the same prognosis as 50 years ago.

We have learned in this volume, since Sugimura's initial discovery of the methionine dependence of a rat tumor in 1959 [13], that methionine is a promising target for cancer. We have seen that methionine restriction (MR) selectively arrests cancer cells in the late S/G_2 phase of the cell cycle [14–17], enabling cell-cycle-based chemotherapy which can selectively eliminate cancer cells in the presence of normal cells in vitro [18] and in vivo [15, 16]. During this period, a recombinant methioninase (rMETase) was highly developed preclinically with large-scale production [19–24] that was modified also by PEGylation [25, 26] and shown safe in primates [27, 28].

The highly selective uptake of MET by tumors demonstrated in [^{11}C]-MET-PET imaging [29] re-emphasizes that MET is a target of high potential for cancer therapy.

Why has MET as a target for cancer therapy sat unexploited for 60 years? Perhaps the lure of the excitement of angiogenesis, tyrosine kinase inhibitors, tumor-targeting T cells, etc. obscured MET as a target to invest in and exploit. Now MET has been shown to be a target to extend life span [30] (please *see* Chapter 19 of this volume). Perhaps this will attract the opinion leaders of cancer research to the promised land of MET-targeted cancer chemotherapy.

References

1. Folkman J (1971) Tumor angiogenesis: therapeutic implications. N Engl J Med 19285:1182–1186
2. Montero AJ, Vogel C (2012) Fighting fire with fire: rekindling the bevacizumab debate. N Engl J Med 366:374–375
3. Kolata G. Hope in the lab: a special report. A cautious awe greets drugs that eradicate tumors in mice. https://mobile.nytimes.com/1998/05/03/us/hope-lab-special-report-cautious-awe-greets-drugs-that-eradicate-tumors-mice.html
4. Sawyers CL (2010) Even better kinase inhibitors for chronic myeloid leukemia. N Engl J Med 362:2314–2315
5. Balachandran VP, DeMatteo RP (2014) Gastrointestinal stromal tumors: who should get imatinib and for how long? Adv Surg 48:165–183
6. Larkin J, Ascierto PA, Dréno B, Atkinson V, Liszkay G, Maio M, Mandalà M, Demidov L, Stroyakovskiy D, Thomas L, de la Cruz-Merino L, Dutriaux C, Garbe C, Sovak MA, Chang I, Choong N, Hack SP, McArthur GA, Ribas A (2014) Combined vemurafenib and cobimetinib in BRAF-mutated melanoma. N Engl J Med 371:1867–1876
7. Hoffman RM (ed) (2016) Bacterial therapy of cancer: methods and protocols. Methods in molecular biology 1409. Walker, John M., series ed. Humana Press (Springer Science +Business Media New York)
8. Rosenberg SA, Dudley ME, Restifo NP (2008) Cancer immunotherapy. N Engl J Med 359:1072
9. Brahmer J, Reckamp KL, Baas P, Crinò L, Eberhardt WE, Poddubskaya E, Antonia S, Pluzanski A, Vokes EE, Holgado E, Waterhouse D, Ready N, Gainor J, Arén Frontera O, Havel L, Steins M, Garassino MC, Aerts JG, Domine M, Paz-Ares L, Reck M, Baudelet C, Harbison CT, Lestini B, Spigel DR (2015) Nivolumab versus docetaxel in advanced squamous-cell non-small-cell lung cancer. N Engl J Med 373:123–135, 2015
10. Brown CE, Alizadeh D, Starr R, Weng L, Wagner JR, Naranjo A, Ostberg JR, Blanchard MS, Kilpatrick J, Simpson J, Kurien A, Priceman SJ, Wang X, Harshbarger TL, D'Apuzzo M, Ressler JA, Jensen MC, Barish ME, Chen M, Portnow J, Forman SJ, Badie B (2016) Regression of glioblastoma after chimeric antigen receptor T-cell therapy. N Engl J Med 375:2561–2569
11. Tran E, Longo DL, Urba WJ (2017) A milestone for CAR T cells. N Engl J Med 377:2593–2596
12. Yano S, Zhang Y, Miwa S, Tome Y, Hiroshima Y, Uehara F, Yamamoto M, Suetsugu A, Kishimoto H, Tazawa H, Zhao M, Bouvet M, Fujiwara T, Hoffman RM (2014) Spatial-temporal FUCCI imaging of each cell in a tumor demonstrates locational dependence of cell cycle dynamics and chemoresponsiveness. Cell Cycle 13:2110–2119
13. Sugimura T, Birnbaum SM, Winitz M, Greenstein JP (1959) Quantitative nutritional studies with water-soluble, chemically defined diets. VIII. The forced feeding of diets each lacking in one essential amino acid. Arch Biochem Biophys 81:448–455
14. Hoffman RM, Jacobsen SJ (1980) Reversible growth arrest in simian virus 40-transformed human fibroblasts. Proc Natl Acad Sci USA 77:7306–7310
15. Yano S, Li S, Han Q, Tan Y, Bouvet M, Fujiwara T, Hoffman RM (2014) Selective methioninase-induced trap of cancer cells in S/G_2 phase visualized by FUCCI imaging confers chemosensitivity. Oncotarget 5:8729–8736
16. Yano S, Takehara K, Zhao M, Tan Y, Han Q, Li S, Bouvet M, Fujiwara T, Hoffman RM (2016) Tumor-specific cell-cycle decoy by *Salmonella typhimurium* A1-R combined with tumor-selective cell-cycle trap by methioninase overcome tumor intrinsic chemoresistance as visualized by FUCCI imaging. Cell Cycle 15:1715–1723
17. Guo HY, Herrera H, Hoffman RM (1993) Unchecked DNA synthesis and blocked cell division induced by methionine deprivation in a human prostate cancer cell line. In: In Vitro Cell Dev Biol, vol 29A, pp 359–361
18. Stern PH, Hoffman RM (1986) Enhanced *in vitro* selective toxicity of chemotherapeutic agents for human cancer cells based on a metabolic defect. J Natl Cancer Inst 76:629–639

19. Tan Y, Xu M, Tan X-Z, Tan X-Y, Wang X, Saikawa Y, Nagahama T, Sun X, Lenz M, Hoffman RM (1997) Overexpression and large-scale production of recombinant L-methionine-α-deamino-γ-mercaptomethane-lyase for novel anticancer therapy. Prot Exp Purification 9:233–245
20. Takakura T, Mitsushima K, Yagi S, Inagaki K, Tanaka H, Esaki N, Soda K, Takimoto A (2004) Assay method for antitumor L-methionine γ-lyase: comprehensive kinetic analysis of the complex reaction with L-methionine. Anal Biochem 327:233–240
21. Takakura T, Ito T, Yagi S, Notsu Y, Itakura T, Nakamura T, Inagaki K, Esaki N, Hoffman RM, Takimoto A (2006) High-level expression and bulk crystallization of recombinant L-methionine γ-lyase, an anticancer agent. Appl Microbiol Biotechnol 70:183–192. https://doi.org/10.1007/s00253-005-0038-2
22. Takakura T, Takimoto A, Notsu Y, Yoshida H, Ito T, Nagatome H, Ohno M, Kobayashi Y, Yoshioka T, Inagaki K, Yagi S, Hoffman RM, Esaki N (2006) Physicochemical and pharmacokinetic characterization of highly potent recombinant L-methionine γ-lyase conjugated with polyethylene glycol as an antitumor agent. Cancer Res 66:2807–2814
23. Kudou D, Misaki S, Yamashita M, Tamura T, Takakura T, Yoshioka T, Yagi S, Hoffman RM, Takimoto A, Esaki N, Inagaki K (2007) Structure of the antitumour enzyme L-methionine γ-lyase from *Pseudomonas putida* at 1.8Å resolution. J Biochem 141:535–544
24. Inoue H, Inagaki K, Sugimoto M, Esaki N, Soda K, Tanaka H (1995) Structural analysis of the L-methionine gamma-lyase gene from Pseudomonas putida. J Biochem 117:1120–1125
25. Sun X, Yang Z, Li S, Tan Y, Zhang N, Wang X, Yagi S, Yoshioka T, Takimoto A, Mitsushima K, Suginaka A, Frenkel EP, Hoffman RM (2003) *In vivo* efficacy of recombinant methioninase is enhanced by the combination of polyethylene glycol conjugation and pyridoxal 5′ phosphate supplementation. Cancer Res 63:8377–8383
26. Yang Z, Sun X, Li S, Tan Y, Wang X, Zhang N, Yagi S, Takakura T, Kobayashi Y, Takimoto A, Yoshioka T, Suginaka A, Frenkel EP, Hoffman RM (2004) Circulating half-life of PEGylated recombinant methioninase holoenzyme is highly dose dependent on cofactor pyridoxal-5′-phosphate. Cancer Res 64:5775–5778
27. Yang Z, Wang J, Yoshioka T, Li B, Lu Q, Li S, Sun X, Tan Y, Yagi S, Frenkel EP, Hoffman RM (2004) Pharmacokinetics, methionine depletion, and antigenicity of recombinant methioninase in primates. Clin Cancer Res 10:2131–2138
28. Yang Z, Wang J, Lu Q, Xu J, Kobayashi Y, Takakura T, Takimoto A, Yoshioka T, Lian C, Chen C, Zhang D, Zhang Y, Li S, Sun X, Tan Y, Yagi S, Frenkel EP, Hoffman RM (2004) PEGylation confers greatly extended half-life and attenuated immunogenicity to recombinant methioninase in primates. Cancer Res 64:6673–6678
29. Xu W, Gao L, Shao A, Zheng J, Zhang J (2017) The performance of 11C-methionine PET in the differential diagnosis of glioma recurrence. Oncotarget 8:91030–91039
30. Orentreich N, Matias JR, DeFelice A, Zimmerman JA (1993) Low methionine ingestion by rats extends life span. J Nutr 123:269–274

Index

Robert M. Hoffman (ed.), *Methionine Dependence of Cancer and Aging: Methods and Protocols*, Methods in Molecular Biology, vol. 1866, https://doi.org/10.1007/978-1-4939-8796-2, © Springer Science+Business Media, LLC, part of Springer Nature 2019

H

I

L

M

N

O

P

R

S

T

Y

MIX
Papier aus verantwortungsvollen Quellen
Paper from responsible sources
FSC® C105338

If you have any concerns about our products,
you can contact us on
ProductSafety@springernature.com

In case Publisher is established outside the EU,
the EU authorized representative is:
Springer Nature Customer Service Center GmbH
Europaplatz 3, 69115 Heidelberg, Germany

Printed by Libri Plureos GmbH
in Hamburg, Germany